PEDIATRICS

for

Students and Practitioners

Second Edition

PEDIATRICS

for
Students and Practitioners

Second Edition

DD Chaurasia

Pediatrician

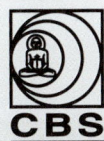

CBS

CBS Publishers & Distributors Pvt Ltd

New Delhi • Bengaluru • Chennai • Kochi • Kolkata • Mumbai

Hyderabad • Jharkhand • Nagpur • Patna • Pune • Uttarakhand

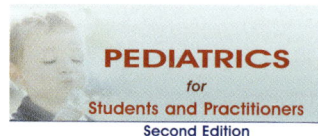

ISBN: 978-93-88725-57-6

Copyright © Author and Publisher

Second Edition: 2021

First Edition: 2000
Reprint: 2005, 2007, 2009, 2010, 2013

Published by Satish Kumar Jain and produced by Varun Jain for

CBS Publishers & Distributors Pvt Ltd
4819/XI Prahlad Street, 24 Ansari Road, Daryaganj, New Delhi 110 002, India.
Ph: 23289259, 23266861, 23266867 Website: www.cbspd.com
Fax: 011-23243014   e-mail: delhi@cbspd.com; cbspubs@airtelmail.in.

Corporate Office: 204 FIE, Industrial Area, Patparganj, Delhi 110 092
Ph: 4934 4934   Fax: 4934 4935   e-mail: publishing@cbspd.com; publicity@cbspd.com

Branches

- **Bengaluru:** Seema House 2975, 17th Cross, K.R. Road, Banasankari 2nd Stage, Bengaluru 560 070, Karnataka
  Ph: +91-80-26771678/79   Fax: +91-80-26771680   e-mail: bangalore@cbspd.com
- **Chennai:** 7, Subbaraya Street, Shenoy Nagar, Chennai 600 030, Tamil Nadu
  Ph: +91-44-26680620/26681266   Fax: +91-44-42032115   e-mail: chennai@cbspd.com
- **Kochi:** 42/1325, 26, Power House Road, Opp KSEB, Ernakulam 682 018, Kochi, Kerala
  Ph: +91-484-4059061-65   Fax: +91-484-4059065   e-mail: kochi@cbspd.com
- **Kolkata:** 6/B, Ground Floor, Rameswar Shaw Road, Kolkata-700 014, West Bengal
  Ph: +91-33-22891126, 22891127, 22891128   e-mail: kolkata@cbspd.com
- **Mumbai:** 83-C, Dr E Moses Road, Worli, Mumbai-400018, Maharashtra
  Ph: +91-22-24902340/41   Fax: +91-22-24902342   e-mail: mumbai@cbspd.com

Representatives

• **Hyderabad**	0-9885175004	• **Jharkhand**	0-9811541605	• **Nagpur**	0-9421945513
• **Patna**	0-9334159340	• **Pune**	0-9623451994	• **Uttarakhand**	0-9716462459

Printed at: Magic International Pvt. Ltd., Greater Noida, UP, India

to
mother of human kind
goddess **Dhandhagarh Devi**

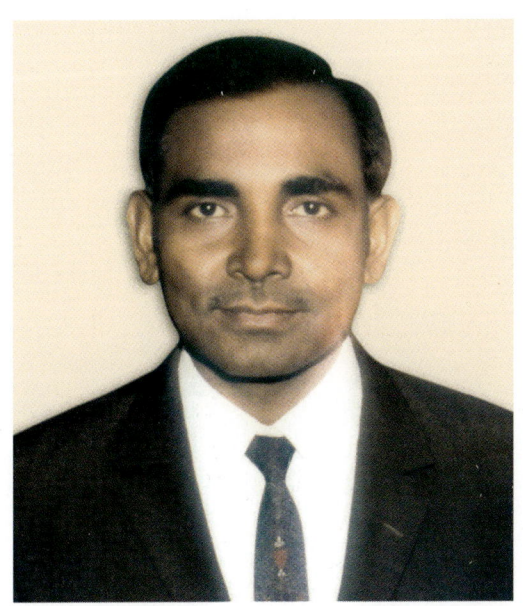

In the memory of
revered uncle ji
Late **Dr BD Chaurasia (1937–1985)**

Preface to the Second Edition

I feel extreme pleasure to present the Second Edition of the book in a complete, up-to-date and concise manner for the requirement of the undergraduate students and pediatricians.

All chapters have been revised and updated in every aspect. New topics are added, well illustrated. Simplicity of the book is maintained with recent scientific literature for the requirement of the students to prepare for various examinations in a short time.

I wish to pay my thanks to all students and pediatricians for their acceptance of my first effort which augmented my desire to do further work in this direction.

I would like to pay my deep regards to my teacher Dr AG Shingwekar, Ex-Professor and Head, Department of Pediatrics, GR Medical College, Gwalior, MP, for his blessing and support.

I would like to thanks Dr Satyam, Dr Suvriti, Dr Vaidehi, Dr Ravindra and Purva of my family for their assistance.

I pay my homage to my uncle late Dr BD Chaurasia, author of *Human Anatomy* by this way of the work for the students.

My heartiest thanks and regards to Mr Satish Kumar Jain (CMD) and Mr Varun Jain (Director), CBS Publishers & Distributors for publishing and distributing the book world-wide.

I am also thankful to CBS Publishers & Distributors. I would like to put on record the sincere efforts of Mr YN Arjuna (Senior Vice-President Publishing, Editorial and Publicity) and his team comprising Mrs Ritu Chawla (GM Production), Mr Parmod Kumar (DTP Operator), Mr Kshirod Kumar and Mr Ananda Mohanty (Proofreaders) and Mr Ram Murthy (Graphic Designer), for bringing out the book in the present form.

DD Chaurasia

Preface to the First Edition

The present book is aimed to provide simple, systematized and complete book on pediatrics for undergraduate students as well as practitioners. The difficulties of students at various steps make me feel to write a complete book which covers all aspects in up-to-date and concise manner. At the beginning of this book chapter on clinical methods in pediatrics has been devoted as child differs in many respects from those employed in the case of adult.

The text is intended to be comprehensive, well described in a simple language. Chapter on growth and development is presented in easy and assimilable form. Diseases of infancy and childhood are described with clinical, etiological, pathological and radiological basis of diagnosis and management with exclusive pediatric approach. The text is illustrated with photographs, diagrams and skiagrams, which help in grasping the subject in easy way. The chapter on practical procedures in pediatrics will provide guide to deal with patient as dispensary, clinic, hospital or at home. Drug dosage in children is presented in inconvenient form along with trade names and preparations available in the market. It will help clinician to write correct prescription for the patient.

A sincere attempt has been made to include only authentic text to keep its standard for which, I am grateful to my teachers and authors of numerous publications, whose knowledge has been freely utilized in preparation of this book. I am very grateful to my teachers of Department of Pediatrics, GR Medical College, Gwalior, Prof (Dr) PS Mathur, Prof Dr Miss RK Taluja, Prof KM Belapurkar, Dr AG Shingwekar (Assistant Professor), Dr YP Thawrani (Assistant Professor) and Dr AK Rawat (Assistant Professor) for their excellent teaching, affection and encouragement.

I pay my deep regards to Prof Meharban Singh, Professor and Head, Department of Pediatrics, All India Institute of Medical Sciences, New Delhi, for his open-hearted encouragement for my first book, which boosted up my desire to write this treatise.

Thanks are also to Dr R Bhojwani, Radiologist, Gwalior, for judicious help in radio-diagnosis and to Shri LM Chaurasia for encouragement and admiration.

I am highly obliged to Shri Dharmvir ji for valuable guidance.

I would be grateful to readers for the suggestions to improve the book.

I am deeply indebted to Shri SK Jain, Shri VK Jain, CBS Publishers & Distributors for publishing the book in desired form and thanks are also to Mr Sunil Dhir from Super Computers for the best laser typesetting, RV Printers, Delhi, is gratefully acknowledged for descent printing.

At last I remember my uncle late Dr BD Chaurasia. This book is my homage to him.

DD Chaurasia

Contents

Introduction

Pediatrics is a Greek word which means 'branch of science which deals with treatment of child'. It is a branch of medicine which deals about health care of child from conception to adolescence. It also includes growth and physical and emotional development of the child.

Children are not merely miniature adults but differ from adult by physiological immaturity, physical and emotional growth and maturation and their dependence upon adults during infancy. The dependence period is long because in human development is slowest among all mammals. They require larger amount of drug per unit of body weight in comparison to adults.

Healthy child is only expected when he/she gets sufficient balanced nutrition and remain protected from disease. Parents, family size, social and economic factors influence him in different ways.

Children below 14 years of age constitute 40% of population and those below five years of age 12% of India's population. They accounts for 50% to total mortality in the country. Major causes of this mortality are acute respiratory tract infection, diarrhea and vaccine preventable diseases. Other diseases account minor part.

Planet earth no longer can accept that in the age of modern technology children should die in millions by the diseases which can be prevented by vaccine or treated by other therapy. So, by preventive, promotive and curative means major part of death can be prevented and morbidity reduced. Greatest care is required to newborn which is vulnerable to suffer from fatal diseases.

Ideally care of child should begin before its coming in conception, such as age of marriage of a lady should be such that she can carry and deliver a healthy child successfully which her genital organs are fully developed as well as birth spacing between two children must be sufficient.

Care of the 'soma' is not the only part but care of 'psyche' is also important during childhood. Environmental factors influence children maximum. Any abnormality may precipitate psychosomatic disorders, which are increasing day by day due to increasing anxiety, tension in the family and society.

Help of informed cooperation of society, loving care and intelligent interest of parents, devotion of health workers, raising necessary funds and materials are the vital ingredient of the cocktail needed to give life to all children of the world.

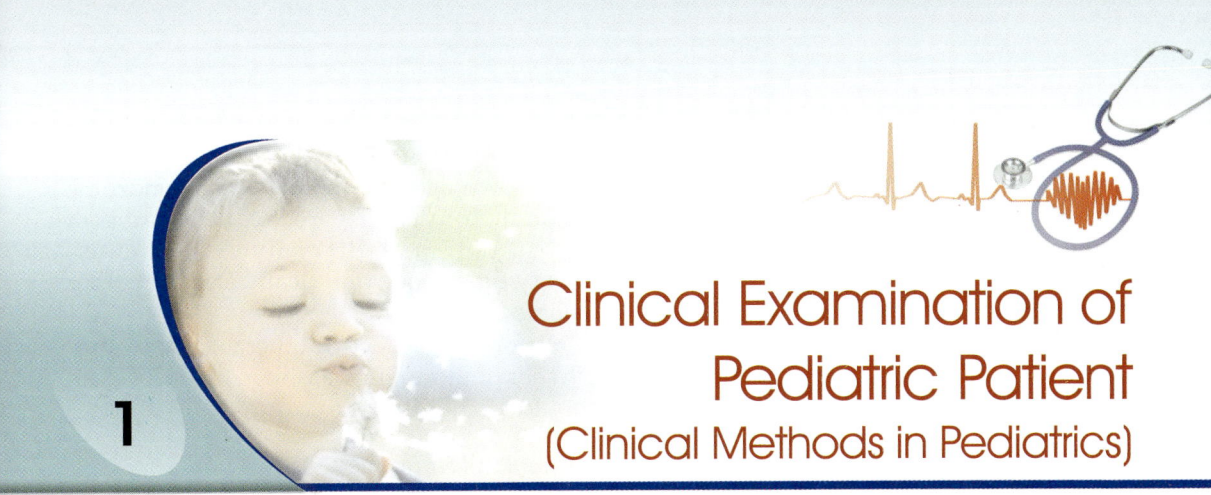

Clinical Examination of Pediatric Patient
(Clinical Methods in Pediatrics)

1

Good history and correct clinical examination is essential for diagnosis of pediatric illnesses. The examination of young children is a matter of difficult art to the unexperienced doctors.

HISTORY-TAKING

The child usually remains in parent's arms during history-taking. Toy, pictures, etc. may be used to create confidence and friendly atmosphere during examination; older child may be interpreted directly for his complaints.

Child cannot express his illness and attendent expression may be biased or incorrect. First listen the complaint told by parents, then put leading questions to fill the gap.

Basic Information

Name, age, sex, father's name, address, occupation of parents, education and religion should be inquired.

Presenting Complaints

First question must be asked 'what is complaint.' Complaints told by parents should be written in their own words not in scientific words. All details of chief complaints must be written in chronological order.

History of Present Illness

Parents should be allowed to give details of sequence of events. When was the child quite well? How long have the symptoms been present? How did they progress or regress? Any treatment taken, etc. Every details of mode of onset, course of the disease, etc. is taken. The symptoms referable to various body systems, e.g. GIT, CVS, CNS should be reviewed in order to identify the site of the disease.

History of Past Illness

Ask about the patient's previous illness and its duration. It may have correlation with present complaints, e.g. history of joints pain and swelling (rheumatism) may be present in cardiac disease. In children suffering from asthma records should be made of similar attacks and their frequency in the past.

Perinatal History

Ask every happening and ailments during antenatal, neonatal or postnatal life.

Antenatal History

History of illness to the mother, e.g. rubella, syphilis, toxemia, diabetes, heart disease, tuberculosis, exposure to radiation, medication, alcohol intake, smoking must be noted.

Natal History

Hospital or home delivery, prolongation of delivery period, any complaint, use of forceps, delayed cry, cyanosis, respiratory distress, convulsions, treatment, resuscitation required, weight at birth, anomalies, etc. should be inquired.

Postnatal History

In immediate postnatal period history of jaundice, delayed feeding, convulsions, umbilical sepsis, cyanosis, loss of weight should be asked.

Dietic History

How long breastfeeding continued, top milk by bottle or other ways, dilution, amount, when semisolid introduced? What types of food (chapati, dal, eggs, etc.) taken? Liking and disliking. It may give clues about cause of malnutrition. Ask in detail of food intake during last 24 hours to calculate approximate calorie and protein intake per day.

Developmental History

Ask about at which age child had first social smile, sitting, standing, neek holding, etc. It gives knowledge of mental retardation and physical retardation. Whether normal or delayed. Indentify whether retardation is in every field or in specific field such as delayed speech with normal motor development suggest deaf mutism while delayed standing and walking with normal social and adaptive development is indication of protein energy malnutrition.

General evaluation of milestones is as follows:

Social smile (4–6 weeks), holds rattle (12 weeks), turn his head (12 weeks), first able to go for rattle (20 weeks), begins to roll from his front to his back (24 weeks), from back to his front (28 weeks). Begins to take an object one hand to another (26 weeks), sits with support (28 weeks), sits without support (32 weeks), stands holding furniture (36 weeks), crawl on abdomen (40 weeks), walk holding furniture (48 weeks), walk with one hand held (52 weeks), walk without help (13 months), creeps upstairs (15–18 months), joins two or three words in sentence (21–24 months), takes some clothes off (24 months). Dresses self (3–4 years).

Family History

Note down age of parents (Down syndrome is common in elder parents), birth order of patient, any hereditary illness in family, history of abortion and death. Death of other sibling.

History of contact of tuberculosis, history of whooping cough, measles in other children should be inquired into.

Immunization Status

Note type and time of vaccination given. Look for scar of BCG vaccination during physical examination.

Socioeconomic History

What is economic status of family, type of occupations of parents, time given to child care by them, education of parent? Ask about relations and behavior to family members, other contacts at home and school should be inquired into his behavior aggressive, negative, etc.

PHYSICAL EXAMINATION

Examination of child should be started as soon as he is brought to the doctor. First try to get confidence and friendly atmosphere created. If one is hurried or rough, the child begins to cry at once and other examination is rendered much more difficult.

No definite pattern should be used to examine him. The unpleasant examination should be postponed to the end. For best cooperation child is examined in different positions which is best suited such as at examination table, mother's lap, standing, etc. Child should be undressed slowly. Cooperation can be gained with the help of toys, bells, friendly atmosphere, etc.

Position

Observe position of child. It helps in diagnosis, e.g. dyspnea in lying flat indicates congestive cardiac failure. The decorticate posture—patient in flexion at the elbow and at the wrist with the thumbs abducted into palm with lower limbs extended.

The decerebrate position is characterized by extended neck, extended shoulder and elbows and pronated forearms with lower limbs in extension (Figs 1.1 and 1.2).

ANTHROPOMETRIC MEASUREMENTS

Weight, height or length, head circumference, etc. should be noted (*see* page 11, details under anthropometric examination).

DEVELOPMENTAL EXAMINATION

Objective assessment of development is required for some patients (*see* page 84).

VITAL SIGNS (Table 1.1)

Temperature, pulse, blood pressure and respiratory rate should be noted.

Temperature (skin temperature) at groin and axilla is recorded by usual thermometer; in infants and preschool children, it is quite reliable. It is 0.5°C lower than rectal (core) temperature. Rectal temperature may be recorded in critically sick children by rectal thermometer which has short bulb.

Temperature record by thermocrystal strips from skin at forehead is unreliable method. Low reading thermometers are used for severely malnourished children.

Look for anemia, cyanosis, edema, lymphadenopathy.

Cry: Listen cry which is also characterstic of some disease.
a. Cat-like cry (cri du chat syndrome)
b. Horse cry (cretinism)
c. Shrill cry (CNS infection)
d. Cry of preterm babies, cry of hungry baby, cry of pain.
e. Weak cry (various debilitating diseases)
f. Cry on handling (meningeal irritation, septic arthritis)
g. Voiceless (vocal cord paralysis)

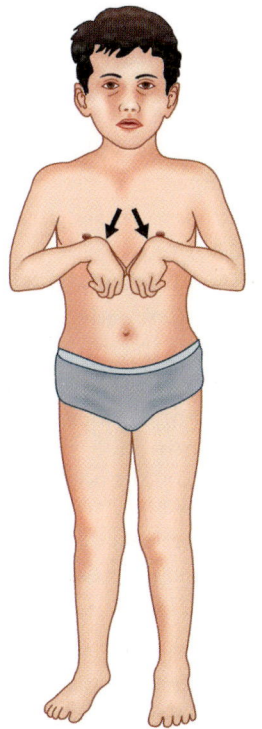

Fig. 1.1: Decorticate posture.

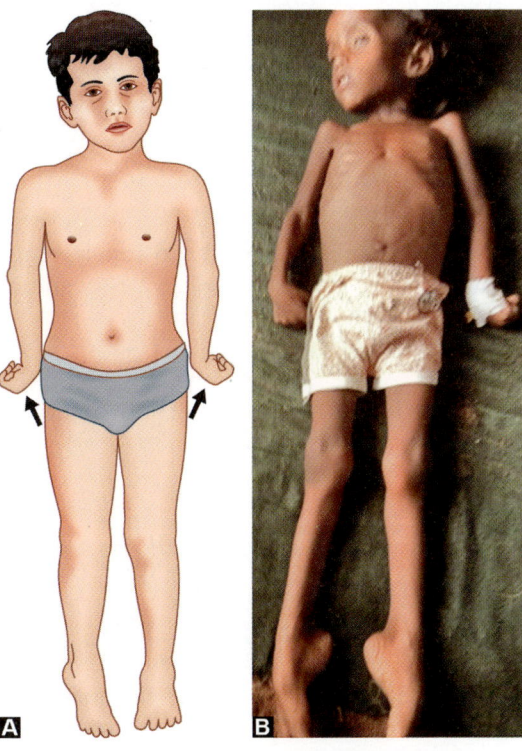

Fig. 1.2A and B: Decerebrate posture.

Table 1.1: Vital signs in children (normal values)

Age	Temp.°C	Pulse	Respiration	BP
Newborn	36–37	140	40	60/40
1 year	36.5–37.5	120	30	70/50
5 years	37 ± 0.2	100	20	90/50
10 years	37 ± 0.2	90	18	100/70
Over 10 years	37 ± 0.2	80	18	110/80

Alertness

Note: Alertness, interest in surroundings, apathy.

Coma

It is a state of profound and prolonged uncons-ciousness from which the individual cannot be aroused except for a short period.

Stages

Stage 1 (stupor): Patient can be aroused for brief period, during which he may make, voluntary and verbal responses.

Stage 2 (light coma): Patient cannot be aroused in spite of painful stimuli. Semi-purposeful movements may be noticed.

Stage 3: Painful stimuli fail to produce response, decerebrate posturing.

Stage 4: The patient is flaccid and apneic, brain stem functions are lost though a few spinal reflexes may be intact.

Nutrition

Note: Nutritional status, loss of subcutaneous fat, asthenia, cachexia, obesity.

Odour

Note: The odours. Some of them are charac-teristic, e.g. fruity smell of diphtheria, smell of ingested toxin (kerosene, etc.)

Gait

See the gait during walking-scissors gait (spastic cerebral palsy), waddling duck-like (proximal myopathy), ataxic, hemiplegic, high stepping, limping, equinus gait, etc.

Head

Note: Size, shape, uniformity, abnormal swelling or depression, fontanelle, palpation and auscultation (Fig. 1.3).

Size and Shape

Confirm microcephaly, macrocephaly or normal by head circumference measurement. Shape may be normal or abnormal. Abnor-malities, may be:

a. Flat occiput: When children lie in one position as in newborn or mentally retarded children.
b. Prominent occiput as in trisomy.
c. Frontal bossing, e.g. in rickets.
d. Acrocephaly: Top of the head is pointed (Alport syndrome).
e. Brachycephaly: It is a short wide head.
f. Plagiocephaly: One side is rounded more than the other as in craniostenosis.
g. Trignocephaly: Metopic suture is pointed.
h. Hot cross bun appearance: Cranial bossing, rounded prominences in the center of parietal and frontal bones cause the head square in shape as in rickets, so four prominences or bosses are separated by grooves. It gives hot cross bun appearance,
i. Scaphocephaly: Head is elongated antero-posteriorly.

Abnormal swellings or depression, e.g. cyst, hematoma, etc. are noted.

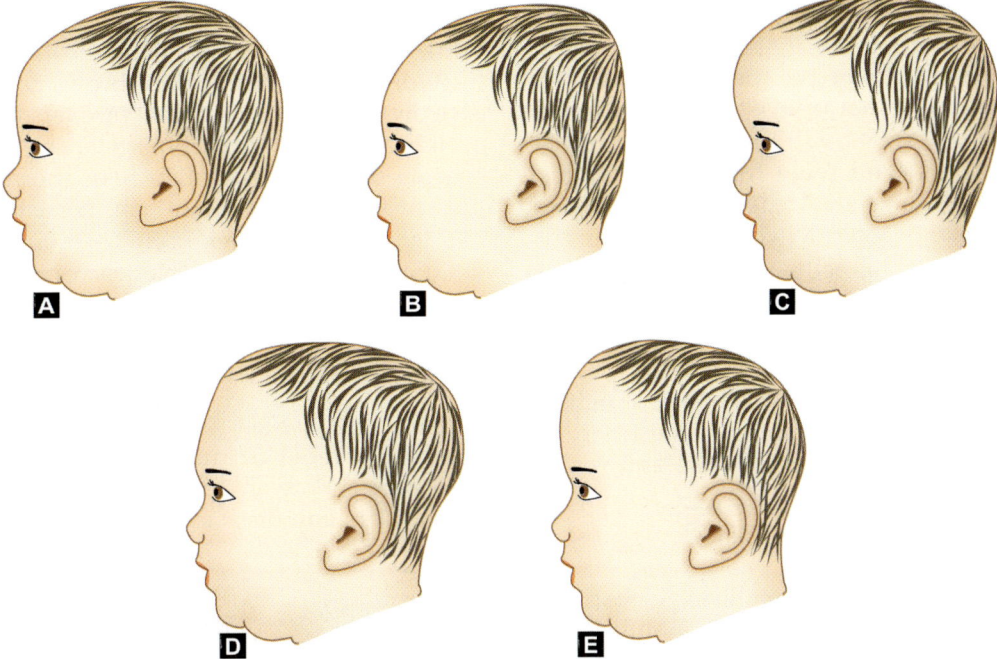

Fig. 1.3: Abnormalities of skull. (A) Normal; (B) Skull with flat occiput; (C) Frontal bossing; (D) Prominent occiput; (E) Short skull.

Fontanelle

Note: Presence or absence, size, fullness and pulsation.

At birth, six fontanelles are present—anterior, posterior, two sphenoidal and two mastoid (Figs 1.4 and 1.5). Most important fontanelles are anterior and posterior.

Size

The anterior fontanelle is 2.5 × 2.5 cm at the age of 3 months. The size is reduced gradually filling the gap and closing at the age of 9–18 months in majority.

The size of posterior fontanelle is that of fingertip at birth and it closes by two months

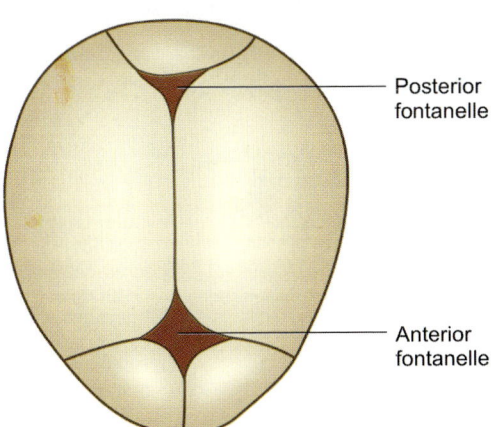

Fig. 1.4: Skull showing position of fontanelles.

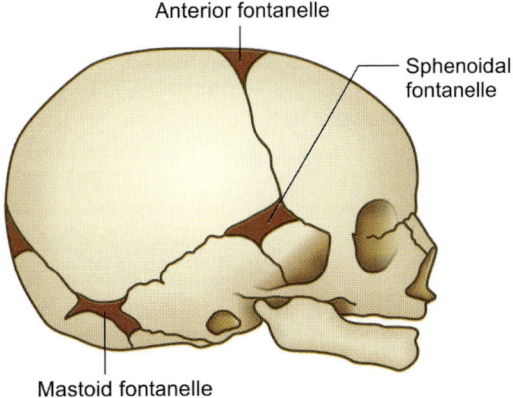

Fig. 1.5: Lateral view of skull (position of fontanelles).

of age. Early closure of fontanelle occurs in microcephaly craniostenosis.

Delayed closure of fontanelle and large fontanelle is seen in hydrocephalus, rickets, trisomy.

Elevated and wide fontanelle suggests increased intracranial tension while depressed fontanelle denotes dehydration.

Normal fontanelle is slightly depressed; physiological bulging is present in crying.

Pulsation

Normally anterior fontanelle may or may not be pulsatile but in increased intracranial tension fontanelle may be tense and without pulsation.

Cranial Sutures

Palpate the suture. Normally in newborn they overlap. But by the age of six months suture line is not palpated. After this age suture is wide as in hydrocephalus.

Palpation

The outer table of skull parieto-occipital region can be indented when pressed like table-tennis ball (craniotabes) seen in rickets, premature infants, hydrocephalus.

Percussion

Tap the skull with one finger not far from suture line of skull. Cracked pot-like sound may be heard in conditions in which sutures are separated, e.g. hydrocephalus.

Transillumination Test

Test is positive in hydrocephaly.

Auscultation

Bruit is heard in hemangioma of face.

Condition of Hairs

Condition of hairs is also noted light colored, sparse, brittle, coarse, dry or lustureless, localized or generalized loss.

Eyes

Look ptosis (Fig. 1.6) or shunken eye (dehydration). Look about eyebrows normal, excessive, any loss. Puffiness or edema over eyelids as in nephritis. Hypertelorism (wide spacing of eyes). Epicanthal folds (normally present up to 3 months of age) persist after this age in mongolism (Fig. 1.7).

Look at conjunctiva, sclera, cornea, iris, pupil and lens. Vision is recorded; fundus should be examined at the end.

Ears

Ears may be low set (when tragus of ear is below the level of outer canthus) as in mongolism. Note any deformity in shape of pinna. Note any discharge from ear, foreign

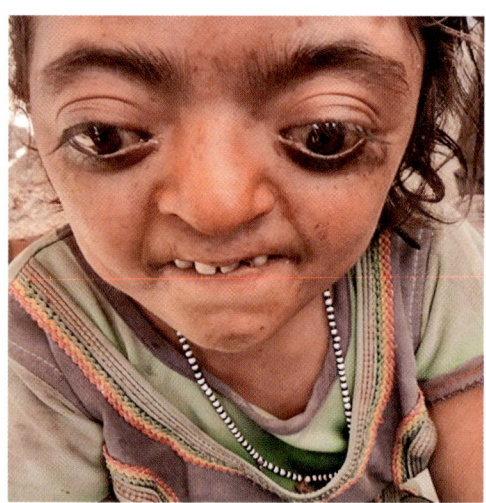

Fig. 1.6: Ptosis in Crouzon disease.

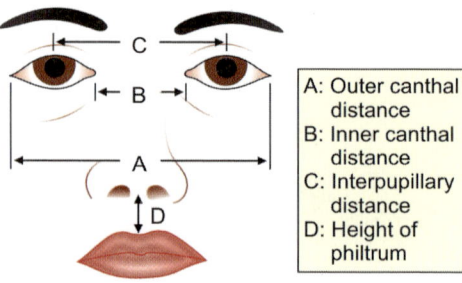

A: Outer canthal distance
B: Inner canthal distance
C: Interpupillary distance
D: Height of philtrum

Fig. 1.7: Measurement of face.

body. Test the hearing. In infant, turning of head in the direction of sound is indicative of hearing function normal.

Nose

Look for mucosa, discharge, polyp or membrane, saddle-shaped nose (hereditary) or due to syphilis.

Lips

The lips are pale in anemia and blue in cyanosis. Note large, broad, flattened or unusually pursed. Note any vesicles.

Mouth

May be small or large. Note any cleft lip, fissure radiating from ends to lips are seen in riboflavin deficiency and in fungal infection.

Tongue

Size may be large as in Down syndrome and cretinism. Scrotal tongue is seen in Down syndrome. Look moisture (dry in dehydration) and color—pale in anemia, blue in cyanosis.

See for any coating and any abnormal movements. Papillae are atrophic in anemia and pellagra, hypertrophic in scarlet fever, black hairy in hemophilias and purpura.

Gums

Normal color is pinkish blue. Color is reddish and gums are spongy in vitamin deficiency. Gums are hypertrophied in dilantin intake for long period and in leukemia.

Buccal Mucosa

Note Koplik spots (small bluish spots surrounded by reddish zone opposite to the molar teeth) are characteristic of prodromal stage of measles.

Look also for thrush and pigmentation.

Palate

Normal palate is slightly curved. See for any cleft, perforation or paralysis. High arched palate is seen in Down syndrome or Marfan's syndrome.

Throat

Throat can be examined both in supine or sitting position. The attendant (mother or nurse) is asked to restrain the child by immobilising his head and holding both the upper limbs. The neck should be slightly extended and crying actually helps to see the throat (Fig. 1.8).

Elder child is asked to say 'Ah' or 'Eh'. Note any enlargement of tonsils (Fig. 1.9), any areas of pus, grey or yellowish membrane which is difficult to remove as seen in diphtheria. Look for peritonsillar abscess.

Pharynx

Look for any fluctuant abscess or retero-pharyngeal abcess.

Teeth

Milk teeth are white in color and have a smooth edge and permanent teeth are of ivory (off white) color and have a serrated edge.

Delay in eruption of teeth may be due to hypothyroidism, cleidocranial dysostosis, rickets. If no teeth erupt up to 2 years of age, it is abnormal. Sometimes newborn has

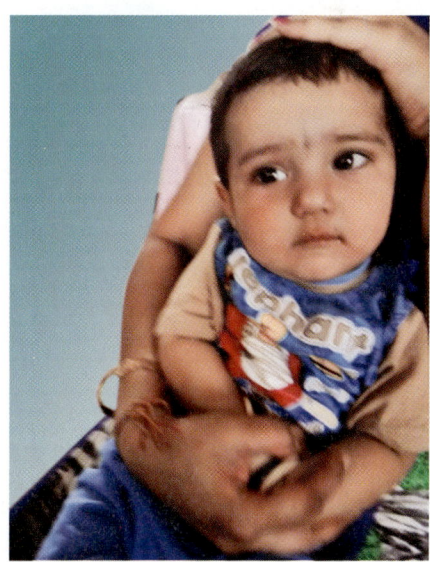

Fig. 1.8: Position and restraining the child for throat examination.

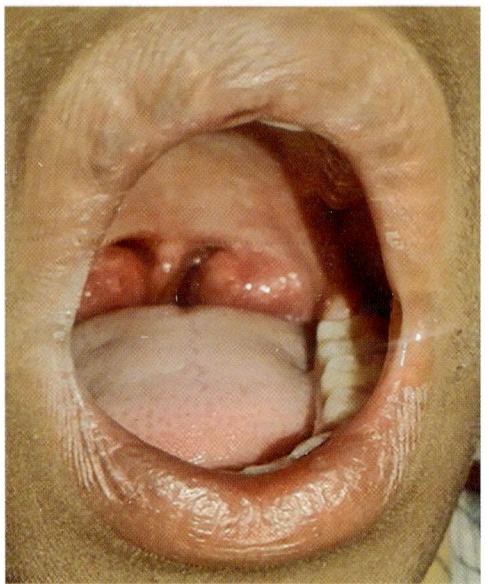

Fig. 1.9: Enlarged tonsils.

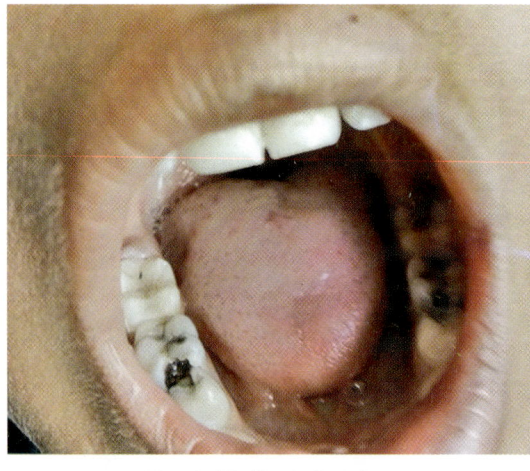

Fig. 1.10: Dental caries.

teeth but this is of no importance. Different abnormal colors observed are: Black (oral iron), yellowish (tetracycline therapy), green (erythroblastosis), red (porphyrias). In carries brown in early stage while black in late stage (Fig. 1.10). Excessive plaques are seen in bad orodental hygiene.

Hands

Cold and sweating (shock), pallor, jaundice best seen on palm. Cyanosis is seen at the fingertips.

In *clubbing* the tissue at the base of nails is thickened and angle between nail and adjacent skin is obliterated which is also detected this way. Look at the finger from side. The vertical height at the proximal edge of the nail (base) is about equal or slightly less than the vertical height at the distal interphalangeal joints normally. In late stage nail loses its longitudinal ridges and becomes convex (Figs 1.11 to 1.13).

Koilonychia is a feature of iron deficiency anemia, is rarely seen in children. Nail becomes soft, thin, brittle and concave (Fig. 1.14).

Clubbing is a feature of cyanotic heart diseases, suppurative condition of lungs, acute bacterial endocarditis.

Look for *palmar erythema, single palmar crease* (Fig. 1.15) and incurved little finger or any congenital deformity (Fig. 1.16). Observe any tremors or abnormal movements such as wriggling of worms (chorea).

Feet

Note any deformity, anomaly, solar creases in newborn (Fig. 1.17).

Skin

Inspect the skin and see the following:
Color: Pallor (anemia), cyanosis see whether it is only at the distal part of body (peripheral) or effects the lips and tongue also (central), jaundice (yellow discoloration), pigmentation (excessive or less).

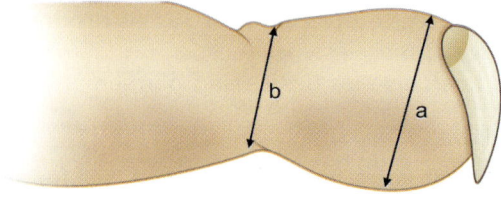

Fig. 1.11: Clubbing of fingers. (a) Height at the base of nail, (b) height at the distal interphalangeal joint.

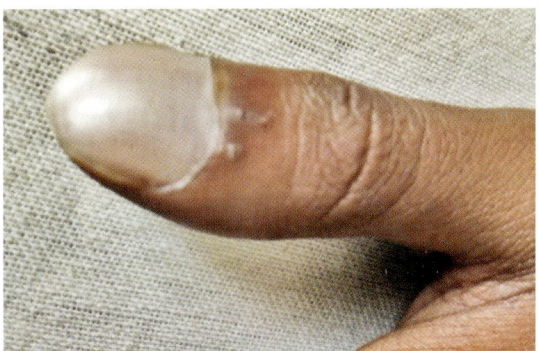

Fig. 1.12: Clubbing of finger.

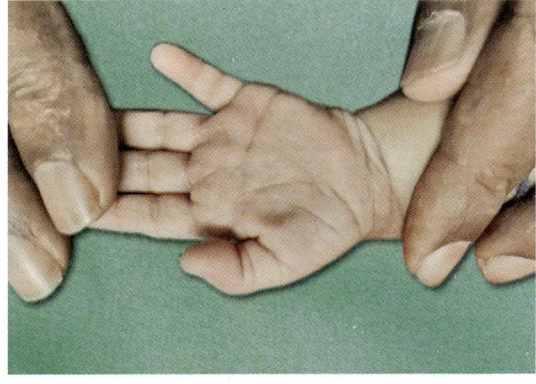

Fig. 1.15: Single palmar crease.

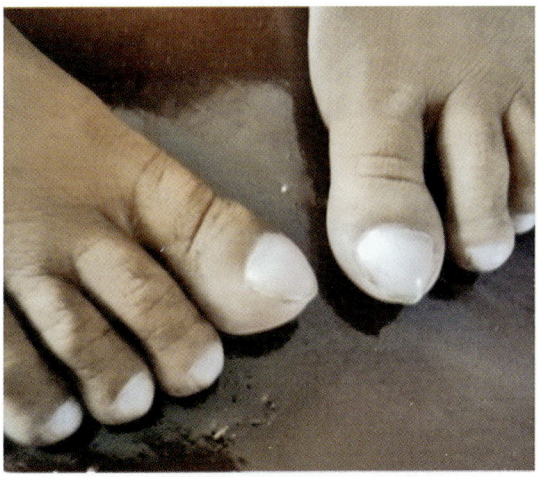

Fig. 1.13: Clubbing of fingers of feet.

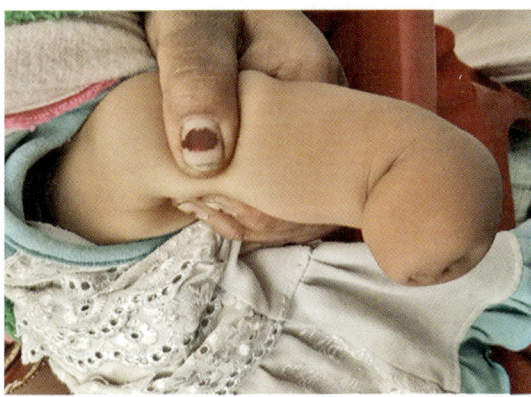

Fig. 1.16: Phocomelia.

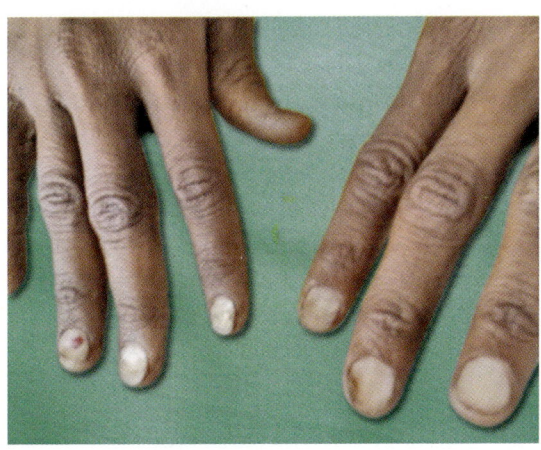

Fig. 1.14: Koilonychia.

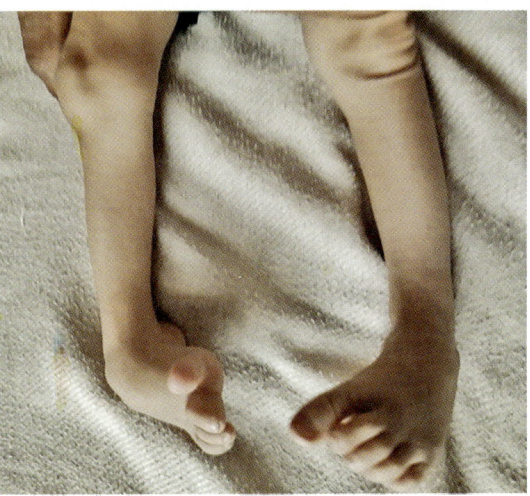

Fig. 1.17: Club foot.

Eruption

a. *Macule:* Flat lesions flush with surface of skin that blanch with pressure while petechiae does not.

b. *Papule:* Thickened elevated lesion of 0.5 mm size.

c. *Vesicle:* Elevated lesion above the skin surface with fluid in them.

d. *Pustule:* Vesicle which contains pus.

e. *Wheal:* Slightly elevated having central position paler than periphery.

Secondary lesions are excoriations, crust formation and squamation, pigmentation, ulceration, scar formation and atrophy.

Palpate the skin: Normal skin is smooth, soft, and moist. See texture-excessive roughness or dryness. Edema—pitting on pressure or nonpitting (filariasis) and its site. Palpate the subcutaneous emphysema.

Elasticity: Pick up skin and let it go. In normal elasticity skin falls quickly back to original state. In dehydration skin does not fall back quickly and remains creased, demonstrated well on anterior abdominal wall (Fig. 1.18A and B).

Palpate also for nevi, hemangioma, pus, blood or lymph or air (crepitus in subcutaneous emphysema).

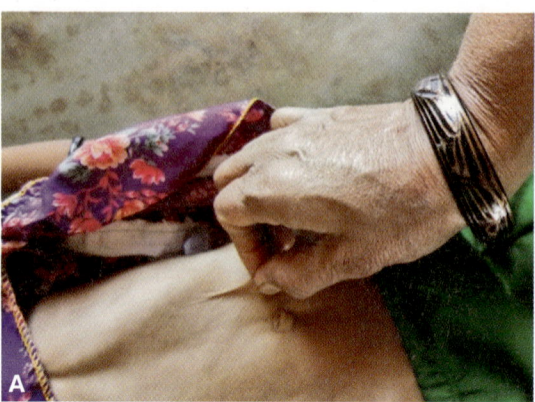

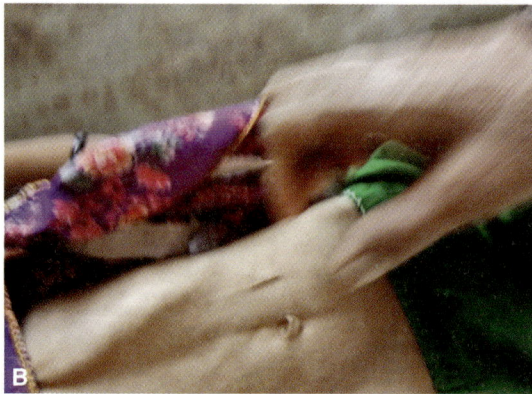

Fig. 1.18A and B: Testing skin elasticity.

Cyanosis: It means bluish discoloration of the skin and mucous membrane due to increased level of reduced hemoglobin in arterial blood or accumulation of abnormal hemoglobin.

It may be central or peripheral. Central cyanosis is generalized though involvement of tongue is characteristic. In peripheral cyanosis tongue remains unaffected and limbs are cold.

In heart failure cyanosis may be mixed type.

Dyspnea: It is a uncomfortable awareness of difficulty in breathing. Whether it is present at rest or on exertion.

Dysuria: It refers to discomfort or pain in micturition.

Edema: It may be generalized anasarca or localized such as ascites, hydrothorax.

Enuresis: Occurrence of involuntary voiding of urine after the age of which volition bladder control should have been established (about 5 years of age).

Hairs

Normal color varies with races. Hairs are thin, hypopigmented and easily pluckable in severe malnutrition. See also loss of hairs.

Neck

Normally neck is visible between the thorax and head, short in Turner's syndrome.

Lymph Glands

Cervical, axillary and inguinal lymph glands should be palpated and described its location, size, shape, consistency, temperature, tenderness, edge, pulsation and their discreteness.

OTOSCOPIC EXAMINATION OF EARS

Ear must be examined to visualize the tympanic membrane, the pinna of the ear is pulled with thumbs and index finger of one hand and back in older children and downwards in infants and newborn. The hands holding the otoscope should rest against the cheek of the child. Restrain the child before examination.

BONES AND JOINTS

Look for chest deformity, localized swelling, sternal tenderness, joint swelling, tenderness, mobility, size and symmetry of limbs.

Look for any deformity such as bowed leg, knock knee, telepes, club foot (Fig. 1.17). Bowed legs are normally seen during first 2 years of life. While sight knock knees are common up to 2–12 years of age.

Spine

Curvature (kyphosis, scoliosis), tenderness range of movements should be looked.

GENITAL AND SEXUAL MATURITY

Assess sexual maturity and look for any genital abnormality (Fig. 1.19).

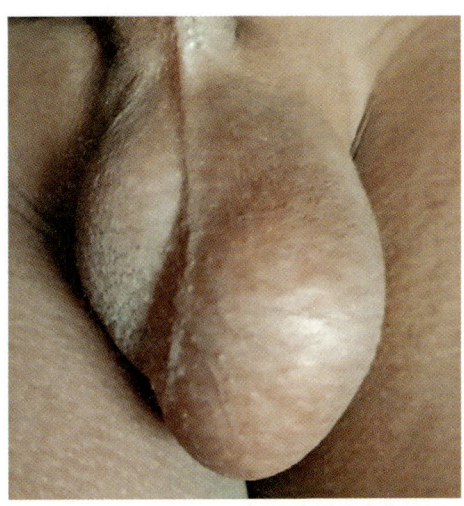

Fig. 1.19: Congenital left-sided hydrocele.

ANTHROPOMETRIC EXAMINATION

Weight

Recording of weight is essential for calculation and assessment of nutrition, calculation of drug dosage and early detection of malnutrition (Fig. 1.20).

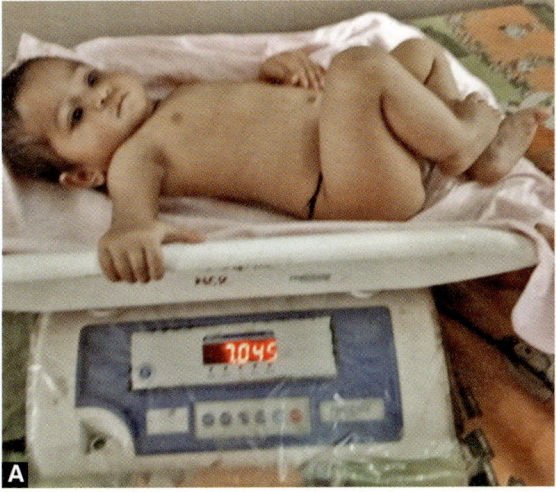
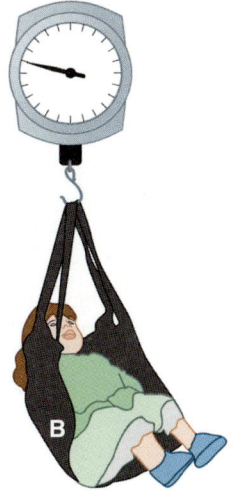

Fig. 1.20A and B: Weight recording.

The weight of child is taken without clothes on beam type of weighing machine, electronic, or other weight machine. For field condition salter spring machine is quite satisfactory because it is convenient to carry. The machine is hung from a hook or held by attendant and baby is placed on sling attached to bottom of hook.

Weight Charts

Serial weights are taken at regular interval and plotted in a graphy form which is known as weight chart. These charts have two curves:

a. The top line denotes mean weight of child reliving in good socioeconomic condition and 50th percentile of Harvard Standard Weight (Table 1.2).

b. Lower line represents mean weight of children of lower socioeconomic condition and 50th percentile of Indian Medical Council Research weight of average Indian child.

The space between two weight curves is described as 'Road to health'; weigh of child falling in between two lines is the normal, below it is malnourished (Fig. 1.21).

Table 1.2: Median weight for different ages

Age	Boys	Girls
At birth	3.3	3.2
3 months	7.0	5.8
6 months	7.9	7.3
9 months	8.9	8.2
12 months	9.6	8.2
2 years	12.2	11.5
3 years	14.3	13.9
4 years	16.3	16.1
5 years	18.3	18.2
6 years	20.5	22.2
7 years	22.9	22.4
8 years	25.9	25.5
9 years	28.1	28.2
10 years	31.2	31.9

Weight in kg = (age in years + 3) × 2

Table 1.3: Grades of malnutrition as per weight

Grades	Percentage of weight of reference standard (Harvard)
Grade I	71–80
Grade II	61–70
Grade III	51–60
Grade IV	50 or below

K infront of grade denotes kwashiorkor

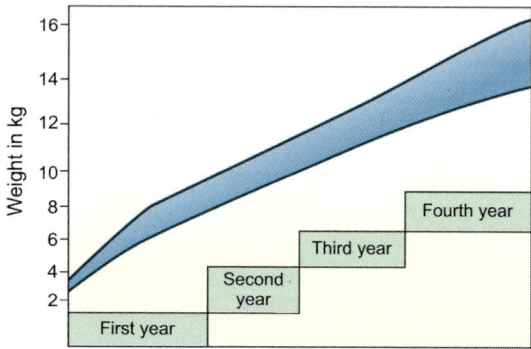

Fig. 1.21: Road to health chart for early detection of malnutrition.

Weight for length is a reliable index of nutritional status. Severity of undernutrition can be assessed as follows as suggested by Indian Academy of Pediatrics (Table 1.3).

Generally boy's weight is more than girls up to age of 10 years. During 12 and 13 years the girl's weight is more than boys due to early pubertal growth spurt.

Length or Height (Table 1.4)

a. **Below 2 years:** Length of the child is measured up to 2 years with the help of an infantometer. The infant is placed supine on the infantometer. Assistant keeps the vertex just touching the fixed vertical plane. The legs are fully extended by pressing over knees and feet are kept vertical at 90°, the movable pedal of infantometer is kept just opposed against the soles and length is read from scale (Fig. 1.22A).

Table 1.4: Normal height (50th percentile of Harvard Standard)

Age	Height in cm (boys)	Height in cm (girls)
At birth	50.6	50.2
3 months	60.4	59.2
6 months	66.4	65.2
9 months	71.2	70.1
12 months	75.2	74.2
2 years	87.5	86.6
3 years	96.2	95.7
4 years	103.4	103.2
5 years	108.7	109.1
7 years	124.1	122.3
10 yqars	140.3	140.3
12 years	148.6	151.9

Length or height (inches) = Age in years × 2.5 + 30

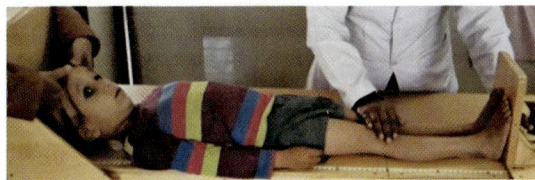

Fig. 1.22A: Measurement of length.

b. **Above 2 years:** Height is measured by stadiometer or simply making the child stand against a wall on which measuring scale is attached or by the rod attached to the lever type of weight machine. Child should stand bare- foot with feet together, back straight, eyes looking straight so that a line joining the external auditory meatus to the lower border of eye socket is parellel to the floor. With the help of wooden spatula or plastic ruler, the topmost point of vertex is identified on wall (Fig. 1.22B).

The change in height is observed in prolonged malnutrition hence this cannot be utilized as a tool to detect early or acute malnutrition.

Sitting Height

Child is made to sit on a firm horizontal place with knees apart and ankle crossed, the

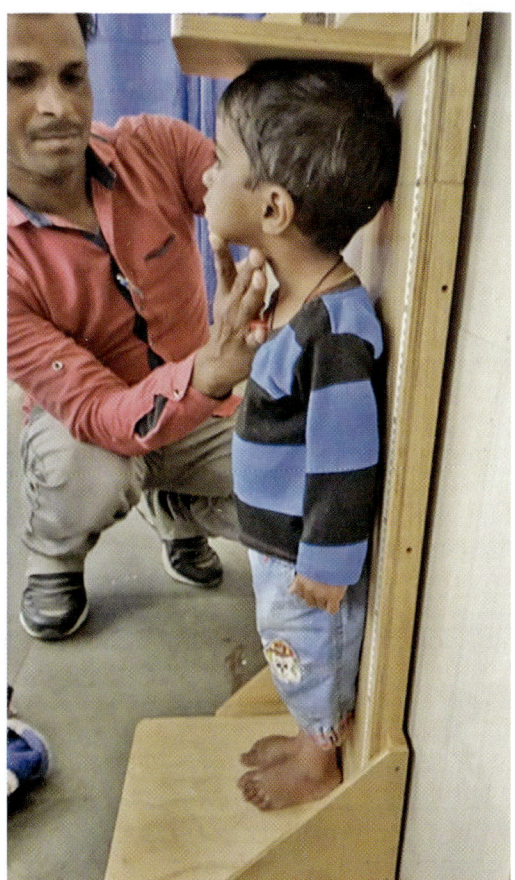

Fig. 1.22B: Measurement of height.

sacrum and dorsal regions are placed opposite to the vertical board or surface and it is measured. In dwarfism height below 3rd percentile and gigantism height is above 97th percentile.

Head Circumference (Table 1.5)

The head circumference is measured best with fiber glass tape with cross tape technique. The tape should encircle over the most prominent part of occiput and supraorbital area at frontal part.

Maximum increase in head circumference occurs in first year of life because rapid rate of growth; while between 1 and 5 years age only 5 cm gain occurs in head size; adult head size is achieved at about 5–6 years of age.

Table 1.5: Head circumference at different ages

Age	10th percentile (cm)	90th percentile (cm)
At birth	32.0	35.5
3 months	38.0	41.5
6 months	40.0	43.5
9 months	42.0	45.0
1 year	43.5	46.5
2 years	45.5	49.0
3 years	46.5	50.3
4 years	47.5	50.9
5 years	48.1	51.5

When head circumference (Fig. 1.23) is less than two standard deviations for the age and sex and height it is called microcephaly (Fig. 1.24) and when it is more than two standard deviations it is called macrocephaly (Fig. 1.25).

Chest Circumference

Chest circumference is measured at the level of nipples anteriorly and inferior angle of scapula posteriorly midway between inspiration and expiration with cross tape technique. The child is in recumbent position.

At birth circumference of head is larger than that of chest circumference while at 6–12 months of age both are equal. After 1 year chest is larger than head. In malnutrition this transition is delayed even up to 3 years of age because growth of brain is less affected by undernutrition.

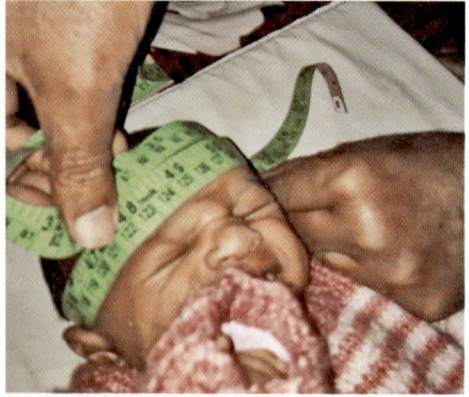

Fig. 1.23: Measurement of head circumference.

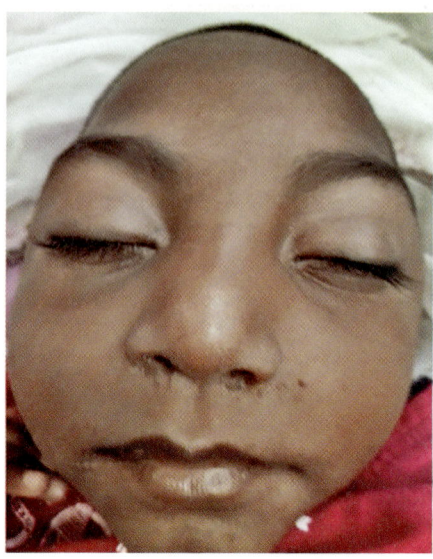

Fig. 1.24: Microcephaly.

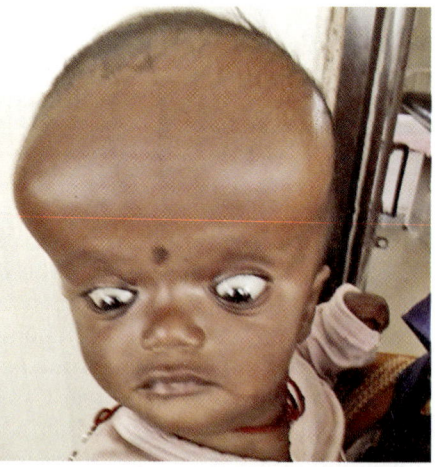

Fig. 1.25: Macrocephaly.

Mid-arm Circumference

Mid-arm circumference is measured by fibre glass or steel glass tape at the midpoint at arm between acromian and olecranon. For the detection of undernutrition, this is an age independent criterion because it remains constant from 6 months to 5 years of age (it remains constant at 16 to 17 cm). If the circumference of arm is below 12.5 cm it is suggestive of moderate to severe malnutrition (Fig. 1.26).

Bangle Test: It is an easy and quick test for assessment of arm circumference (Fig. 1.27).

A fibre glass ring of 4 cm diameter is slipped up the arm. If it passes above the elbow, it suggests that upper arm is less than 12.5 cm and child is malnourished.

Shakir Tape: It is an easy test which can be done by paramedical workers.

Tape of fibre has a red (<11.5 cm), yellow (11.5–12.4 cm) and green shades (>12.5 cm).

Skinfold Thickness: Measure over triceps or subscapular region by Herpenden's calipers. Normally, it is 10 mm or more; less than 6 mm indicates severe malnutrition.

Quack Test: Quack stick is a meter rod with two sets of markings. Expected height for particular mid-arm circumference is read on the arm. Undernourished child has more height than normal for particular mid-arm circumference.

CH:CR Ratio: At birth trunk is longer than limbs but afterward limb grows in length more than the trunk. Therefore, ratio of crown heel length (standing height) with crown rump

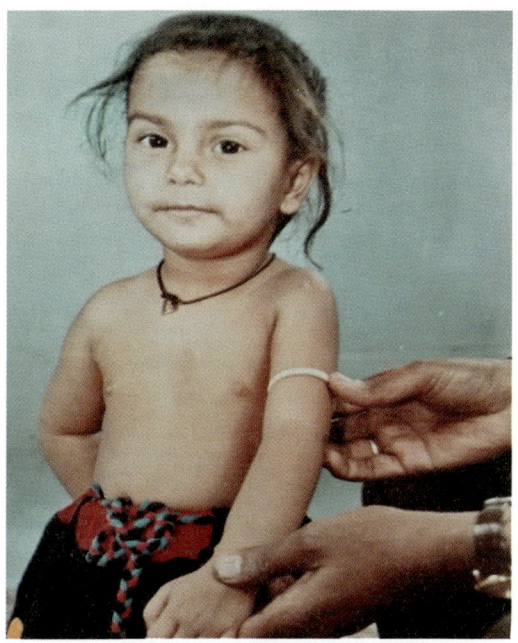

Fig. 1.27: Arm circumference by bangle.

ratio (sitting height) is at birth 1.7:1, at 4 years 1.4:1, 10–12 years 1.1:1.

In cretinism and achondroplasia CH:CR ratio is more while in arachnodactyly it is less. In pituitary dwarfism it is normal.

RESPIRATORY SYSTEM

Peculiarities in Children

1. Narrow air passage in children results in easy blockage by plugs, mucus, inflammatory edema, etc. Even small degree of airways obstruction can induce an obstructive process. That is why wheezing is common complaint in young children and infants and small areas of segmental collapse are common due to blockage of bronchi by pus or mucus.
2. Mucous membrane of whole respiratory tract is in continuity hence diseases of lungs closely linked to that of nasal sinuses.
3. In infants below 2 years transverse section of thorax is circular.

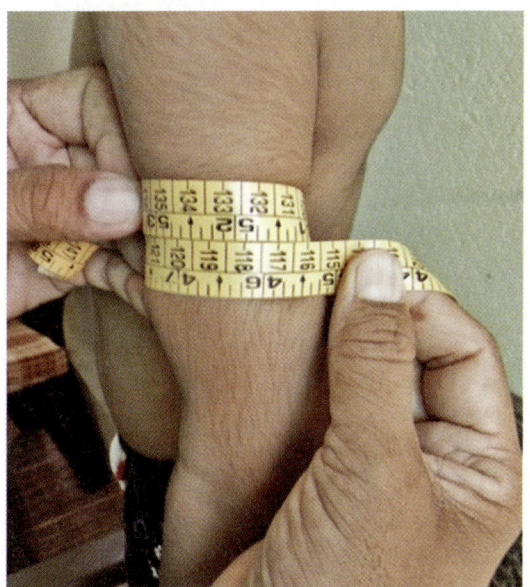

Fig. 1.26: Measurement of mid-arm circumference.

4. In infants, the respiration is purely abdominal (diaphragmatic) because the ribs are horizontal. Children therefore are more liable to pneumonia after abdominal operation because child resists breathing due to pain and secretions in the lungs tend to accumulate which may become infected and cause pneumonia. Moreover, expelling the secretions by coughing is intensely painful due to abdominal wound.

5. Chest wall is soft with incompletely calcified ribs easily sucked in chest wall is highly elastic so fracture of ribs is rare.

6. Mediastinum is mobile, rarely fixed with adhesions.

7. Lymphatic system well developed. Hilar lymph nodes enlarge readily.

8. Nasal air passages are most important for newborns because they are nose breathers and nasal obstruction may result in severe respiratory distress.

9. Percussion over manubrium may be impaired due to enlarged thymus. The chest in children is more resonant than adult.

10. The breath sounds are hollow and puerile or harsh vesicular in children. Due to small thorax the adventitious sound may be conducted from one side to opposite side.

11. A relatively short and open eustachian tube in infants and young children is responsible for higher incidence of otitis media.

12. Lung changes are most often found in upper lobe due to aspiration during infancy because during feeding and post-feeding period infant is often recumbent.

13. History of contact for tubeculosis and history of measles and whooping cough must always be taken.

Areas of examinations of chest for description purpose are as follows:

Front: Supraclavicular, infraclavicular, mammary and inframammary areas.

Side: Superior, middle and inferior axillary areas.

Back: Suprascapular, interscapular, scapular, infrascapular and basal areas.

Respiratory system is examined under: (i) Inspection; (ii) Palpation; (iii) Percussion; and (iv) Auscultation.

It is better to do percussion at the end because it may frighten the child.

Inspection

Chest is examined by standing at the head or foot side of the patient with eyes at the level of chest.

SHAPE OF THE CHEST

Normally, shape of the chest is round up to 2 years, after 2 years of age, it is oval because anteroposterior diameter increases.

In chronic obstructive disease as in asthma oval shape becomes rounded in shape in elder child.

Look for abnormalities of shape of chest as under:
  i. Depression of the sternum (pectus excavatum)
  ii. Protrusion of sternum (pigeon chest)
  iii. Swelling ol costocondral junctions (ricketty rosary as seen in rickets)
  iv. Deep groove at the site of diaphragmatic attachment
  v. Bulging on any side. Look for deformity—spine, ribs, clavicle, scapulae.

Look for hypoplastic nipple (Down syndrome) or widely spaced nipple (Turner's syndrome).

Symmetry: Note whether symmetrical or not, or any bulging present.

Movements of chest: Look for rate and rhythm.

Rate: Count the rate of respiration per minute. It is increased or slowed down. Pulse respiration ratio is normally 1:4 but in pneumonia it becomes equal.

Rhythm: Respiration is irregularly irregular in newborn, transitory apnea may be seen normally. Look for inspiration or expiration. If inspiration is unduly delayed it is suggestive of laryngeal or tracheal disease. While delayed expiration is suggestive of bronchial or pulmonary disease, e.g. asthma.

Signs of Dyspnea

Flaring of ala nasi, retraction of suprasternal notch, intercostal spaces and subcostal region.

Expansion and Symmetry

Diminished or no movement and expansion is seen in pleural effusion, pneumothorax, collapse.

In Cheyne-Stokes breathing respiration gradually gets deeper and deeper till maximum then falls again until pause of complete apnea occurs then again deepening and reduced respiration. It is a feature of increased intracranial pressure, renal and cardiac diseases.

In paradoxical respiration which occurs in diaphragm paralysis due to injury to phrenic nerve or poliomyelitis—chest collapse on inspiration and the abdomen becomes prominent on expiration.

PALPATION

Findings of inspection to be confirmed.

Position of Trachea

Put the index finger and ring finger on the sternal attachment of the sternocleidomastoid. Feel the trachea with middle finger at the suprasternal notch.

Normally, trachea is slightly deviated towards the right, marked deviation occurs on same side due to pulling force, e.g. collapse, while deviation towards other side may be due to pushing force, e.g. pleural effusion, pneumothorax.

Cardiac Impulse (Apex Beat)

Palpate the maximum cardiac impulse. It is usually at 5th left intercostal space just inside midclavicular line.

Apex beat is changed in lung disease. In scoliosis apex beat is changed.

Movements

Fix the fingertips of either hand at the patient's side and making the tip of the thumbs just meet in midline of posterior of chest. Ask the child to take deep breath or see when he takes deep breath in between when he is crying. The distance of departure of the thumbs from the midline indicates the extent of expansion of each half of the chest. Diminished movement suggests effusion or collapse or consolidation of lung on affected side.

Vocal Fremitus

Palm of the hand should be applied flat on chest then patient is asked to say 'one', 'ninty nine', or 'ek do tin'. Compare on other side, normally where heart encroaches on left lung it is diminished.

Vocal fremitus is diminished in pleural effusion because collapsed lung fails to convey the vocal fremitus. It is increased when lung is consolidated or contains large cavity near surface.

Palpate for any swelling or tenderness at chest.

PERCUSSION

Direct Percussion

With one finger over the chest wall it is easily done on infant and newborn.

Indirect Percussion

The middle finger (pleximeter) of the left hand is placed firmly on the part which is to be percussed. The other fingers should not touch the chest wall since they may dampen the resonance. The back of middle phalanx is then struck with the tip of middle finger of right hand (percussion finger). The intensity and quality of sound produced and feeling of resistance imparted to the pleximeter finger is observed. Start at the top of chest and compare with same area on opposite side and proceed downward. Pleximeter finger should be kept parallel to the expected line of dullness.

Normal resonance is heard over lungs while tympanic note is heard at stomach and dull note at liver and heart.

Hyperresonance is heard due to pneumothorax while dull note is heard during consolidation, fibrosis, collapse and pleural effusion.

Limit of Liver Dullness

Normally found on the 10th intercostal space on the midclavicular line and 8th rib on midaxillary line and 10th rib at back on right side.

Auscultatory Percussion (Fig. 1.28)

More reliable and sensitive than ordinary percussion. The examiner stands or sits on other side of the sitting patient. Examiner percusses over the front of chest over the manubrium by tapping lightly with distal phalanx of middle or index finger of dominant hand while listening with the diaphragm piece of stethoscope over the posterior side of chest. Compare both sides from apex to base. In the end, paravertebral areas are auscultated for detection of mediastinal or hilar lymph nodes enlargement.

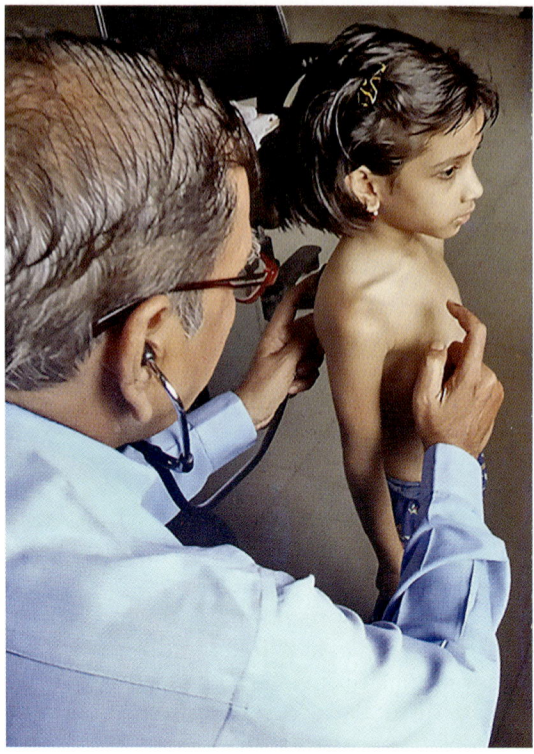

Fig. 1.28: Method for auscultatory percussion.

AUSCULTATION

For auscultation of child stethoscope with smaller diaphragm and bell is better because it covers small area at a time. Infant and young children can be examined in whatever position—put to mother's breast or given feeding, bottle, etc. or while mother or father supports the child upright against the security of their shoulders.

Crying child is auscultated when he takes deep breath during crying and vocal fremitus and resonance can be assessed during crying.

Characteristics of breath sounds are described as follows:

a. Normal breath sounds
b. Vocal resonance
c. Adventitious sounds.

Breath sounds are vesicular and bronchial.

Vesicular

Normally heard all over the lungs, best heard at axilla and infrascapular areas. The inspiratory sound is high intensity rustling sound which is produced by air entry through alveoli and heard during entire period of inspiration. The expiratory sound is heard immediately after the inspiratory phase without pause but it is heard during the earliar part of expiration. The inspiratory phase is twice longer than expiratory phase (Fig. 1.29).

Bronchial

Bronchial breathing is heard commonly when stethoscope is placed over the trachea and upper part of front of chest. Also in small infants posteriorly second thoracic intercostal space. Inspiratory sound is of higher pitch and has an aspirate quality and not heard throughout the inspiratory phase. There is a pause between inspiration and expiration. The inspiratory sound is harsher than expiratory sound and heard throughout the expiration (Fig. 1.30).

Bronchial breathing is heard apart from normal areas in case of consolidation, large cavity or sometime in effusion.

Breath sounds are diminished over areas with reduced air entry, e.g. in pleural effusion, pneumothorax, collapse of lung.

Vocal Resonance

Ask the patient to say 'ek', 'do', tin or 'one' 'ninty nine' and listen to the chest with stethoscope or during crying compare with opposite side.

It is diminished in condition in which air cannot pass through the air passages, e.g. obstruction of bronchi or in condition when voice is not conducted to the chest wall as in massive pleural effusion or pneumothorax, etc.

Vocal resonance is increased when sounds are heard as if they are close to the ear. Words are heard more distinctly or as if originating in ears or even whisper by patient is heard. Increased vocal resonance is feature of consolidation or cavity.

Adventitious Sounds

Crepitations: These are discontinuous or bubbling sounds commonly heard at the beginning of inspiration. They may be fine, coarse or medium. They are features of bronchitis, bronchiolitis, while fine creptations are commonly heard at the peak of inspiration and are feature of early stage of pneumonia.

Rhonchi: Prolonged, uninterrupted sounds arising in bronchi and due to partial obstruction of lumen of bronchi due to mucosal swelling, secretions and constriction of smooth muscles. They may be feature of childhood asthma, bronchiolitis or eosinophilia (Fig. 1.31).

Pleural rub: Pleural rub is a leathery sound having rubbing character and associated with inspiration and expiration and is produced by rubbing together of inflamed pleural layers.

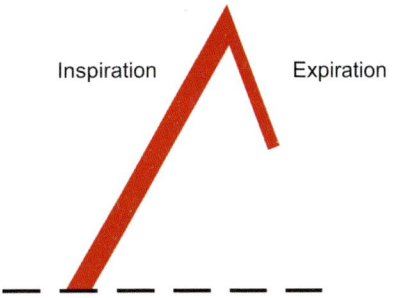

Fig. 1.29: Vesicular breathing.

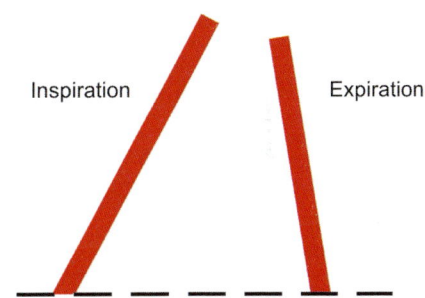

Fig. 1.30: Bronchial breathing.

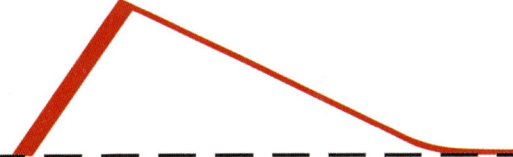

Fig. 1.31: Vesicular breathing with wheezing.

Note

Throat sounds due to secretions at the throat may confuse crepitations. They are generalized and disappear after coughing or suction of throat. Put the chest piece of stethoscope near the mouth—throat sounds may be heard.

GASTROINTESTINAL SYSTEM

Peculiarities in Children

i. Shape of abdomen is protuberant (pot belly) and soft in infant

ii. Liver is palpable up to 2 cm and soft in consistency and is normal throughout childhood.

iii. Spleen tip may be felt during first 3 months of life.

For description, abdomen is divided in compartments as seen in Fig. 1.32.

Inspection

Normally, abdomen has a full contour. In early life it may be little protuberant because of the physiological lumbar lordosis and thin musculature of abdominal wall.

Abnormally, it may be scaphoid, flat or protuberant, causes of protuberant abdomen are:

1. Flatus (gas), fluid (ascites), faeces, fat, in obese children.
2. Due to laxity of abdominal wall rickets, celiac disease and hypothyroidism.
3. Intestinal obstruction.
4. Hirschsprung's disease.

Flat abdomen: Normally in thin children, malnutrition, failure to thrive and anorexia nervosa. In newborn, flat abdomen is suggestive of diaphragmatic hernia. Complete absence of muscles seen in Prune-Belly syndrome.

Localized Swelling

See any localized, e.g. linear, spleen enlargement, pyloric stenosis lump, Wilm's tumour etc.

Abnormal Pulsation

Pulsation at epigastrium may indicate pulsations of the liver or enlargement of right ventricle or in thin subject.

Movements

See movements of abdominal wall. Diminished or absent in guarding of muscles as in peritonitis. Paradoxical (collapsing in inspiration) in diaphargmatic paralysis.

Striae

White striae indicate recent weight loss or steroid therapy, purplish in Cushing's syndrome or slate colored discoloration in Addison's disease.

Distended Veins

Seen at epigastrium in obstruction of inferior vena cava. Blood flow is below upward while in portal hypertension direction of blood flow is away from umbilicus (Fig. 1.33).

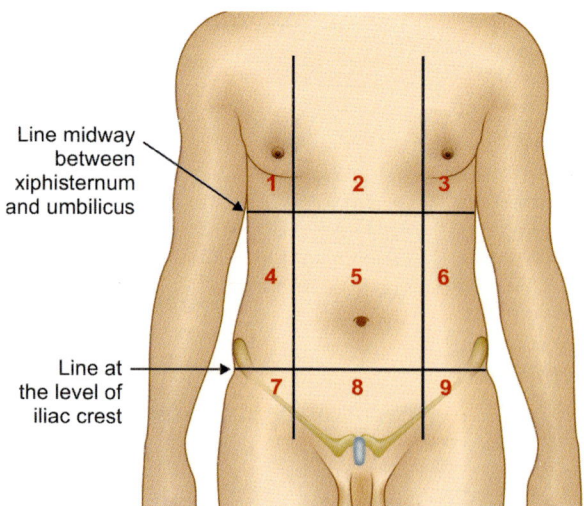

Line midway between xiphisternum and umbilicus

Line at the level of iliac crest

1: Right hypochondrium
2: Epigastrium
3: Left hypochondrium
4: Right lumbar
5: Umbilical region
6: Left lumbar
7: Right iliac region
8: Hypochondrium
9: Left iliac region

Fig. 1.32: Abdomen is divided into nine regions.

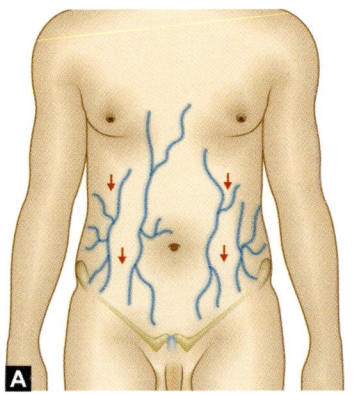 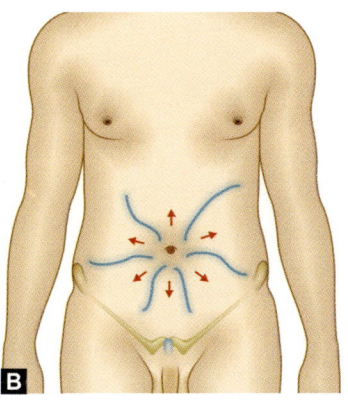 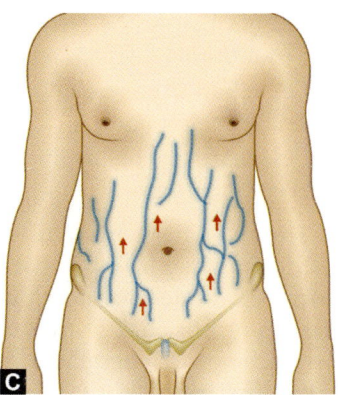

Fig. 1.33: Superficial veins on abdominal wall showing direction of blood flow: (A) Superior vena cava obstruction; (B) Portal hypertension giving rise to caput medusae; (C) Inferior vena cava obstruction.

Peristaltic Movements

Peristaltic movements are normally visible in thin child. Abnormally excessive peristaltic movements over left upper quadrant of abdomen are seen in pyloric stenosis.

Normally, movements are left to right but in large intestinal obstruction movements are right to left.

Movements are better seen if some feed is given to child.

Diastasis of rectus muscle is seen in midline in a linear form while exstrophy of the muscle seen just above symphysis pubis.

Umbilicus: Look for hernia, discharge, granuloma or polyp.

PALPATION

It is most important part of examination. Examine when child is asleep or best examine in the mother's lap. Dipping technique is used if massive ascites is present.

Tone

Note the tone of the abdominal wall. It is soft, firm or tense. Board-like rigidity indicates peritonitis, diffuse firmness muscular spasm as in tetanus or chest disease. Localized firmness at midline as seen in full bladder. Very soft abdomen is feature of Prune-Belly syndrome.

Mass

Palpate for any mass, e.g. caecum.

Pain or Tenderness

Normally, abdomen palpation is painless. See any tenderness or painful area. When tenderness is seen on withdrawal of the fingers it is called rebound tenderness as seen in peritonitis.

Palpation of Mass of Congenital Pyloric Stenosis

Give some water or feed. Palpate with left hand from left side of the baby at a point midway between the umbilicus and costal margins along the right lateral border of the rectus muscles.

Palpation of Liver

Standing right side of patient place the right hand flat on abdomen.

Start palpating from right iliac fossa and move upward. During inspiration edge is palpable. It will be felt as the regular border which rides beneath the hands trace it towards epigastrium and to the right side.

Note the tenderness, consistency, its surface and edge; lower border is normally palpable.
- 3–3.5 cm below the costal margins up to 6 months of age.

- 0–3 cm below the costal margin between 6 month to 4 years of age.
- Less than 2 cm below the costal margin 4–10 years of age.
- Less than 1 cm below the costal margin over 10 years of age.

These enlargments of liver taken in midclavicular line. If upper border is below the normal it is downward displacement while if upper border is above, it is upward displacement. Generalized increase in size is called hepatomegaly.

Pulsatile liver is seen in tricuspid incompetence or stenosis or constructive pericarditis.

Spleen

Spleen is located on left side; in newborn, it may be palpable normally. It is usually not palpable unless it is enlarged at least three times its size.

Feel for spleen standing on right side of the patient. Place the flat of hand (left) over the edge of costal margin and firmly below ribs and lateral abdominal wall medially as the patient breathes in. Start palpation with right hand. The edge of the enlarged organ will be felt against the finger of right hand. If it is not palpable in supine position place the patient in right lateral position. Keep your hand over the left lower ribs on mid scapular line pushing spleen forward. Now right hand is used to palpate the spleen starting from right lower quadrant to left upper.

Auscultate for friction rib over spleen.

Kidneys

It is done by bimanual palpation. Place the left hand posteriorly at the flank pushing the kidney forward while with other hand anteriorly below the costal margin push it backward, upward and inward.

If abdominal wall is relaxed and patient takes deep inspiration if kidney is enlarged or displaced it is felt to move downwards and then on expiration upwards.

In newborn kidneys are palpable normally.

Other Abdominal Masses

Look for any other abdominal mass and describe its size, shape, location, consistency and movement with respiration bimanually palpable, intra-abdominal or in the abdominal wall, attachment to liver, spleen, kidney, etc.

PERCUSSION

Normally, the abdomen is tympanic on percussion except on solid organs as liver or gall bladder. Highly tympanic note is heard in intestinal obstruction or paralytic ileus.

Dull note may be due to free fluid in abdominal cavity or tumours.

Methods to Detect Free Fluid

i. **Fluid thrill**: Patient is lying supine. Ask the third person to place the edge of the hand vertically on the midline of abdomen. The examiner now places the palm of the hand on one side of abdomen and taps with the finger on opposite side of flanks. If free fluid is present, one can feel a fluid wave created by tap.

ii. **Shifting dullness:** Patient is on supine position. Place a finger on the flank parallel to midline. Percuss over an area of dullness. Now ask the patient to roll off on opposite side without taking pleximeter finger off. Wait for a time till fluid has settled at the dependent position. Percuss again. Percussion will now give a tympanic note over the same place where it was dull on percussion when patient was supine.

AUSCULTATION

Normally various tinkling sounds are heard. They are increased in obstruction or decreased or absent in paralytic ileus or peritonitis.

Listen systolic murmur at groin in renal artery stenosis.

Genitalia

Examine scrotum, testes and penis and see any abnormality: Examine female genital organs. Look for secondary sexual character.

Anus and Rectum

Anus is examined in left lateral position; look for any abnormality. Rectal examination is better to do with little finger. Empty rectum suggests megacolon or mass (intussusception).

CARDIOVASCULAR SYSTEM

Peculiarities in Children

1. Foramen ovale closes immediately after birth but potential opening remains for months or years.
2. Ductus arteriosus functional closure occurs within minutes after birth, while anatomical closure occurs in weeks.
3. Ductus venosus obliterates within weeks.
4. Heart size relatively large at birth but grows less rapidly than rest of the body and appears to become smaller.
5. Position of apex beat is at 4th left intercostal space in midclavicular line in young child.
6. Percussion of heart border is of greater value than adult owing to thinness of chest wall.
7. Pulse is rapid and difficult to feel among infants due to increased vagal tone.
8. In infants, 1st and 2nd heart sounds at apex are equal in intensity, later in childhood 1st heart sound is louder at apex; 2nd sound is louder at base.
9. Second sound louder over pulmonary than aortic area (*vice versa* in adult).
10. Third sound at apex common and physiological.
11. Sinus arrhythmia common. Functional systolic murmur and venous hum are common in children.
12. Right ventricular hypertrophy is common in newborn while left ventricular hypertrophy in adult.
13. Blood pressure is difficult to determine; may require narrow (3 cm) cuff but reading with small cuff higher than with large. Flush method or Doppler system may have to be used to record blood pressure in infants.
14. Jugular venous pressure is difficult to take due to short and obese neck.
15. Heart rate fluctuates within normal limits.

Arterial Pulse

Feel the radial artery; apart from it temporal, femoral, dorsalis pedis artery should be felt.

Rate

In infant cardiac rate of newborn is rapid and with wide fluctuations. Normal values are as follows:

Age	Pulse rate/min.
Newborn	70–109
Up to 1 year	80–160
2 years	80–130
4 years	80–120
6 years	75–115
8 years	70–110
10 years	70–110

Also auscultate the heart; look for pulse deficit (ectopic and auricular fibrillation).

Sinus arrhythmias in which pulse rate is higher during inspiration and less during expiration is common or physiological in children.

Rhythm

See whether it is regular or irregular. Rhythm of heartbeat in newborn is often irregular and related to respiration. When the infant is asleep there may be period of apnea and slow cardiac rate which speeds up with respiration.

Volume

Volume of pulse is appreciated by the lift on the fingers as the pulse wave passes through.

Tension

Tension is estimated by noting the intensity of pressure required to obliterate the pulse. It represents pulse pressure.

Character

Character is difficult to determine in younger children (normal, bounding, collapsing or water hammer type, plateau).

Blood Pressure

Proper cuff size is essential. It can also be recorded by flush method. Cuff is wrapped around the arm and limb is raised vertically and held above the head till palm becomes pale. Now pressure in the cuff is raised beyond the expected systolic pressure in this position. The arm is then brought down to the side on the cot and cuff is gradually deflated. The point at which the palm becomes flushed is indicative of systolic pressure. Diastolic pressure cannot be recorded.

Doppler method is best to record blood pressure in newborn and infant.

Venous Pulse

Look at the neck veins. For measurement of jugular venous pressure patient is kept propped up in bed at an angle of 45°. Mean height of venous columm is measured by observing vertical height to which the distended and pulsating portion of veins rise above the sternal angle. Raised pressure occurs in right heart failure.

Child is in Trendelenburg position at an angle 45° with the help of plastic ruler. JVP is measured in relation to angle of Louis (Fig. 1.34).

Inspection and Palpation

i. *Deformity in chest wall:* Note any deformity, bulging or depression, in bony case. It may be due to cardiomegaly or displacement of mediastinum.

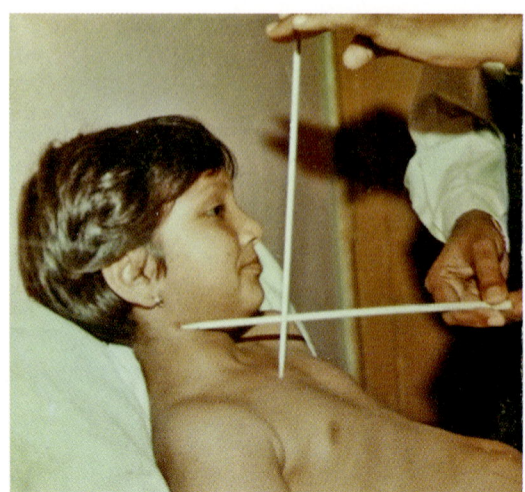

Fig. 1.34: Method of evaluation of jugular venous pressure (JVP).

ii. *Veins on chest wall:* Note if veins are prominent. Direction of flow is noted. Direction is above downward in mediastinal tumour or growth and below upward in inferior vena cava obstruction.

iii. *Apex beat:* Apex beat corresponds to the lowermost and outermost portion of cardiac impulse. It is up to 2 years in the 4th intercostal space in or just medial to midclavicular line while later on it is in 5th space at or just medial to midclavicular line.

Note its character. It is heaving when it lifts the palm on palpation of precordium. Look pulsations at 2nd space due to pulmonary artery enlargement or other parts of chest.

Look for precordial bulging of chest wall due to ventricular enlargement.

Neck Veins

Examine, with the child at an angle of about 45° (not sitting erect). In healthy person the level of the column of blood in the jugular vein is not seen because it is never above the level of manubrium sterni as in heart failure. Pulsations are difficult to see in children due to short neck and problem of cooperation of child.

Thrill

See for any palpable 'purring' sensation called thrill under the palm over the precordium. It is a feature of organic heart disease and absent in functional murmur.

PERCUSSION

Used as a mean to detect changes in heart size. Percuss with plexor finger parallel to the heart border on the right and left side and parallel to the ribs on first and second interspace. Start away from the heart and proceed towards it until percussion note changes.

Heart size is increased in pericardial effusion.

AUSCULTATION

Child should be examined both in sitting and supine position. Start auscultation from mitral area and move in all four areas—mitral, tricuspid, aortic, pulmonary and also in second intercostal space and back (Fig. 1.35).

The finding in each of the major areas of precordium are described under the following headings.

Heart Sounds

- First and second heart sounds
- Splitting and spacing of heart sounds
- Opening snap
- Triple rhythm
- Third and fourth sounds.

First heart sound is short and sharp (lup) while second heart sound is described as 'dup'. Splitting of second heart sound is normal. Third heart sound is normal in children best heard at apex in lateral position. Increased intensity is associated with constrictive pericarditis.

Opening snap is a clicking sound heard only in systole best on precordium suggestive of mitral stenosis.

Triple rhythm may be due to third heart sounds or a gallop rhythm. Fourth heart sound similar to third heart sound is best heard at precordium at apex caused by filling of left ventricle late in diastole due to atrial contraction.

Adventitious Sounds

Murmurs

i. See whether they are functional or organic, time of occurrence (systolic, early systolic, diastolic immediate diastolic, delayed diastolic, mid-diastolic or continuous murmur.

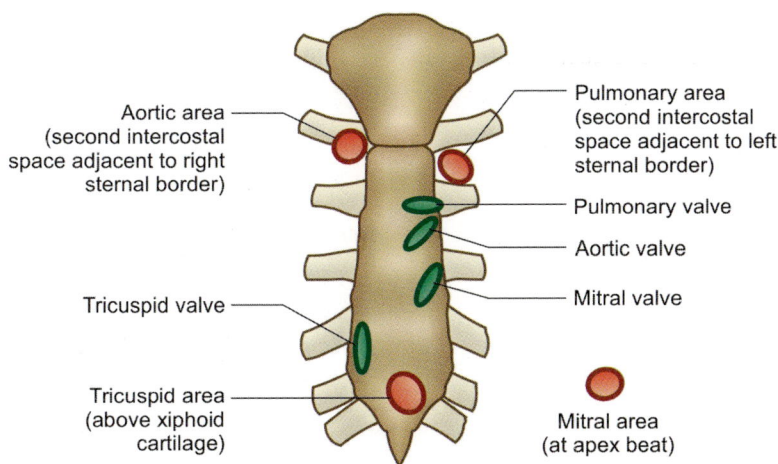

Fig. 1.35: Auscultatory areas of heart.

ii. **Intensity:** Intensity is not related to the seriousness of the disease. It is graded as follows: *Grade I*: Soft, not heard in all positions, no thrill. *Grade II*: Soft, heard in all positions, no thrill. *Grade III*: Loud, no thrill. *Grade IV*: Loud, thrill present. *Grade V*: Louder murmur with thrill. *Grade VI*: Loudest, heard even without stethoscope, thrill present.

iii. **Change with respiration:** Ask the patient to take deep breath and hold the breath for a few seconds and listen the intensity of murmur. Murmurs orginating on right side of heart increase in intensity during inspiration.

iv. **Direction of spread:** The murmur is said to spread if it is heard some distance away from the point of maximum intensity. It is suggestive of organic disease.

v. **Character of murmur:** Rough and low pitched murmur due to obstruction in blood flow, soft and high pitched (regurgitant murmur).

CENTRAL NERVOUS SYSTEM

Peculiarities in Children

1. Sensory system almost impossible to investigate accurately until child is old enough to cooperate but effect of painful stimuli noted.
2. Several primitive automatic reflexes (Moro reflex, etc.) disappear up to the age of 5–6 months. Persistence suggests brain damage.
3. Developmental history and examination is essential for evaluation of central nervous system.
4. Deep tenden jerks are brisk during infancy; plantars may be normally extensor in infants up to 2 years.
5. Abdominal and cremasteric reflexes develop about 3–4 months of age.
6. Fundus examination shows pale disk in normal infants. Papilledema appears only after 3 years of age when sutures have closed.

7. Examination of skull is essential for CNS evaluation.

History: Ask about obstetric history, fall or injury, family history of convulsions, onset of symptoms and its course.

HIGHER FUNCTIONS

1. **Level of consciousness:** Consciousness can be defined as the state of awareness including responsiveness to stimulation and ability to recall past events.
   Assess whether the child is fully conscious, drowsy, confused, semicomatosed or in coma. The child may be awake but gives a blank staring look. There is no response to social interaction (coma vigile).
2. **Orientation:** Ask simple questions about time, place and recent, past events: 'Where he is?' etc., it can be tested in older child. Orientation is altered in toxic state.
3. **Emotional status:** Assess emotional behavior look for hyperactivity, short span of attention, impulsiveness.
4. **Speech:** Note its presence or absence— failure to speak any word by 18 months and failure to make meaningful sentences by 3 years age are abnormal. Mutism may be evidence of deafness, mental retardation or autism.
   Look for sensory or motor aphasia or disorders of articulation such as stammering, lalling. Ascertain whether disorder is in expression (talking) or receptive (understanding) or inability in reading. In global aphasia both receptive and expressive speech are effective.

Intelligence

See growth and development.

Memory

Give him few numbers, e.g. 5, 6, 7, 8, ask to count forward and backward. Backward repetition is effected in lesion of brain.

Name the city, flower, food. Ask him to repeat the items from memory.

Delusions and Hallucination

False belief is called delusion while hallucination is false signal or impression from the organ of special senses.

CRANIAL NERVES

Cranial Nerve I (Olfactory Nerve)

In children, testing of smell is very difficult. Ask child to close his eyes. Present some common objects for smell, e.g. toothpaste, coffee, tea. In infants, change of facial expression is only clue. Exclude chronic rhinitis before testing.

Cranial Nerve II (Optic Nerve)

 i. Vision
 ii. Acuity
 iii. Field
 iv. Fundus.

Vision

 i. Make a menacing gesture as if we are going to poke the eye. A consistent blink response indicates cortical vision while inconsistent blink response means vision is intact but interpretation of vision is defective (parietal lobe lesion).
 ii. If child follows a moving light or objects, intact cortical vision is confirmed.

Visual Acuity

 a. In toddler, rough assessment of visual acuity is done by looking his response to small common objects.
 b. After the age of 5 years, simplest is the vision screening by 'EV chart or in elder by Snellen chart.

Field of Vision

Formal perimetry is possible at school age and if children are cooperating with perimetry gross evaluation is possible as soon as infant follows object and develops visual fixation. common test object, e.g. colorful toy (red black) brought to the eye from sides separately. Note if the child responds for approached object from one side and not from other side.

In another test when child is looking towards examiner's eye placed at some level, examiner takes his hands to the periphery of the visual field with index finger extended and diagonally opposite direction. He fixes one of the fingers and then asks the child to show which finger moved. This is repeated at different points in the perimeter of the field.

Fundus Examination

Better done at last. Better pupillary dilatation is done by instillation of 10% phenylephrine eye drops for 5 minutes. Examine with ophthalmoscope. See optic disc which is relatively pale in infants, distinct is white with sharp distinct margins in optic atrophy. Disc is dirty pale with blurred margins in post-papilledematous optic atrophy.

Look for papilledema, papillitis, chorioretinitis, hypertensive retinopathy, retinal hemorrhage, cherry red spot, retinitis pigmentosa, choroidal tubercles.

Color Vision

It is difficult to evaluate below 3 years. Give common numbers 'Xs' or 'Os' and triangles, ask him to name or trace. Elder children are tested with modified Ishihara chart. Defective color vision may be due to optic nerve lesion.

Oculomotor (Third Nerve)

It supplies all the extraocular muscles of the eye except external rectus and superior oblique. Look for following signs for its testing (Table 1.6).

 i. Diplopia
 ii. Ptosis
 iii. Dilated and fixed pupil. Loss of light and consensual reflex. Pupil is larger in size in children than the adult and its diameter up to 5 mm is normal.
 iv. The eye is displaced outwards and downwards.

Table 1.6: Effects of paralysis of eye muscles

Muscle	Cranial nerve	Diplopia when child looks	Eyeball deviation
Internal rectus	Third	Towards nose	Outwards
Superior rectus	Third	Upward and outward	Downward and inward
Inferior rectus	Third	Downward and outward	Upward and inward
Inferior oblique	Third	Upward and inward	Downward and outward
Superior oblique	Fourth	Downward and inward	Upward and outward
External rectus	Sixth	Toward temple	Inward

Trochlear (Fourth Nerve)

The downward movement of eye is impaired and diplopia is noticed on looking at horizontal line.

Abducent (Sixth Nerve)

Paralysis causes internal squint and inability to move the eyeball outwards and diplopia occurs on looking outwards.

Fifth Cranial Nerve (Trigeminal)

The trigeminal nerve has motor and sensory components. There are three divisions of trigeminal nerve—ophthalmic, maxillary and mandibular (Fig. 1.36). First two are sensory and third is motor and sensory.

Test

Motor

i. Ask the patient to clench the teeth and palpate the masseters and the temporalis muscles.
ii. Ask him to open and close the mouth, if one side is paralyzed the jaw will be deviated to the nonparalyzed side when mouth is opened.

Sensory

a. Touch and temperature are tested as usual on face.
b. Corneal reflex. Blow in the child's eye causes a blink or touch in cornea with small cotton piece causes blink. Test both sides.

Reflex

Ask the patient to open the mouth. Gently place a finger at the tip of mandible and tape

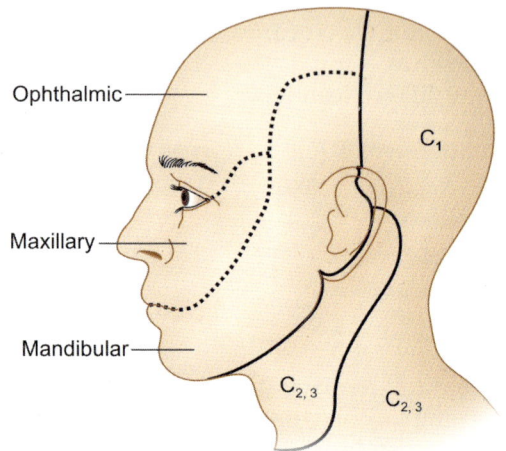

Fig. 1.36: Sensory nerve supply of face (3 divisions of trigeminal nerve).

with percussion hammer. Masseter muscle contracts.

Taste

Loss of sensations occurs over anterior two-thirds of tongue only when peripheral part of nerve is damaged.

Seventh Nerve (Facial Nerve)

a. It is purely motor nerve. It supplies all the muscles of face and scalp except levator palpebrae superioris.
b. Chorda tympani which runs part of its course with facial nerve carries sensations from anterior two-thirds of the tongue.
c. Autonomic afferent fibres to lacrimal gland and submaxillary and submandibular salivary glands also run with the facial nerve.

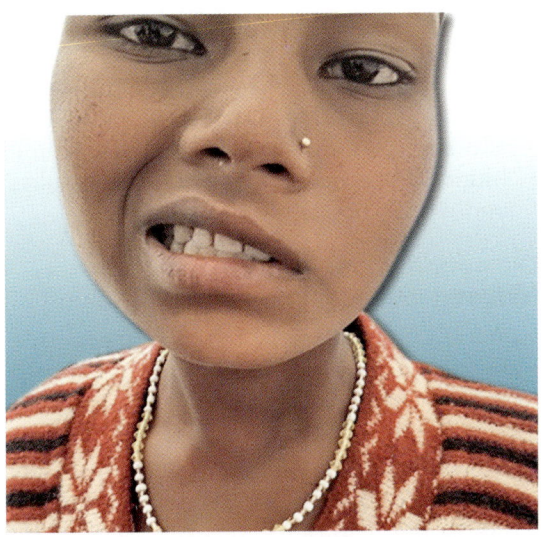

Fig. 1.37: Left-sided facial palsy.

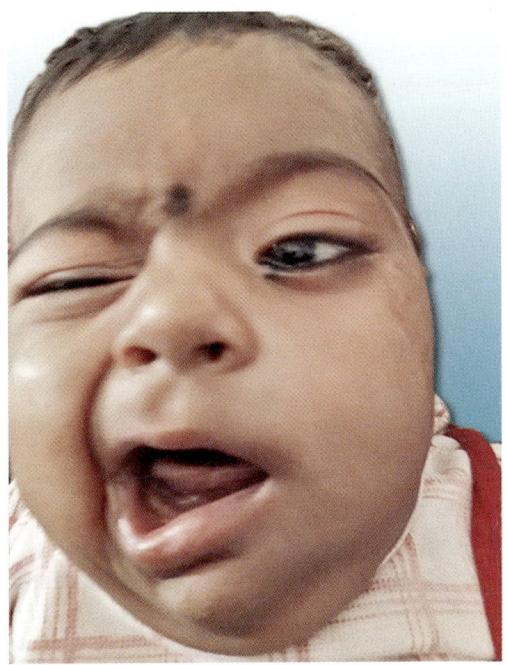

Fig. 1.38: Left-sided facial palsy.

Test

a. Ask the child to close the eyes as tightly as 'possible' he cannot close on effected side.
b. Ask the child to whistle; he cannot.
c. Ask the child to blow up one cheek and push out air against closed lips. It is easy to push out the air out of paralyzed side.
d. Ask him to wrinkle the forehead; he cannot.
e. Ask him to show his teeth and smile. The face is flat on one side and the pull is toward the unaffected side (Fig. 1.37).

In infant and young children observe face during crying (Fig. 1.38).

Taste Sensation

Hold the tip of tongue with moist filter paper dry one half of tongue with filter paper and place drops of salt (NaCl) or sugar (dextrose) on outstretched tip by means of dropper or cotton applicator and ask the patient to indicate by finger clues or head nods (Fig. 1.39).

Now wash the tongue. Next taste tested, bitter is tested at last.

Lacrimation and salivation is effected on effected side if proximal part of the nerve is effected during its course.

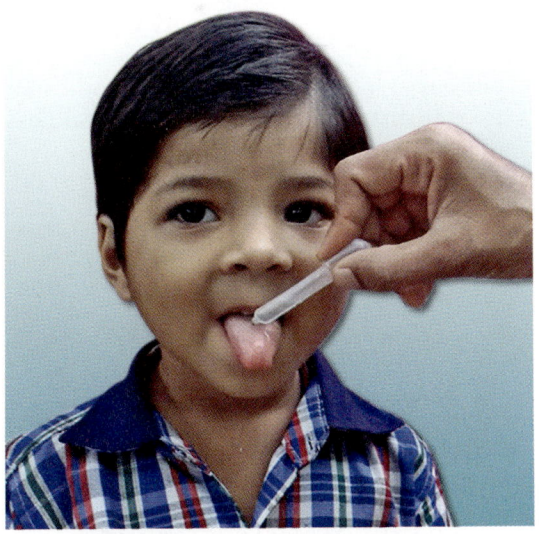

Fig. 1.39: Testing for taste sensation.

Supranuclear Lesion

Only lower part of face is paralyzed and upper part (frontalis and the part of orbicularis oculi) escapes due to ipsilateral represen-tation in cerebral cortex.

	Upper motor neuron	Lower motor neuron
1.	Wrinkling of forehead not effected	Effected
2.	Upper part of face is not effected. Ask to close eyes. He can close	Effected
3.	Taste not effected	Effected

Vestibulocochlear Nerve (Eighth Nerve)

a. **Test for hearing (auditory component):** It is difficult to test for hearing in children up to 3–4 years of age and mentally retarded child. There is some clue in patient history, e.g. failure to respond to normal sounds, delayed speech.

Child is at mother's lap facing examiner. Make some noise on one side near the ear and see the response. Intensity is increased gradually to judge the threshold. Examine one ear at a time. Audiometry is indicated to confirm and partial high tone weakness (Fig. 1.40).

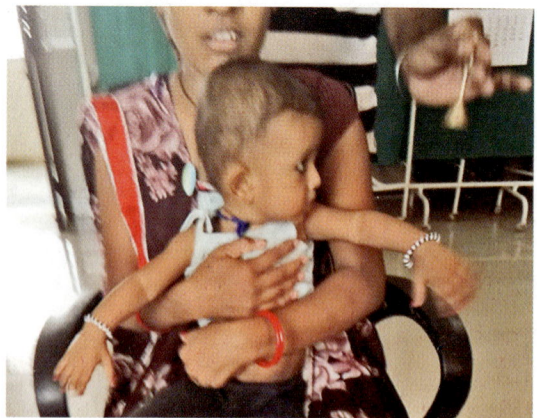

Fig. 1.40: Test for hearing.

b. **Vestibular:** Vestibular dysfunction is rare in childhood.

Child cannot explain vertigo. Clues are unexplained—crying, try to bury his face and not wanting to open the eyes. Vomi-ting with change of posture or imbalance and nystagmus is found.

Glossopharyngeal, Vagus and Accessory Nerves (Ninth, Tenth and Eleventh Nerves)

Glossopharyngeal carry sensory fibres from posterior one-third of tongue and motor to middle constrictor of pharynx and stylo-pharyngeous.

Vagus is motor to soft palate, pharynx and larynx. Its parasympathetic portion supplies the respiratory, cardiovascular and gastrointestinal muscles.

Paralyses of these nerves are tested as follows (in paralyses):

1. Stridor, nasal or hoarseness of voice in unilateral paralysis while aphonia in bilateral paralysis.
2. Loss of swallowing reflex with drooling and choking.
3. Nasal regurgitation when swallowing liquids due to palatal paralysis.
4. Ask the patient to say 'Ah' and see the uvula. No movement of palate on effected side. Uvula is drawn towards normal side.
5. Gag reflex: The stimulus is produced by touching the base of the tongue or pharyn-geal wall with tongue blade. Normally, retraction of tongue and elevation of pharyngeal wall occur. In paralysis it does not occur.
6. Loss of sensation in posterior one-third of the tongue.

Accessory Nerve (Eleventh Nerve)

a. Ask the patient to shrung the shoulder against resistance. Neck retraction towards opposite side.
b. Infant keep the head slightly rotated towards affected side.

Hypoglossai Nerve

Motor nerve supplies tongue.

Test

i. Atrophy and fibrillation of the tongue.
ii. Ask the patient to protrude the tongue. It is deviated towards affected side.

Motor System

Examine upper limbs, trunk and lower limbs in that order.

1. **Posture:** Paralyzed limb is kept in state of extension and external rotation. Look for decerebrate rigidity or posture.
2. **Abnormal movements:** Look for tremors, chorea, athetosis, dystonia or myoclonus.
3. **Fibrillation and twiching:** Due to slow degeneration of anterior horn cells or motor nuclei of cranial nerves.
4. **Nutrition:** Circumference of the limbs should be measured at identical points identified at bony land marks (anterior superior iliac spine, olecranon). Compare it to other side and look for wasting. Hypertrophy means enlarged muscle mass with good tone (as in athletes.) Pseudohypertrophy muscle mass is enlarged due to fatty infiltration of muscles. Muscles are weak.
5. **Muscle tone:** Tone is examined by following ways: (i) See any abnormal posture; (ii) Palpate the muscle, soft or flabby; (iii) Put major joint on passive movement through their full range and see the resistance; (iv) By shaking the unsupported limb for range and fuidity of movement. Compare both sides.
   It may be increased (spasticity) or decreased (flaccidity) or normal.

Muscle Power

Assess the strength of young child by looking at his activity of routine work and by some tests as follows:

Test	Muscle
1. Ask the patient to get up from supine and stand	Back, leg, hip and proximal leg muscles
2. Ask to walk on tip—toes and on heel	Gastrocnemias soleus and tibialis anterior
3. Support or lift the child with examiner's hands in the child's axilla	Shoulder muscle
4. Observe respiration, ask to blow	Intercostal muscle
5. Ask the patient to flex the elbow with palm facing upwards	Biceps
6. Extend the arm	Triceps

In elder child individual muscle group is tested actively and passively with or without gravity and with or without resistance and graded as follows:

Grade:

0 : Complete paralysis.
1 : Flicker of contraction possible.
2 : Movements possible if gravity eliminated
3 : Movements against gravity but not against resistance
4 : Movements possible against some resistance.
5 : Normal power.

Muscle weakness occurs in both upper and lower motor neuron paralysis but absent in extrapyramidal disorders.

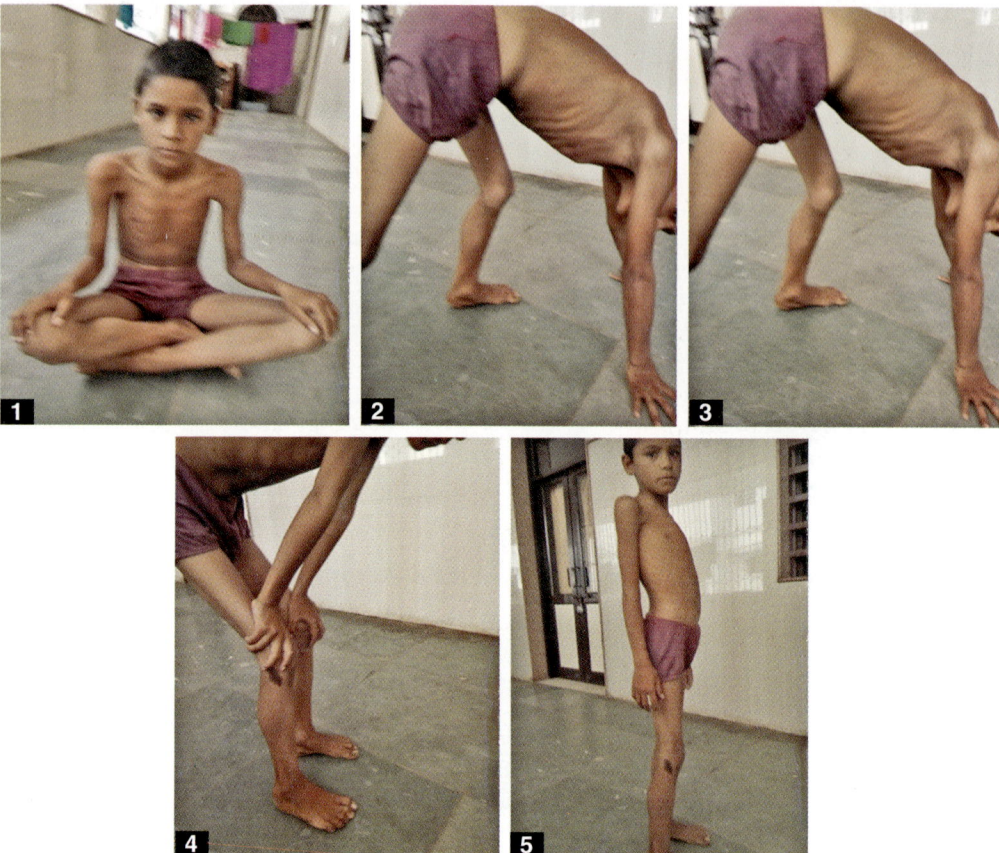

Fig. 1.41: Gower's sign (1–5).

Gower's sign: Ask the child to stand up from lying down. In getting up, he first rolls to the prone position, kneels and then raises himself to standing by pushing with his hands against shins, knees and thighs. It is positive in moderate to severe muscular dystrophy (Fig. 1.41).

Coordination

Impairment of skilled movements is found in disorder of upper motor neurons and in cerebellar disorder.

Test for Coordination

i. **Finger nose test:** Ask the patient to touch the nose with the finger, then touch the tip of examiner's finger held in space and touch his nose again.

ii. **Rapid alternating movements:** Ask the patient to supinate and pronate the hands rapidly.

Irregular and slow performance is seen in cerebellar disorder. Normally, child above 5 years of age should be able to do rapid alternate movements.

iii. The patient flexes the elbow against resistance by examiner, now examiner withdraws the resistance. In cerebellar lesion arm may hit his face uncontrollably.

iv. Ask the patient to extend his arm in front of him slightly separately. Tremors, chorea, etc. identified.

v. Ask the patient to run, ride cycle, walk on line with heel or toe.

vi. Patient is lying prone with the knee flexed 90°. Now hold the toes down firmly and tap the Achilles tendon; see the response. Normal response is plantar flexion.

Interpretation

Exaggerated response: Pyramidal lesion, increased in myopathies, absent in peripheral nerve lesion.

Clonus

Having the child lie down, the knee flexed slightly and ankle resting on left hand so that tendon of Achilles tendon is slightly stretched. With the finger of right hand a sudden jerk is given to flex the foot, clonus is felt by right hand. Response; Forced alternating contractions and partial relaxation. Foot will go through plantar flexion, dorsiflexion movements repeatedly.

SENSORY SYSTEM

Superficial Sensory

Touch: Child's eyes should be closed and examiner touches the skin with cotton wool. The child has to indicate 'yes' when he feels. First complete on one side then proceed on other side.

Pain: Some stimulus is given as by tip of pen. Ask to say 'sharp' or 'dull', not just say 'yes'. Also see facial expression and withdrawal of limbs.

Temperature: Two tubes are filled with cold and hot water. Touch the skin with one then other. Ask to respond by saying hot or cold. Note: There is an overlap of innervation near midline from two sides. Spinal cord segment does not correspond to level of vertebra.

Level of anesthesia is calculated as follows:

Vertebra	C_1	C_7	T_{10}	T_{12}	L_1
Spinal segment	C_1	C_8	T_u	L_3	end of cord
Assess the dermatomes also.					

REFLEXES

Deep Tendon Reflexes

Biceps (C_5–C_6): The patien's arm is held with elbow in flexion and supported by hand of examiner. The thumb of the supporting hand is held over the insertion of biceps tendon and thumb is tapped with a reflex hammer. Note contraction of biceps (Fig. 1.42).

Triceps (C_6–C_7): With the arm flexed 90° at the elbow the forearm is supported by examiner. A tap over the triceps tendon causes contraction of triceps with or without extension of elbow (Fig. 1.43).

Supinator (C_5–C_6): With the arm between pronation and supination and forearm supported by examiner the styloid process of radius is lapped. Normally, there is flexion of forearm and supination (Fig. 1.44).

i. Patient sits at the edge of the table, legs hanging free and loose.
ii. Patient lying supine, the knees are supported by examiner's hand relaxed and flexed 30°–40°.
iii. In newborn, flex the knee and foot flat over the examiner's abdomen.

Tapping the patellar tendon produces contraction of quadriceps resulting in extension at the knee.

Knee jerks (L_2–L_4): These may be tested in various positions (Fig. 1.45).

Ankle jerks (S_1–S_2): Patient lying supine with his hip flexed and externally rotated and the knee flexed with the foot lying over the anterier aspect of other leg. Press sole of foot and tap tendon Achilles. Normal response is plantar flexion.

Deep Sensory

Test for sense of position, sense of movements and vibration to sense and stereognosis.

Cortical Sensory

a. **Two-point discrimination:** Two pinpricks up to 1 cm apart can be normally appreciated. Explain the patient when eye open what is one or two. Now ask to close his eye and touch two pinpricks and ask 'one' or 'two'.

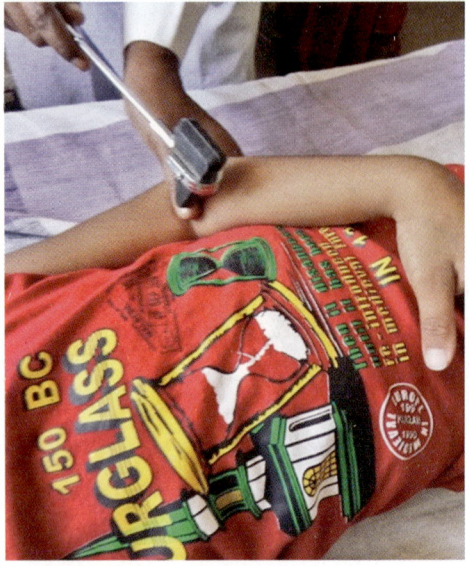

Fig. 1.42: Elicitation of biceps jerk.

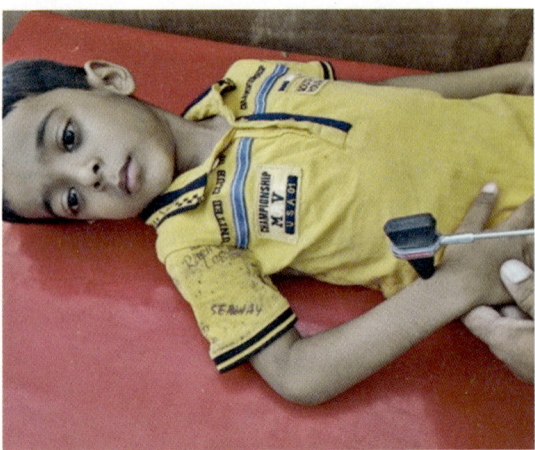

Fig. 1.44: Elicitation of supinator jerk.

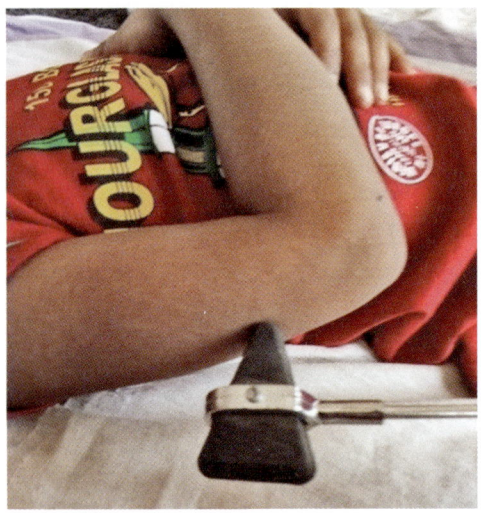

Fig. 1.43: Elicitation of triceps jerk.

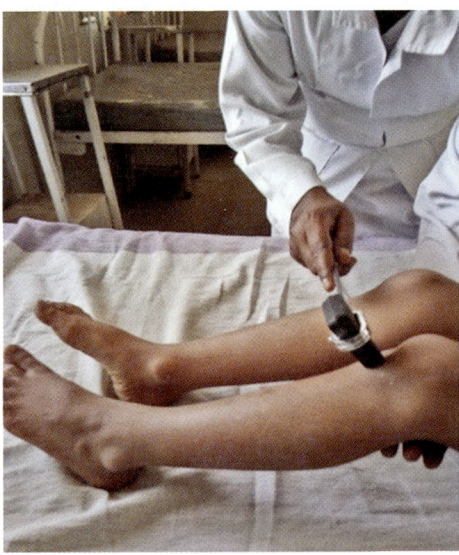

Fig. 1.45: Elicitation of knee jerk.

b. **Texture discrimination:** Ask the child to close the eyes and examiner touches two points on two parts of body (both cheeks, both hands, etc.). Ask him to name which area is touched. If he recognises that the cheeks are touched but not recognises the hands were touched. It suggests extinction of distal stimulus.

c. **Stereognosis:** Ask the child to close his eyes. Place some common objects such as coin, key, etc. and ask to name.

Interpretation: Loss of stereognosis and two points discrimination suggest parietal lobe syndrome.

Superficial Reflexes

1. **Corneal and conjunctival reflex (5, 7 cranial nerves):** Touch the cornea or

conjunctiva with cotton wool, response is prompt closure of eye.

2. **Abdominal reflexes (D_4–D_{12}):** Stroke with a pencil or key on four quadrants from periphery "towards umbilicus; see contraction of underlying muscles.
3. **Cremasteric reflex (L_1–L_2):** Stroke the medial aspect of upper thigh and watch for ipsilateral contraction of cremasteric muscle.
4. **Anal reflex (S_3–S_4):** Perianal area is stroked and anal response observed. Anal tone should be palpated.
5. **Plantar reflex or Babinski response (L_5–S_1)** (Fig. 1.46).

Test: Scratch the outer border of soles with blunt instrument (e.g. handle of knee hammer, key, ball pen) starting from the heel and carry the stimulus over the base of the metatarsals ending near the back of great toe.

Response: Normal plantar flexion of great toe and other toes also flex and adducted. In some entire leg may be withdrawn.

Abnormal: Dorsiflexion of great toe often associated with fanning of other toes is indicative of pyramidal lesion. There may be dorsiflexion of ankle and withdrawal of entire extremity. Babinski is positive if the great toe dorsiflex with or without fanning of other toes.

Babinski is positive normally up to 2 years age probably due to lack of myelination of spinal cord. Other way to elicit Babinski response are:
a. Pressing firmly with the thumb and striking along the anterior border of tibia.
b. Squeezing the calf.
c. Flexing and twisting any toe.
d. Striking the big toe along the lateral side.

Glabellar tap reflex: Tapping of nasion is followed by blink response; after 3–4 taps response disappears due to habituation. Persist in degenerative disorder of CNS.

Palmomental reflex: Scratch or tap the thenar eminence of hand. Normally no response. In frontal lobe lesion mentalis and orbicularis oculi muscles contract.

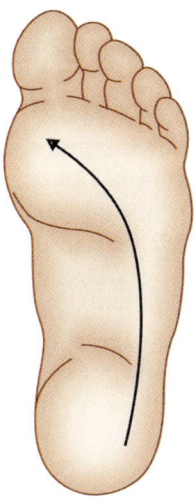

Fig. 1.46: Plantar reflex: Direction of scratch.

Signs of Meningeal Irritation

Neck Rigidity

i. Ask the child to touch his chest with chin and to turn the head from side to side. In case he is unable to do, place your one hand under his head and raise it. It can be rotated side to side. Resistance to flexion and rotation of neck is sign of meningeal irritation.
ii. In struggling patient, suspend the head beyond the edge of the table and then test for neck rigidity.

Kernig sign: Examiner flexes the hip and knees fully and then trying to extend with flexed hip. In case of spinal meninges irritation this extension is arrested by the spasm of hamstring. It is doubtful up to 6 months of age.

Examination of autonomic nervous system: Measurement of blood pressure, body temperature, absense of sweating is tested by painting a portion of skin with iodine and covering it with starch paper. Starch does not turn blue in area of anhydrosis, sphincter disturbances, changes in salivation, lacrimation and sweating.

Examine: Gait and skull as described earlier.

HISTORY TAKING OF COMMON SYMPTOMS OF DISORDERS OF CHILDREN

Fever

- Onset acute or insidious fluctuation less than 1°C during 24 hours.
- Character—continuous, remittent, fluctuations exceeds 2°C (intermittent).
- Severity—low grade, high grade.
- Associated with chills or rigors—child can not express chills, mother can observe rigors as shaking movements. *Intermittent fever* is present for several hours in a day but remain normal at rest of the time.
- Temperature normal daily (quatidian)
- Every alternate day (tertian)
- After every two days (quartan)
- History of drugs such as antipyretic may alter the pattern of fever.
- Duration: How long child is suffering from fever?

Cough

Cough refers to the violent and noisy expulsion of air from lungs.
- Acute or chronic
- Duration of cough: When did cough start?
- Barking or brassy
- Accompanied with wheezing.

Relationship with food, associated with history of allergy, heart disease, asthma, tuberculosis.
- Paroxysmal cough followed by long noisy inspiration in whoop.
- Cough in followed by vomiting
- Expectoration present or dry cough.
- Child may swallow expectoration and no history is given.
- Any history of foreign body inhalation.

Pain in Abdomen

Acute or recurrent, site of pain localized or generalized, nature of pain stabbing, colicky or dull, behavior when become worst or appears to be sitting down, way of feeding.

Generalized pain organic causes are less likely.

Diarrhea

Defined as recent increased frequency and reduced consistency of stool. Passing of fluids is more important than frequency.

Many breastfed babies pass frequent stools after each feed in a day but stool does not contain fluid, it is not diarrhea.

Ask about number, color of stool (green in starvation diarrhea), mixed with blood or mucus or not, associated with abdominal pain, abdominal distension, duration—more than 2 weeks (chronic diarrhea), is associated with vomiting, fever, weight loss, increasing thirst (dehydration). History of worms in stool.

Stool—pale, frothy and fowl smelling (steatorrhea), white fatty stool (giardiasis).

Persistent diarrhea after gastroenteritis is suggestive of secondary lactose intolerance.

Feeding history, e.g. taking ice cream, oliguria, anuria, or history suggesting dehydration.

Vomiting

Forcible expulsion of contents of the stomach from mouth.

Causes in newborn are different than young children.

Ask—acute or recurrent, frequency, relationship with feeding color and character of vomitus, abdominal pain or discomfort, drooling, history of food poisoning, history of trauma, weight loss, association with diarrhea.

Dyspnea

It is an uncomfortable awareness of difficulty in breathing.

History should be taken—present at rest or on exertion, degree of exertion to produce, aspiration of foreign body, history of asthma, trauma, heart disease and drugs.

Convulsions

Convulsions are involuntary motor, sensory autonomic or psychic phenomenon with some change in sensorium.

Ask about onset—sudden or gradual, local or generalized, where they begin, fashion, they migrate, how long did attack last? Fever was associated or not, history of sleep after attack, passing of urine or defecation during attack, vomiting, loss of consciousness.

In recurrent convulsion, ask about minimal gap between two convulsions, aura preceding convulsions, temporary paralysis after convulsions (todd's paralysis).

Failure to Thrive

Failure to thrive means infants and children who fail to gain weight proportional to length or height or even loss. Take about his feeding history in detail, how is his appetite, does he eat enough and yet not gaining weight, asks about daily intake and calculate calories, problems related to feeding.

History of worm infestation, chronic diarrhea, family history of tuberculosis, physically handicapped, e.g. cleft palate, cervical palsy, adverse factors in family environment, child abuse or neglect history of chronic coexisting symptoms.

Constipation

Term refers to passage of small hard dry stools that contain mainly solid and minimum water and frequency of defaecation does not mean constipation in real sense.

It is present since birth or occurred later, what was usual habit, any change from it, is related to diet, relation with drugs laxative or purgative, associated with defaecation, abdominal pain, color of stool, is there vomiting, fecal incontinence, history of passage of worms?

Hematuria

Appearance of blood in urine.

Ask about *total* hematuria (lesion above bladder) *initial* (lesion in urethra), or *terminal* (lesion in urinary bladder or its neck or prostate).

Any history of drug taken, disuria, recent trauma, periorbital edema, pain in abdomen, history of existing systemic infections, preceding upper respiratory infection, any bleeding disorder in patient and in family members.

Hoarseness

Duration, how did it start, gradual or sudden, does it follows prolong crying, history of trauma, lethargic, feeding, problem, delayed milestones (cretinism), pyrexia (laryngitis), foreign body inhalation.

Joints Pain

Arthritis denotes inflammation of a joint manifested by pain, heat, tenderness and swelling, *arthralgia* mean only pain in joints without inflammation.

Ask as pain in joint—single or member of joints, one joint (history of trauma) movement causes limitation of function, fever, history of bleeding disorders, bleeding from other sites (gums). If multiple joints are involved, ask about fleeting or flitting (rheumatic arthritis), fever, previous history of sore throat, drugs taken, ask about symptoms related to cardiovascular system disorders.

Headache

Headache means unpleasant sensations in the region of cranial vault.

Ask about when did it start, intensity any definable sensation, location, period it lasts, factor make it worst, or better, any change due to change in environment, any association with vomiting, dizziness, visual disturbance or sweating, vision (myopic), any neck stiffness, drowsiness, irritability, fever, personality and behavior changes, whether headache precedes menstrual period (elder girls).

It is persistent or recurrent, symptoms of sinusitis and hypertension.

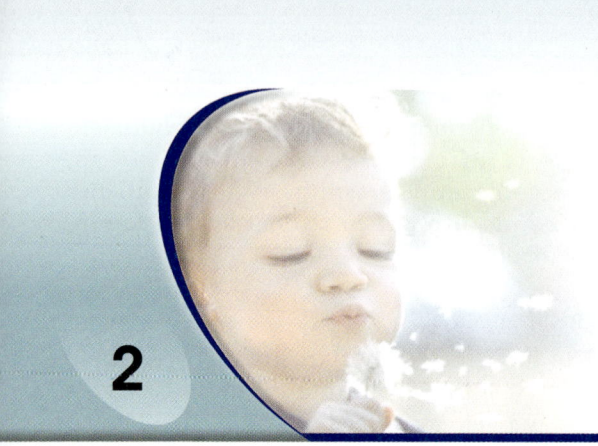

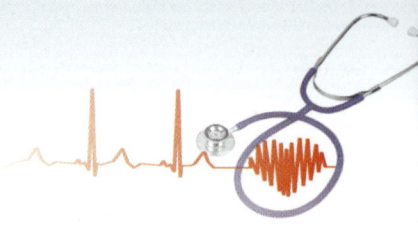

2

Neonatology

Neonatal period: Neonatal period extends up to 28 days of life.

Perinatal period: Extends from 28th week of gestation to 7th day of life.

Gestational age: It is calculated from 1st day of last menstrual period to the date of birth in complete weeks.

Low birth weight (LBW): Babies with birth weight 2500 gm or less are called low birth weight babies.

Term babies: Babies with gestational age between 37 and 41 weeks are called term babies while babies with gestational age <37 weeks (up to 36 weeks) are called preterm and more than 42 weeks are called post-term babies.

Classification (*Refer to* Fig. 2.31)

Small for date (intrauterine growth retardation, small for gestational age or light for date): Babies with a birth weight of less than 10th percentile or two standard deviations below the mean birth weight for the gestational age.

Appropriate for date: Babies with birth weight between 10th and 90th percentile or between two standard deviations of the mean birth weight.

Large for date: Babies with birth weight more than 90th percentile or more than two standard deviations of the mean birth weight for the gestational age.

EXAMINATION OF NEWBORN

Newborn is examined on the lines given for examination of children but special points concerning the examination of newborn are as follows:

i. History of pregnancy and delivery should be taken in detail and scoring at the time of delivery.

ii. Symptoms and signs of illness are minimal in newborn even in the presence of serious and life-threatening illness.

iii. Congenital malformations should be recognized specially, although many times it is not possible at birth.

Normal Full-term Newborn Infant

1. **General:** Fairly active movements of extremities. Normal sleep. Few tremors of limbs and jaw particularly with activity and while crying.

   Abnormal: Limp, very irritable, pallor or central cyanosis

2. **Weight normal:** 2.5 kg in India

3. **Height average:** 50 cm

4. **Circumference of head:** 34–35 cm

5. **Chest circumference:** 3 cm less than head circumference

6. Ratio of crown to public symphysis—pubic symphysis to sole of feet = 1.7/1 to 1.9/1

7. **Respiratory rate:** 30–50/min

8. **Heart rate:** 70–180/min

Attitude: Attitude of flexion in full term.

Head: Rounded head in premature infants and infants born after breech delivery; slight asymmetry at birth with overlapping of suture. Fontanel small.

Excessively large or small size of head, large fontanel.

Eyes: It is easy to make the infants open their eyes by tilting them gently forward and backward. No tears. Sclera appears slightly bluish.

Excess tearing due to obstruction of nasolacrimal duct, purulent discharge, large cornea, coloboma of eyelids and iris, cataract absent red reflex.

Nose: Normal—patent both sides; no discharge.

Ears: Ear cartilage is firm, fully curved with good elastic recoil.

Mouth, Tongue, Palate, Teeth: Normal—no defect; occasionally one or two teeth may be present.

Chest and Lungs: Rounded with anterio-posterior diameter equal to transverse diameter. Mostly abdominal type of respiration.

Heart: The size is relatively large compared to rest of the chest.

Abdomen: Abdomen is usually prominent is newborn. Liver is palpable 2–3 cm below costal margin; respiratory movements are mostly abdominal; tip of spleen and lower end of kidney palpable normally; cut end of cord without granuloma or discharge.

Genitalia: Male—testes descended; Female—large labia minora in premature.

Skin: Normal 'pink'. Peripheral cyanosis particularly in cold; mottling is normal.

Extremities and spine: Symmetrical, look for number of fingers and toes. Simian crease, spina bifida, pilonidal sinus, tuft of hairs.

Neurological: Active symmetrical movements of all extremities, feeding, reflexes.

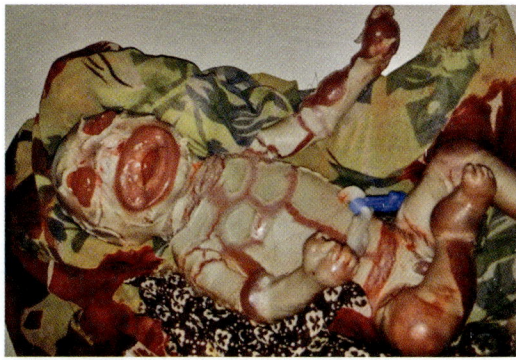

Fig. 2.1: Collodion baby. The skin appears like cello-tape and tightly stretched, eversion of eyelid, lips (eclabium), and fish-like oral opening.

Skin: Examine for jaundice, cyanosis, patachia, birth marks, hemangioma, rashes, sign of dysmaturity, ichthyosis collodion baby (Fig. 2.1).

The skin appears like cellotape

And tightly stretched, eversion of eyelid, lips (eclabium)

And fish-like oral opening

Neonatal Reflexes

A number of neonatal reflexes has been described out of which only a few important ones are being discussed here.

Moro's reflex: The baby is lying supine. Infant's head is gently raised above the end of bed and then released suddenly. Rapid release of head initiates the reflex. Alternatively hold the hands and raise the baby a little. Rapid release of the hands causes a sudden movement and initiates the reflex. A positive reflex consists of abduction and extension of arms and opening up of hands which is followed by closing of fists and abduction of arms. His knees and hips also flex (Fig. 2.2).

Significance: Absence of Moro's reflex in a newborn or its persistence after 5 months suggests CNS injury and insufficiency. Hyperactive reflex shows tetanus, tetany or CNS infection.

Its absence in one arm (unilateral) indicates fracture of humerus or clavicle or brachial

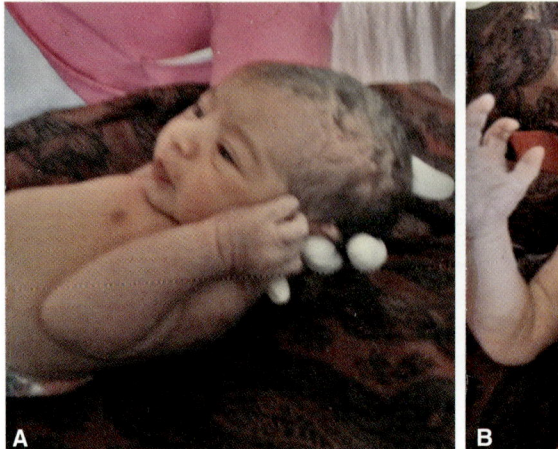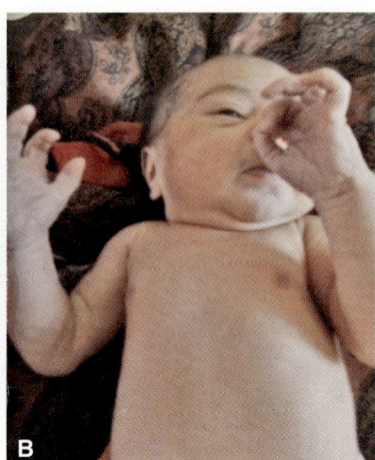

Fig. 2.2A and B: Elicitation of Moro's reflex.

palsy. Absence or diminished response in one lower limb indicates lower spinal trauma, hip dislocation, fracture of leg bone(s) or meningomyelocele.

Reverse Moro's reflex: If there is no response in first five days and then child responds by extending and externally rotating the arms and then fixing in rigidity in the same position. It is present in 'kernicterus' due to basal ganglion damage.

Tonic Neck Reflex

Place the baby supine on bed; turn his head to one side. The ipsilateral arm and leg extended while contralateral arm and leg flex. This reflex is prominent between 2nd and 4th months. Persistence of the reflex beyond 9 months or a constant tonic neck posture are abnormal and usually indicate spastic cerebral palsy (Fig. 2.3).

Sucking and rooting reflex: Introduce a finger or teat in baby's mouth. Vigorous sucking movement starts which is easily felt and seen. This is associated with swallowing also (sucking reflex) (Fig. 2.4).

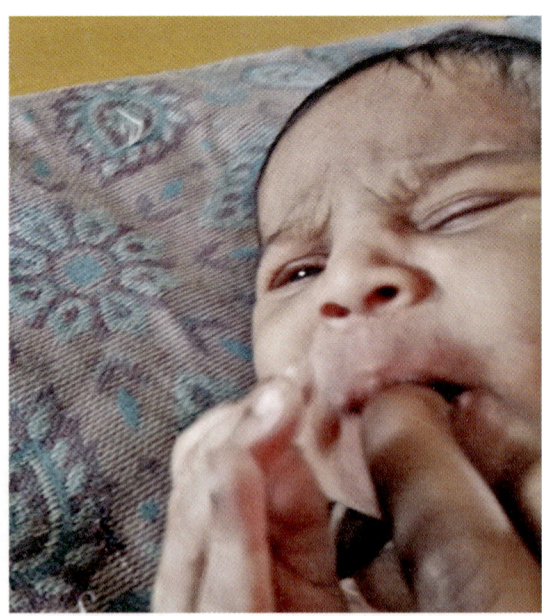

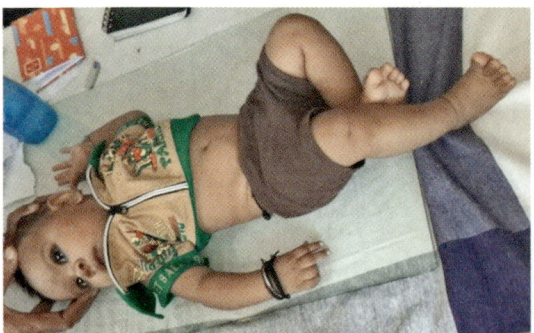

Fig. 2.3: Tonic neck reflex.

Fig. 2.4: Elicitation sucking reflex.

When baby's cheeks come in contact with mother's breast nipple, he moves his mouth towards stimulus to reach the nipple. This reflex helps him finding out the nipple without being directed to it (rooting reflex).

Glabellar Tap

When the examiner gently taps the glabella (junction between nose and forehead), blinking of both eyelids of neonates takes place (Fig. 2.5).

Crossed Extension

If foot is stroked with the leg held extended at knee, there is flexion, abduction and extension of the opposite leg.

Placing, stepping and walking reflex Placing reflex is elicited by bringing the anterior aspect of tibia against the edge of table. Child lifts the leg up to step onto the table as if there is alternate flexion and extension seen is attempted walking (Fig. 2.6).

Grasp Reflex

When the baby's palm is stroked the examiner's finger, the baby's finger closes and grasps it. The grasp reflex persists up to age

of 12 weeks. Beyond this age if it persists it indicates brain damage (Fig. 2.7).

The Babinski's sign and Chvostek's sign may be present in a normal term neonate.

Normal Abnormalities of Newborn

Normal abnormalities are minor peculiarities seen in newborn which become alright spontaneously and need no treatment.

 i. *Toxic erythema or urticaria neonatorum:* It is seen in first 2–3 days as red area with central pallor over face, spreading towards trunk and extremities. This is thought to be due to irritation of delicate

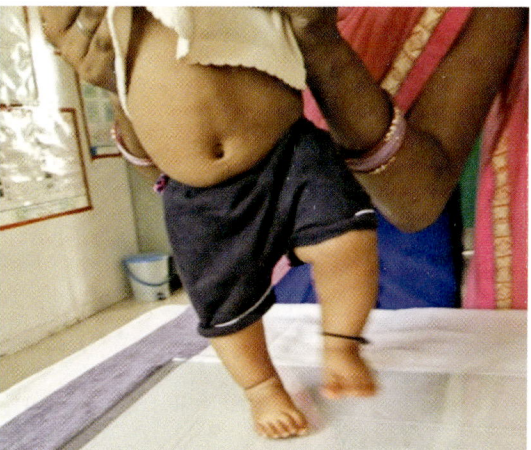

Fig. 2.6: Stepping reflex.

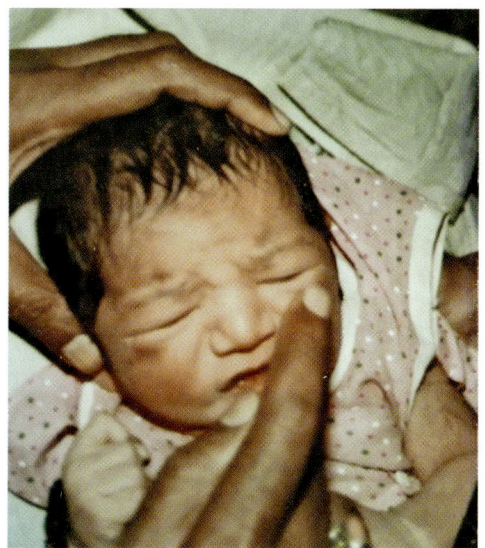

Fig. 2.5: Elicitation of glabellar tap.

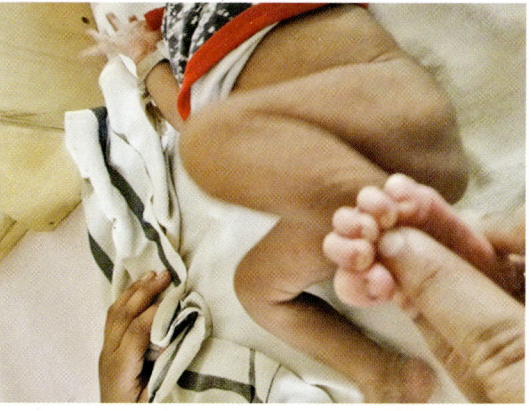

Fig. 2.7: Elicitation of grasp reflex.

skin by various things like clothes, soaps, etc.

ii. *Miliaria:* These are yellowish white spots on nose, cheeks and skin and caused by retention of sebum.

iii. *Peeling skin:* Dry skin with peeling is seen in post-term and sometimes in full-term babies.

iv. *Salman patches (naevus simplex):* These are pinkish gray capillary hemangioma commonly located at the nape of neek, upper eyelids, forehead and root of the nose; disappear spontaneously within few months.

v. *Mongolian spots:* These are blue patches of irregular shape usually seen over sacral area and buttocks less commonly over back and extremities.

vi. Herlequin color change.

vii. *Subconjunctival hemorrhage:* Semilunar subconjunctival hemorrhage, usually towards the outer canthus of eye seen in few newborns. Blood gets resorbed within few days.

viii. *Epstein Pearls:* White spots on one or both sides of median raphae of hard palate.

ix. *Sucking callosities:* These are small rounded cornified plaques at the centre of upper lip. It is thought to be due to sucking efforts of baby *in utero.*

x. *Tongue tie:* Frenulum linguae may be broad membrane or thick fibrous band.

xi. Physiological phimosis in all males.

xii. *Hymen tags:* Mucosal tags at the margin of hymen.

xiii. *Umbilical hernia:* May manifest after 2 months. Disappear by 2 years of age.

xiv. *Vaginal bleeding:* Nonpurulent secretion or bleeding is seen in female babies due to maternal hormones, requiring no interference.

APGAR SCORE

It was first introduced by Virginia Apgar. This provides a gross quantitative expression at

Table 2.1: Apgar scoring system

Criteria	0	1	2
1. Respiration	Nil	Slow	Crying
2. Heart rate	Nil	<100/m	>100/m
3. Tone	Flaccid	In between	Flexed
4. Reflex response	Nil	Grimace	Cry
5. Color	Pale or blue	Peripheral cyanosis	Pink

Note: Absent heart rate and respiration are of greatest importance.

birth. One minute score predicts immediate neonatal outcome while 5 minute score predicts future mental prognosis (Table 2.1).

Method

There are total 5 objective signs seen. In the total score each is given 0, 1, 2. Total score is 10.

Interpretation

Score is assessed at one minute and five minutes.

Score   8–10: Excellent condition
5–7: Moderate depression
Less than 5: Severe asphyxia

RESUSCITATION

Neonatal Resuscitation

Neonatal resuscitation means to revive or restore life to a baby from state of asphyxia.

Ninety percent of newly born babies make the transition from intrauterine to extrauterine life without difficulty. They begin spontaneous and regular respiration with little or no assistance. Approximately 10% of newborn require some assistance to begin breathing at birth. About one percent of newborn may need extensive resuscitation for their survival.

Adequate ventilation is more important than additional oxygen; quick action with bag and mask is more important than intubation. This period of resuscitation is very important (Golden five minutes).

Steps for Successful Resuscitation

Preparation for Birth

1. A warm room with temperature ≥25°C, draught free
2. A clean, dry and warm delivery surface
3. A radiant warmer/overhead lamp with 200 watt bulb if available.
4. Two clean and warm clothes for baby towels.
5. A folded piece of cloth
6. A newborn size self inflating bag and infant masks in two sizes—size 'l' for normal weight baby and 'O' for small baby.
7. A suction device, machine, mucus suction
8. Oxygen (if available)
9. A clock (with second hands).

- All pieces of equipment must be cleaned and checked, appropriate size. Volume of bag should not be more than 250–500 ml and generate pressure of at least 35 cm of water (Fig. 2.8).
- Mucus extractor: The trap should be enough (20 ml) to prevent aspirated fluid going into the resuscitator's mouth. Suction should not exceed a negative pressure of 100 mmHg or 130 cm of water.
- Test the function of bag and mask for ventilation.
  - Fit mask onto the bag and deliver test breathes the palm of the hand. You should check pressure in the palm as the bag is squeezed (Fig. 2.9).
  - Form a seal between the mask and palm of the hand. Squeeze the bag enough for the pop off (pressure release) valve to open and make a sound as the air escapes.
  - Check that the bag re-inflates when released after squeezing the bag.

Assessment at Birth

Baby should be delivered on the mother's abdomen or make sure there is warn, clean towel or clothes on the bed to place the baby on. Note the time of birth and keep the baby warm as a first priority. The baby has to be dried with a warm and clean towel (better

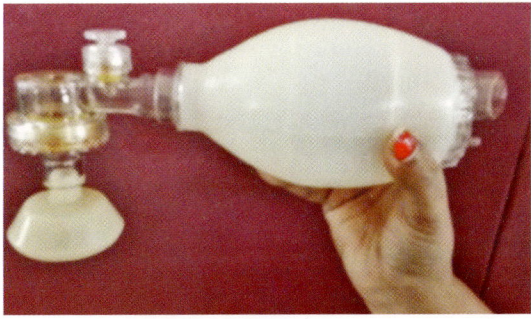

Fig. 2.8: Bag and mask.

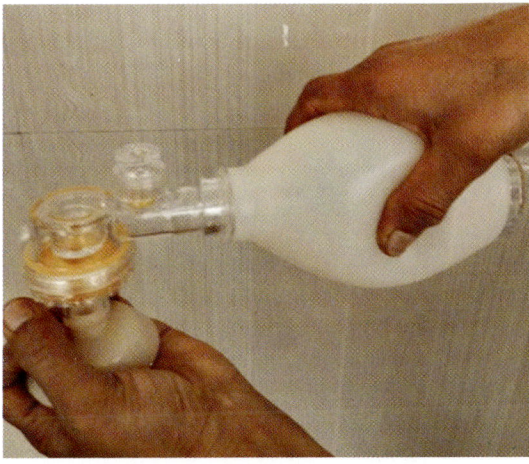

Fig. 2.9: Testing bag and mask.

cotton towel). The wet towels or clothes should be replaced after drying and baby wrapped in clean, dry and warm towel.

After the birth baby remains wet with the amniotic fluid which if not dried can lead to heat loss and temperature of body falls rapidly.

Breathing and warmth go together and breathing should be assessed whilst drying the baby. Drying also provides sufficient stimulation for breathing to start.

If meconium is present

Meconium is the faeces passed by fetus *in utero* it is greenish to brownish in color.

When meconium is present on baby surface and baby is not crying you should immediately start suction.

First do suction from mouth by inserting the tube of suction devise no more than 5 cm beyond the lip. Apply suction while with drawing the tube. Suck from your mouth when mucus extractor is used (Fig. 2.10). Stop suctioning where secretions are clear.

Even if the baby does not breathe. Then dry the baby.

- Do suction first from mouth then nose both side
- Do not do suction vigorously or deeply (more than 5 cm in mouth and more than 2 cm in nose) as it can produce a vagal response, causing the heart rate to slow down or breathing to stop.

Always apply suction while withdrawing the tube.

Do suction from both nostrils placing the tube about 2 cm inside each nostril.

a. Assess the baby's breathing: Chest moves equally on both sides with no difficulty (30–60 times in a minute)
   i. If baby is crying or chest rising regularly between (30–60 times in a minute)—no need of resuscitation.
   ii. Baby is gasping or not breathing—start resuscitation.

Steps of Resuscitation (Flowchart 2.1)

If baby requires resuscitation tie and cut the cord. Transfer the baby warm, clean and dry surface.

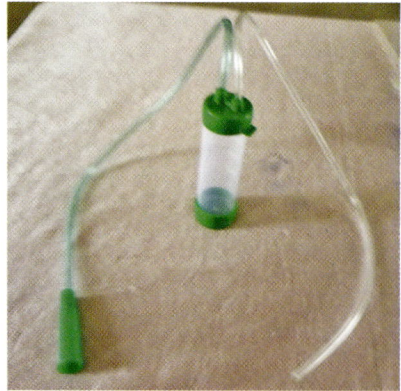

Fig. 2.10: Mucus extractor.

Flowchart 2.1: Neonatal resuscitation

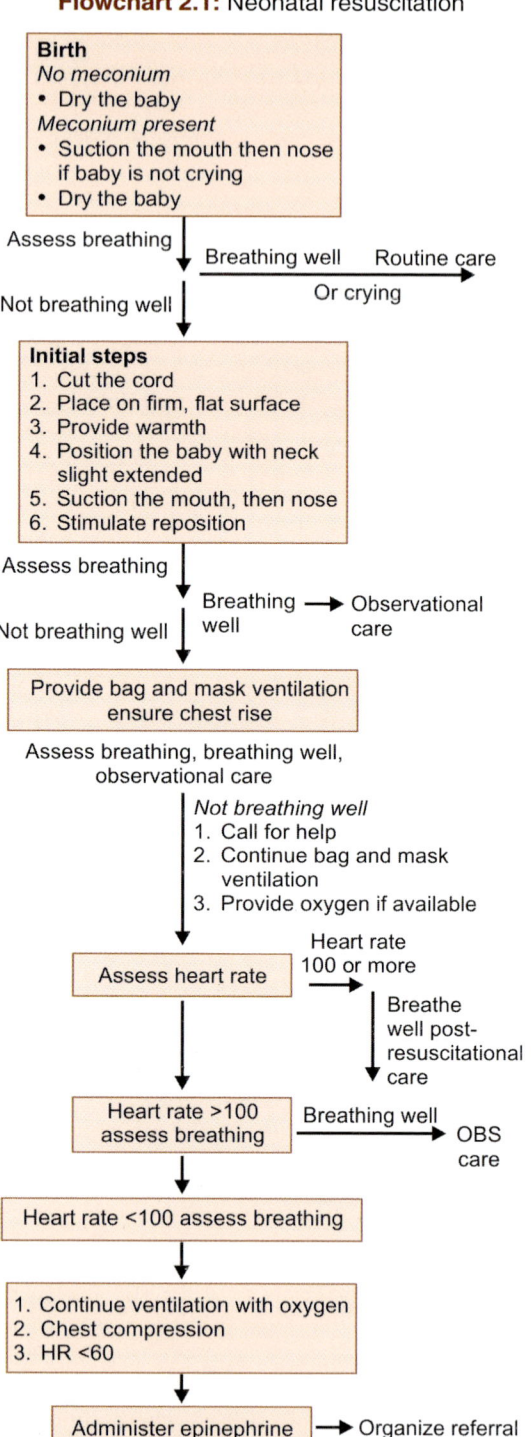

a. Provide warm environment: Shut down all windows and switch off fan of room before birth.

b. Place the newborn under overhead lamp with 200 watt bulb placed 50–60 cm above surface, or

c. Place the newborn under radiant warmer.

d. Open the baby's airway: Position the head. Place the baby on its back. Put a folded piece of cloth under the baby's shoulder so to maintain the head in slightly extended position (Fig. 2.11). It will open airway. Hyperextension and hyperflexon will close the airway.

e. Suction the mouth and the nose—suction first the mouth and then nose.

f. Stimulation—both drying and suctioning stimulate the newborn.

If the baby does not cry at birth, stimulate for breathing such as:

- Slapping or flickering the soles of the feet.
- Rubbing the newborn's back or limbs gently.

g. If the baby is still not breathing: Ventilation with bag and mask.

If baby is not breathing well at the end of 30 seconds after above steps, start the ventilation with bag and mask.

- Position the baby to maintain a open airway with the help of shoulder roll. Position your self at side or back of head to a for better resuscitation.

Position of bag and mask on face: The mask should be placed on the face so that it covers the nose and mouth. Appropriate size of mask in chosen (Fig. 2.12). The mask is held on the face with the thumb and index and/or middle fingers encircling the rim of mask by left hand. Hold the bag on right hand (right-handed person) or vice versa.

Initiation of Ventilation

Start ventilation by squeezing the bag to deliver breath. Adequate pressure required to squeeze the bag just sufficient to produce gentle chest rise (Figs 2.13 and 2.14).

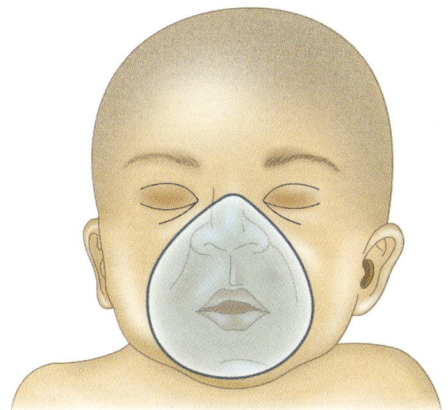

Fig. 2.12: Correct position of mask.

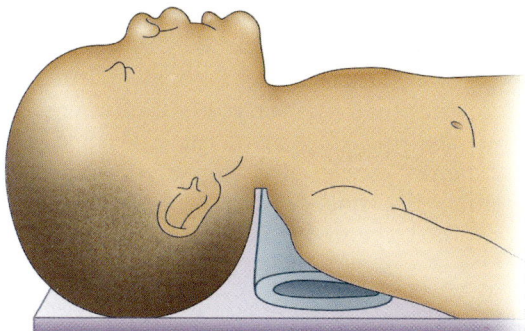

Fig. 2.11: Shoulder roll.

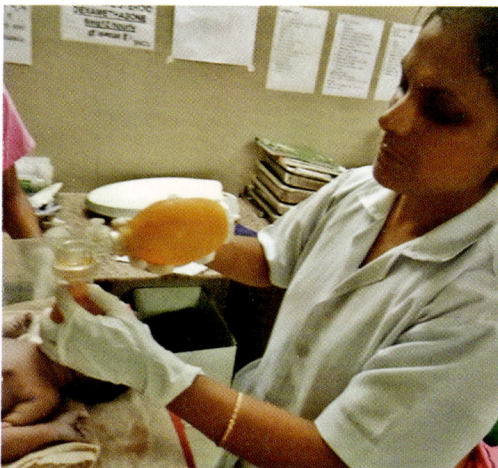

Fig. 2.13: Ventilation with bag and mask.

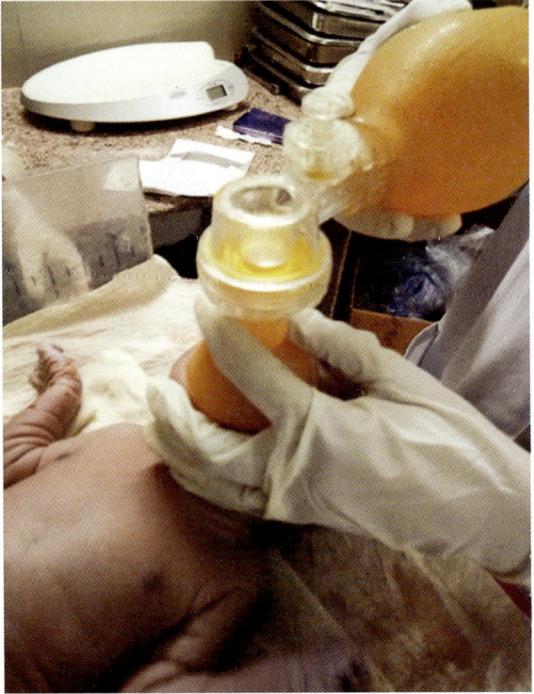

Fig. 2.14: Ventilation with bag and mask.

Avoid over inflation

- How often should you squeeze the bag:
  - During intial phase breaths should be delivered at the rate of 40 to 60 breathe per minute. It can be maintained by:

Say yourself	Do at that time
Breathe and	Squeeze the bag
Two three	Release the bag
Breathe and	Squeeze the bag
Two three	Release the bag

Ensure chest rise: Ensure chest movement when you squeeze the bag. If not adequate check the seal—inadequate? airway blocked? proper pressure is not given? Correct it.

- Improvement of indicated by spontaneous breathing which is after 30 seconds of adequate ventilation. But some baby requires prolong ventilation. If baby is crying or breathing regularly with no grunting at the rate of 30–60/minute, stop the ventilation.

- Evaluate heart rate by feeding the umbilical cord pulse or listening to the heartbeat with stethoscope. Count the beats for 6 seconds and multiply by 10. It gives heart rate in minute.
  Heart rate above 100 is normal.

If heart rate is normal but baby is still not breathing well continue bag and mask ventilation. Reassess after 30 seconds until the baby is breathing well. If not, continue ventilation and refer to advance care.

If heart rate is slow, continue bag and mask ventilation and reassess heart rate after 30 seconds and refer to advance care. If no improvement such baby may require chest compressions, endotracheal intubation and medications.

Post-resuscitation care: It includes:
- Warmth
- Chest breathing, temperature, color, CFT
- Observe
- Monitor blood sugar
- Watch for any complications
- Initiate breastfeeding if baby is well

Resuscitation with positive pressure ventilation and chest compressions

Babies who have heart rate below 60 per minute despite stimulation and 30 seconds of positive pressure ventilation, probable have very low oxygen levels and significant acidosis. As a result, the myocardium is depressed and unable to contract strongly enough to pump blood to the lungs to pick up the oxygen that you have now ensured is in the lungs. Therefore, you will need to mechanically pump the heart while you simultaneously ventilate the lung until the myocardium sufficiently oxygenated to recover adequate spontaneous function. This process also helps to restore oxygen delivery to the brain.

Chest compression: Sometimes refers to as external cardiac massage consisting of rhythmic compressions of the sternum that compress the heart against the spine, increase intrathoracic pressure, circulate blood to vital organs of the baby.

Compressing the sternum compress the heart and increases the pressure in the chest, causing that to be pumped up to arteries, when pressure on sternum is released blood enters the heart from the veins.

Person: Two people are required to administer effective chest compressions, one to compressing chest and to continue ventilation.

Second person may be same person who came to monitor heart rate, breath sounds during positive pressure ventilation.

Techniques: Two techniques are used to perform chest compressions.

1. **Thumbs technique:** Where two thumbs are used to depress the sternum, while the hands encircle the torso and finger support the spine (Fig. 2.15).

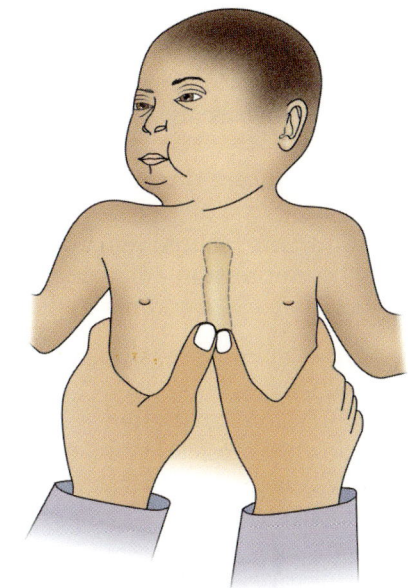

Fig. 2.15: Chest compression thumb technique.

   Pressure is applied to the lower third of the sternum while use between the xyphoid and line drawn between nipple.

   Then place your thumbs or fingers immediately above the xyphoid.

   Method: This technique in done by encircling torso with both hands and placing the thumb on sternum and finger under the baby's back supporting the spine.

   Thumb can be placed side by side or, on small baby one over the other.

   The thumb will be used to compress the sternum, while your fingers provide to the support needed for back. The thumb should be flexed at first font and pressure applied vertically to compress the heart between sternum and the spine.

2. **Two-finger technique:** Where the tips of the middle finger and either the index finger or ring finger of one hand are used to compress the sternum, while the other hand is used to support the baby's back (Fig. 2.16).

   Method: In this technique, the tips of your middle finger and either the index or ring finger of one hand are used from compres-

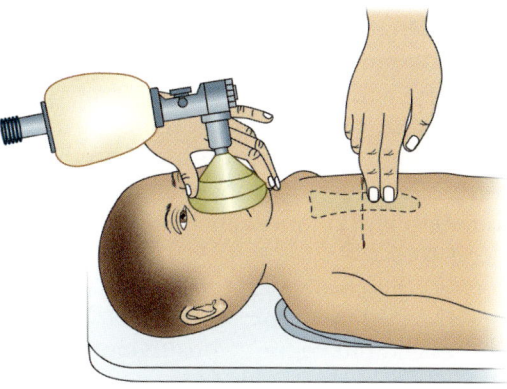

Fig. 2.16: Chest compression two-finger technique.

sions (use right hand in right-handed and left hand in left-handed person).

Position the 2 fingers perpendicular to chest and press with your fingertips.

Your other hand should be used to support the newborn's back so that the heart is more effectively compressed between sternum and spine. With the use of second hand supporting the back you can more easily judge the pressure and the depth of compression.

How much pressure to use?

Use pressure to depress to a depth of about one-third of the anterio-posterior diameter of chest. And then release the pressure to allow the heart to refill.

So, one stroke means downward stroke and release.

Thumb and finger should remain in contact during both compression and release—chest compression may cause trauma to the baby.

Coordination of compression with ventilation

Chest compression must always be accompanied by positive pressure ventilation. These two must be coordinated such a way that on ventilation interposed after every third compression.

For 90 compressions—30 breathes per minutes.

The person doing the compression should take the counting out loud from the person who is doing ventilation.

The compressor should count.

Breathe and two-three breathe and while the person ventilating squeeze during "Breathe and" and release during "two-three".

Stop compression—after 30 seconds of ventilation and compression feel the pulse at base of cord.

Listen the chest with stethoscope if rate more than 60 beats per minute stop chest compression but continue positive pressure.

- If heart rate rises above 100 beats/minute and baby begin to breathe spontaneously. Withdraw positive pressure ventilation.
- If heart rate remains below 60 per minute, then insert an umbilical catheter and give epinephrine.

Endotracheal Intubation

Indication

1. If there is meconium and baby has depressed respiration, muscle tone, or heart rate.
2. If positive pressure ventilation in not resulting in adequate clinical improvement.

3. If chest compressions are necessary, intubation may facilitate coordination of chest compression and maximize the efficacy of each positive pressure breath.
4. If epinephrine is required to stimulate the heart.

Medication

Epinephrine

If heart rate remains below 60 bpm despite administration of ventilation and chest compressions (at about 3 minutes age) place umbilical venous catheter and a dose of 0.6 ml of epinephrine is given into the catheter followed by normal saline flush. If there is no improvement in heart rate repeat the dose every 3 to 5 minutes.

Blood volume expander. Recheck effectiveness of ventilation chest compression, endotracheal intubation and epinephrine delivery, if no improvement then consider that baby is in shock and if there is evidence of blood loss.

Treat the hypovolemia with isotonic crystalloid solution such as:

- 0.9% NaCl (normal saline)
- Ringer lactate
- O Rh negative packed red cells of severe fetal anemia is expected.

Dose: Initial dose 10 ml/kg in a rate of over 5 to 10 minute. If minimal improvement in initial first dose, give another 10 ml/kg through intravenous route (e.g. umbilical vein).

If no improvement after above measure consider congenital airway malformation, pneumothorax, diaphragmatic hernia or congenital heart disease.

If heart rate is absent in spite of all above technique for a minimum 10 minutes discontinue resuscitation consider referral.

LOW BIRTH WEIGHT BABIES

Low birth weight (LBW) babies: Babies with birth weight of 2500 gm or less, irrespective of the period of gestation, are classified as low birth weight. These include: (i) Preterm; and

(ii) Term small for date (intrauterine growth retardation).

Nearly 75% of neonatal deaths and 50% of infant's death occur among LBW babies and LBW babies are prone to malnutrition recurrent infections and neurodevlopmental handicaps.

Definitions: Two parameters are considered for assessment of newborn.
1. Birth weight of baby—normally babies weight more than 2500 gm.
2. Gestation or maturity of the baby.
   Preterm <37 completed weeks
   Term 37–41 completed weeks + 6 days
   Post-term >42 completed weeks

Types of LBW
1. Preterm
2. Intrauterine growth restriction (IUGR)

PRETERM BABIES (PREMATURE BABIES) (IMMATURE, TRUELY PREMATURE, BORN EARLY)

Definition: Baby born less than 37 completed weeks of gestation is called preterm baby.
   Incidence is 8–10% of total babies born

Extremely preterm	<28 weeks
Very preterm	28–<32 weeks
Moderate to late preterm	32–<37 weeks
LBW	<2500 gm
Very low birth weight (VLBW)	<1500 gm
Extremely low birth weight (ELBW)	<1000 gm

Risk Factors
1. History of previous premature birth
2. Mothers age <18 years and >35 years
3. Being underweight or overweight before and/or during pregnancy.
4. Multiple pregnancy
5. Conceiving through *in vitro* fertilization (test tube babies)
6. Multiple miscarriage history
7. Physical injury or trauma

8. Uterine, cervical or placental abnormality
9. Poor nutrition.

Causes of Prematurity
Spontaneous: Premature onset of labour
a. Cause is uncertain (mostly)
b. Poor socioeconomic status of mother
c. Maternal disease: Toxemia of pregnancy, antepartum hemorrhage, anemia, acute systemic maternal illness, cervical incompetency, bicornuate uterus.
d. Multiple pregnancy
e. Congenital malformation

Induced: Induced labour before term due to danger to fetal life, e.g. in maternal diabetes mellitus, placental dysfunction, fetal hypoxia, antepartum hemorrhage and severe iso-immunization.

Clinical Features
Preterm babies are common in very young and unmarried mothers. Previous history of past labour should be obtained. If past history of preterm is associated with 3–4 times, more risk in further pregnancies.

Measurements
Size of the babies is small in comparison to normal baby. Crown heel length is <47 cm. Head is relatively large. Head circumference exceeds the chest circumference more than 3 cm. Chest circumference is usually less than 30 cm. Weight is less than 2500 gm.

General Activity
General activity is sluggish. Neonatal reflexes such as Moro, sucking and swallowing are sluggish. Generalized hypotonia results in extended posture. Cry is weak.

Face and Head
Face appears small because of large head size, fontanelles are large, sutures are widely separated. Craniotabes present poor or deficient ear cartilage results in poor recoil. Hairs

appear fine, fuzzy and scanty. Eyes appear protruding due to shallow orbit. Chin is small. Buccal pad of fat absent. Optic nerve is unmyelinated; usually visualization of it difficult.

Skin: Skin is thin, gelatinous, shiny and excessively pink with prominent lanugo and very little vernix caseosa (Fig. 2.17). Breast nodules are absent or small (Figs 2.18 and 2.19); subcutaneous fat is deficient. One or just a few creases on soles seen (Figs 2.20 and 2.21). Nails are soft, edema may be present.

Genital: In male testes are undescended and scrotum is poorly developed. In female labia majora is not covering labia minora and clitoris is hypertrophied (Figs 2.22 to 2.25) .

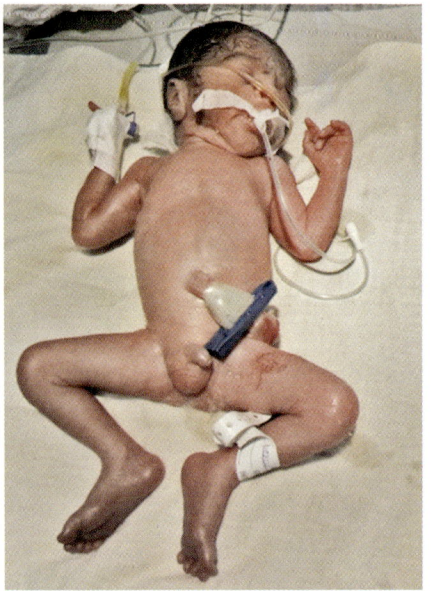

Fig. 2.17: Premature baby.

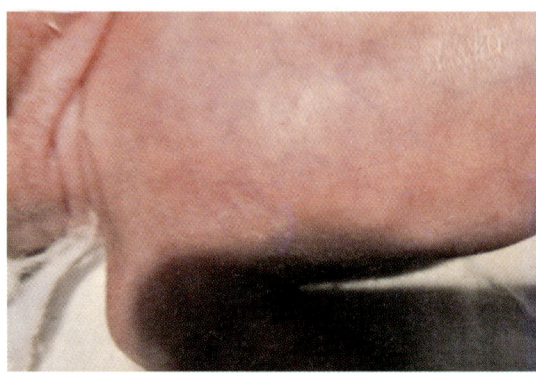

Fig. 2.19: Nipple of preterm baby.

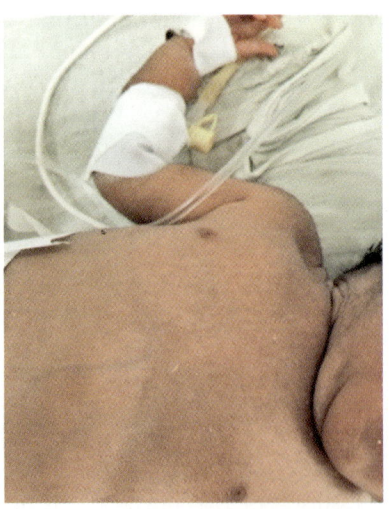

Fig. 2.18: Nipple of term baby.

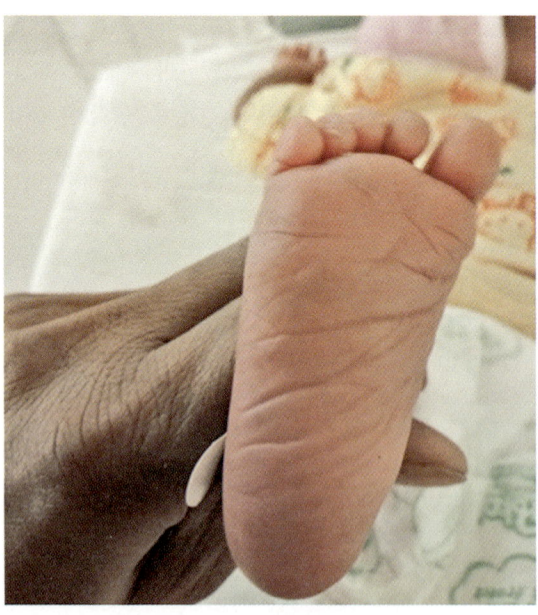

Fig. 2.20: Sole of term baby.

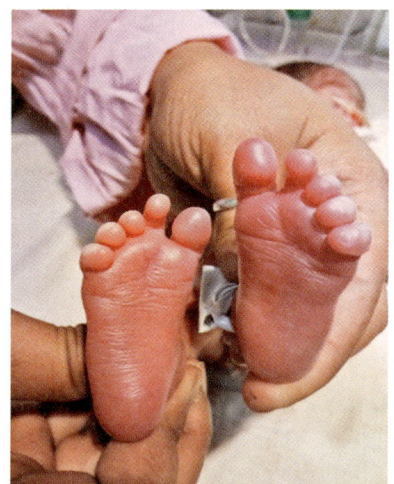

Fig. 2.21: Soles of preterm baby.

Others: Abdomen is large; kidney and spleen are often palpable. Liver and kidney are also palpable.

Physiological Handicaps: Immature baby is functionally and anatomically immature. Thus, he is physiologically handicapped in following ways:

i. *Nervous system:* The preterm babies are lethargic and inactive with poor reflexes.

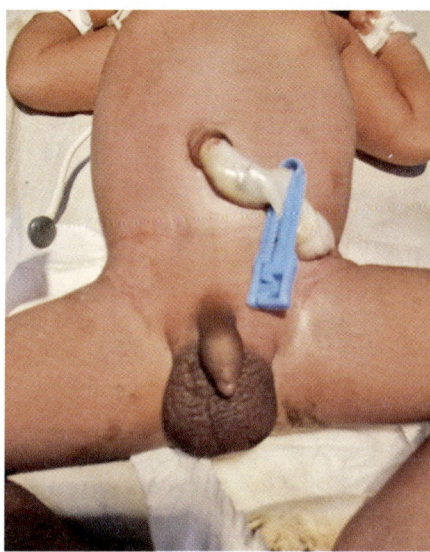

Fig. 2.24: Genitalia of male term baby.

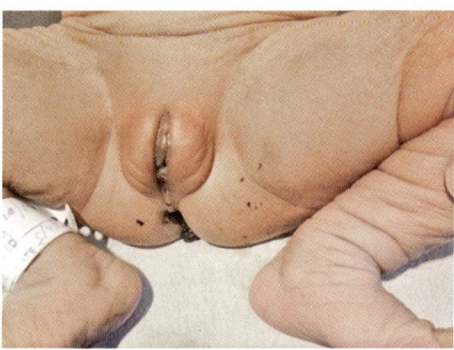

Fig. 2.22: Genitalia of female term baby.

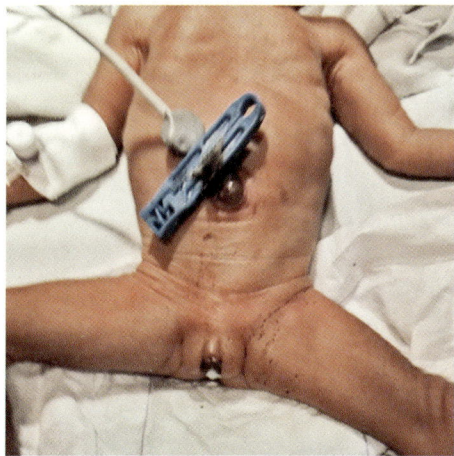

Fig. 2.23: Genitalia of female preterm baby.

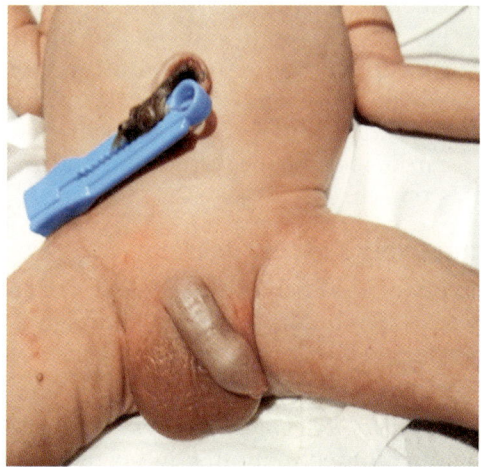

Fig. 2.25: Genitalia of male preterm baby.

Resuscitation is difficult. Brain damage may occur at lower serum bilirubin level.

ii. *Respiratory system:* Resuscitation difficult. Apneic attack common.

Hyaline membrane disease is common in preterm babies.

iii. *Cardiovascular system:* The closure of ductus arteriosus is often delayed.

iv. *Temperature regulation:* Hypothermia is more common in preterm babies because their large surface area resulting more heat loss, deficient fat (insulation), deficient brown fat in preterm which is responsible for heat production. Apart from it poor general activity resulting less heat production, thermic response are weak due to less food consumption, less oxygen consumption.

v. *Metabolic:* Preterm babies are prone to develop hypoglycemia, hypocalcemia, hypoproteinemia and acidosis.

vi. *Renal immaturity:* More prone to develop acidosis.

vii. Increased susceptibility to infection due to lower level of IgG and lesser capacity to synthesize IgM antibodies

viii. Hyperbilirubinemia is more common in preterm babies due to functional immaturity of liver.

ix. Anemia

x. Feeding difficulties are more common due to poor incoordinated sucking and swallowing. Regurgitation and aspiration common due to incompetent cardio-oesophageal sphincter and small stomach.

Management of LBW Babies

Delivery of LBW babies—the delivery of anticipated LBW baby should be conducted in hospital with established newborn case facilities.

LBW babies weighing >1800 gm (>34 weeks) should be shifted to mother in postnatal care area. Mothers of these babies are counseled and educated on regular basis by health providers, e.g.

1. Kangaroo mother care
2. Assessment of temperature by touch technique.
3. Breastfeeding and expression of milk
4. Recognition and reporting of dangerous signs
5. Any queries related to LBW babies.

If unable to feed with breast or *katori* spoon must be shifted soon to SNCU/NBSU.

LBW babies <1800 gm (34 weeks)

The babies are cared at SNCU till they are shifted to mother.

Resuscitation

Problems

Preterm babies have immature lungs so.

Difficulty in ventilating

Vulnerable to lung injury by positive pressure ventilation.

Management

Gentle resuscitation—small tidal volume with small bags for positive pressure ventilation, use of CPAP.

Thin skin and large surface area causing rapid heat loss.

Management: Take extra care for to avoid hypothermia.

Temperature control: Chances of hypothermia is due to higher surface area to body weight ratio, low glycogen store, low subcuteneous fat.

Management

In the hospital

- Overhead radiant warmer
- Incubator
- Regular monitoring of axillary temperature at least in every 6–8 hours.

At home

- Baby should be nursed next to mother and room should be kept warm.

The baby should be well clothed with woolen sweater, shocks hands with mittens and head with cap.

A blanket should be used to cover. Mother is trained about cold stress and additional warmth if it happens.

- Kangaroo mother care (Fig. 2.26)
- Warm chain maintenance (Fig. 2.27).

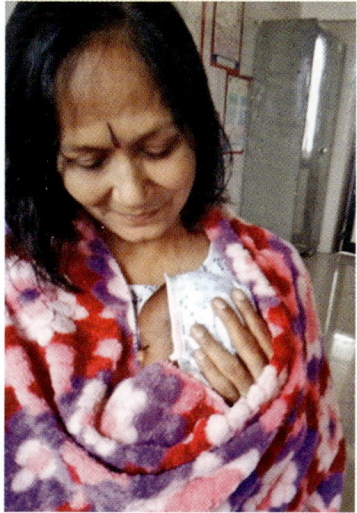

Fig. 2.26: Kangaroo mother care.

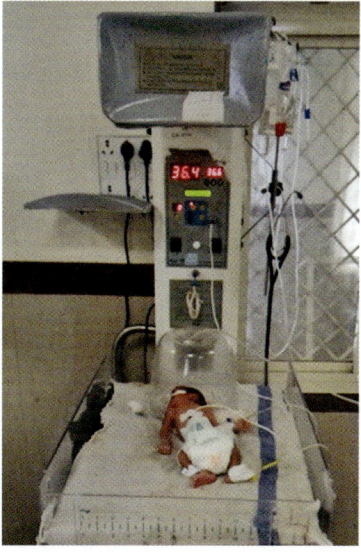

Fig. 2.27: Radiant heat warmer.

Feeding

Early feeding of LBW can be initiated as early as for his immediate survival and long-term benefits.

1. Types of feeding, quantity of feeding
2. Frequency of feeding, modality of feeding.

Types of feeding

1. **Mother's milk** (breastfeeding). Mother milk is best for LBW infant. It should be insured that baby

   Should get hind milk which comes towards the end of feeds so the baby should be fed to adequate time on each breast. Hind milk is rich in fat and provide more energy.

Quantity of feeding (Table 2.2)

Daily fluid requirement of:

Stable growing LBW babies—150 ml/kg up to 180 ml/kg/day

If babies <1500 gm/<32 weeks—60–150 ml/kg/day

Frequency: LBW should be fed every 2 hourly starting as soon as possible.

Tropic Feeds (Minimal Enteral Nutrition)

Expressed breast milk in a small volume 12–24 ml/kg/day is delivered intragastric and started early in sick babies. The feeds enhance gut growth, hormonal secretion and motility and reduce hospital stay.

Mode of feeding (Table 2.3)

Gavage feeds (Fig. 2.28)

Method

1. For gavage feeding of LBW 5–6 french size polythene catheter is required.
2. At the time of feeding the outer end of the tube is attached with a 10 ml syringe (without plunger).

Table 2.2: Volume of fulids to be given							
Birth weight	Day of the life and fluid requirement in ml/day						
	1	2	3	4	5	6	7
<1500 g	80	95	110	125	140	150	150
>1500 g	60	75	90	105	120	135	150

Table 2.3: Mode of providing feeds

Age	Categories of neonates		
Birth weight (gm)	<1200	1200–1800	>1800
Gestation (weeks)	<30	30–34	>34
Initial	Intravenous fluid Try gavage feeding	Gavage	Breastfeeding if unsatisfied *Katori*, spoon feeds
After 1–3 days	Gavage	*Katori* feeding Spoon feeding	Breastfeeding
Later 1–3 weeks		*Katori* feeding Spoon feeding	Breastfeeding
After some more time (4–6 weeks)	Breastfeeding	Breastfeeding	Breastfeeding

3. Milk is filled in syringe and is allowed to tickle by gravity (Fig. 2.28).
4. Baby should be fed in the left lateral position for 15–10 minutes to avoid regurgitation.

Katori–spoon feeds: Babies with a gestation of 30–32 weeks or more may not be good at sucking or coordinated sucking or swallowing. But they can swallow the feeds. So, feeding with *katori* and 'palady' or spoon is safe in LBW babies.

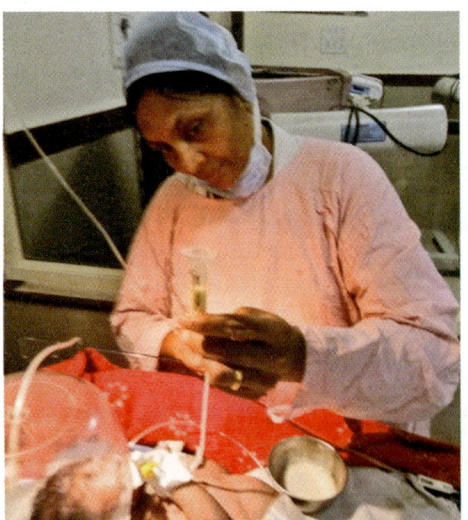

Fig. 2.28: Gavage feeding.

Take the expressed milk in the *katori* or cup. Place the baby in semiupright position. Fill the spoon with milk a little sort of brim and place at the lip of the baby in corner of the mouth and the milk flow into baby's mouth slowly avoiding spilling. The baby will swallow the milk well. Repeat the process till the required amount of milk is given.

Breastfeeding: Method is same but in LBW babies sucking will be slow and takes longer time.

Intravenous fluids (LBW): Intravenous fluid requirement is as follows.

First day   60–80 ml/kg

Daily increase 15 ml/kg till 150 ml/kg is reached.

Adequacy of Nutrition

- Weight pattern of the baby is seen. A preterm LBW loses 1–2% weight per day amounting 10% total weight loss during the first week and then regained by 14th day.
- Once birth weight is regained the LBW baby should gain 1–1.5% of baby weight daily. Increasing weight loss or inadequate weight gain means:
  - Inadequate feeding
  - Cold stress
  - Excessive insensible loss of water.

Jaundice

Functional immaturity of the liver and other factors related to prematurity causes increased production and poor conjugation of bilirubin.

These babies are at risk of developing neurotoxicity at lower level.

Early interruption, phototherapy is required.

Brain Injury

Babies born before 28 weeks of gestation have fragile capillaries, they are at risk of intra-ventricular hemorrhage.

To minimize the risk of feeding, fluids and drugs should be administered slowly, minimal handling should be followed.

Apnea

Due to immaturity of respiratory centre they have apneic spells. Monitoring and stimulator drugs or assisted ventilation required.

Anemia

Physiological anemia aggravated by various factors. Treat the anemia according.

Retinopathy of Prematurity (ROP)

Cause: Immature retina is very susceptible to oxidant damage resulting blindness.

Prevention: Oxygen level monitored by pulse oximeter. It should not be more than 94%.

Hearing Loss

The risk of sensoneural hearing loss increases as the gestation and birth weight decreases.
- Drugs aminoglycosides, frusemide also cause hearing loss.
- Asphyxia, severe jaundice, prolonged ventilator support, sepsis and meningitis are risk factors.

Hypoglycemia: Immature metabolic pathways predispose them to develop hypoglycemia.

Prevent hypoglycemia by early feeding and two hourly feeding schedule.

Prevention of infections: Infections are prevented by decreasing invasive intervention, maintaining temperature, minimal handling, promoting breastfeeding and KMC and maintaining hand hygiene.

Use of appropriate antibiotics are required at first sign of infection.

Nutritional Supplements

Vitamin K—all LBW <1000 gm should be given 0.5 mg IM and >1000 gm should be given 1 mg IM.

Vitamin D—400 IU daily supplementation until 6 months of age.

Multivitamin drop—0.3 ml/day from 2 weeks of age.

Calcium and phosphorus
<1500 gm　Calcium: 120–140 mg/kg/day
　　　　　　Phosphorus: 60–90 mg/kg/day

Continued till 40 weeks of post conceptional age optimal preparations having the calcium and phosphorus in 2:1 should be used.

Iron—supplementation 2–3 mg/kg/day at 6–8 weeks and as early as 2 weeks in <1500 gm babies is effective in preventing anemia of prematurity. It is continued till one year of age.

Prevention of Premature Births

It is difficult to prevent because risk factors are not always identifiable, some ways are as:

Female education: Improved education spacing between two children.

Antenatal steroids: These prevent complications related to preterm delivery.

Institutional deliveries attended by trained personnel, safe transport, timely intervention and drugs.

Vaccination in LBW: BCG, OPV (0 dose), hepatitis B is given.

If sick LBW—vaccination at time of discharge.

If not sick as per schedules.

Discharge planning

- Weight gain recorded on three consecutive days. Vaccination done.
- Length, height, head circumference noted
- Temperature control, feeding, KMC, danger sign should be explained to parents.
- Dexamethasone 6 mg IM every IM 12 hours (4 doses) or
- Betamethasone 12 mg IM every 24 hours (2 doses). To all mothers of preterm labor before delivery.

Prognosis: Prognosis of LBW is inversely related to birth weight and period of gestation, who survives—90% babies have no neurodevelopmental handicaps.

INTRAUTERINE GROWTH RESTRICTION (IUGR)
(SMALL-FOR-DATES: SFD)

Definition

When the weight of baby is less than 10th percentile for the period of gestation it is called small-for-date baby.

Incidence

30–40% in India.

Classification

i. *Malnourished small-for-date babies:* These are malnourished. Growth retardation is due to reduction in size of cells, whereas number of cells are unaffected.
ii. *Hypoplastic small-for-date babies:* Number of cell population is reduced. The baby is proportionately small in all parameters including head size (Fig. 2.29).
iii. Mixed SFD babies.

Causes

A. Maternal factors:
   i. Malnutrition and anemia.
   ii. Chronic systemic diseases, heart, renal hypertension, pulmonary hypertension.
   iii. *Maternal medication:* Diazepam, tetracycline.
   iv. Miscellaneous causes

a. Low socioeconomic status
b. Maternal age below 16 years and above 55 years
c. Tobacco smoking and chewing
d. Addictions (alcohol, LSD, opium)
e. High altitude

B. Placental factors:
   i. **Placental insufficiency:** Toxemia, aging placenta in postmaturity, placental separation, placental infarction.
   ii. **Placental infections:** Syphilis, toxoplasmosis, cytomegalovirus infections, malaria.
   iii. **Multiple pregnancy**: Twin to twin transfusion.

Fetal factors

i. Endogenous causes: Genetic and chromosomal disorders, trisomy, Turner's syndrome
ii. Exogenous causes: Infections: Rubella, syphilis, toxoplasmosis, radiation injury.

Characteristic Features (Fig. 2.29)

i. Babies are low birth weight.
ii. Vernix caseosa is absent on skin. Skin is dry scaly or cracked. Subcutaneous fat is reduced.
iii. Nails and umbilical cord are yellow or green.
iv. Skull bones are firm and hard.
v. Hairs and ear cartilage developed fully.
vi. Testes are descended, crease at soles and palm are well developed. Baby is quite active and alert than normal newborn; he is long, thin and undernourished, easy to feed.

TYPES OF IUGR (*Refer to* page 346)

Complication

i. Hypoglycemia
ii. Brain damage
iii. Asphyxia
iv. Meconium aspiration pneumonia
v. Hypothermia

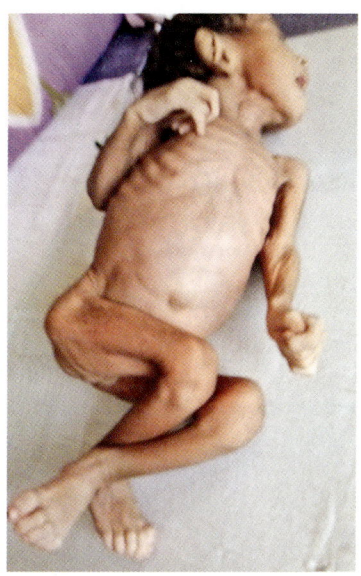

Fig. 2.29: Intrauterine growth restriction.

Diagnosis

   i. Manifest clinical feature of dysmaturity.
  ii. History of pre-eclamptic toxemia generally arouse suspicion.
 iii. Diagnosis of potential hypoglycemia is done by estimation of blood glucose within 2 hours of birth.

Management

   i. *Feeding:* First feed is given within 1st hour of birth to prevent hypoglycemia 30 ml per kg increased to 150 ml per kg milk is given.
  ii. *In utero aspiration or birth asphyxia:* Suction of throat and watch for temperature, respiration, color and seizures for 12–24 hours. Prophylactic antibiotics given if indicated. Exclude surgical emergency causing respiratory distress.
 iii. *Hypoglycemia:* 50% glucose in one-third dilution with distilled water is given 1–2 ml per kg. Intravenous as bolus followed by 60–120 ml/kg continuous intravenous drip for 48 hours. Then 5% dextrose for 24 hours and hydrocortisone is indicated.

   iv. Congenital malformations are detected and dealt.
    v. Temperature regulation and prevention of infection is done as above.

Prognosis

Directly related to birth weight in preterm, 75% of all neonatal deaths occur in these babies.

POST-TERM BABIES
(POST-MATURE, POST-DATED, BORN LATE)

Infants born after a gestation of 42 weeks or late are called post-term.

Clinical features of post-mature babies include increased body length, hard skull bones, small fontanelle and narow sutures. But these are suggestive not conclusive. Vernix caseosa disappears from skin leading to maceration of unprotected skin to its desquamation and formation of deep sole creases. Infant appears thin and dysmature.

Loss of subcuteneous fat, long nails, greenish yellow stained umbilical cord and meconium stained vernix are suggestive. But these signs may be observed in babies which are not post-mature.

Baby is alert at birth and shows advanced neurological development. In intrauterine life, passage of meconium poses grave hazards of respiratory distress due to meconium aspiration.

Management

After birth of postmature child oropharyngeal suction is done to ensure clear airway. Early feeding with glucose and milk feeds are important to correct possible hypoglycemia and prevent brain damage.

Placental functions are assessed for fetal well-being in every case if pregnancy advances beyond 41 weeks.

LARGE-FOR-DATES BABIES
(HEAVY-FOR-DATES, OVERGROWN BABIES)

These include babies in which birth weight is more than 90th percentile or more than

2 standard deviations from the mean weight for gestation.

Causes

i. Genetic or constitutional
ii. Maternal diabetes mellitus and pre-diabetes
iii. Transposition of great vessels
iv. Hydrops fetalis
v. Cretinism
vi. Overgrowth syndromes
   a. Administration of progestins during pregnancy
   b. Adrenal hyperplasia
   c. Thyrotoxicosis syndrome
   d. Cerebral gigantism.

Management

The infant must be fed early and blood glucose should be monitored first 72 hours because overgrown babies are associated with hypertrophy of islets of pancreas.

NEONATAL JAUNDICE

Epidemiology

- About 60% of term and 80% of preterm neonates are clinically jaundiced in first week of life.
- In most cases it is benign, in about 5–10% cases have significant jaundice requiring treatment.

Jaundice is yellow discoloration of skin and sclera. Seen on sclera, face, nasolabial folds, tips of nose in early stage later on in trunk, abdomen, extremities, palm and soles.

At the skin it is easily recognized by blenching the skin.

After the breakdown of hemoglobin bilirubin is released. It is called free bilirubin (unconjugated compound) which is lipid soluble but water insoluble. Free bilirubin bound to serum albumin and result this unconjugated bilirubin-albumin complex. This complex is soluble in plasma but cannot be filtered through renal glomerulus.

Above unconjugated bilirubin-albumin complex is seperated at hepatic cell membrane from its albumin and is taken up in the cell. Here the bilirubin is conjugated with glucuronic acid to form water-soluble bilirubin glucuronide with the help of enzyme called glucuronyl transferase. The conjugated bilirubin is then secreted across the epithelium of small bile ducts into bile canaliculus and is transported to the duodenum.

In newbom, binding capacity to free bilirubin is less than elder. Apart from that, excess production of free bilirubin occurs as in hemolytic process. Lipid solubility of free bilirubin allows to enter to the basal ganglia of the brain through blood–brain barrier giving rise to kernicterus. But albumin bound cannot pass blood–brain barrier (Flowchart 2.2).

In preterm babies enzyme glucuronyl transferase is deficient due to hepatic immaturity hence chances of hyperbilirubinemia (free) are more.

Where jaundice is due to conjugated serum bilirubin, there is no risk of kernicterus because the conjugated bilirubin cannot pass blood–brain barrier.

Common Causes

i. Physiological
ii. Immaturity
iii. Blood group incompatibility
iv. G6PD deficiency
v. Infections—both intrauterine and postnatal
vi. Subcutaneous bruising and cephalhematoma
vii. Drugs
viii. Breast milk jaundice.

Causes and increased by factor that

i. Increases the load of bilirubin to be metabolized by liver.
   a. Hemolytic anemia.
   b. Shortened red cell life due to immaturity, transfused cells.
   c. Increased enterohepatic circulation
   d. Infections

Flowchart 2.2: Neurotoxicity

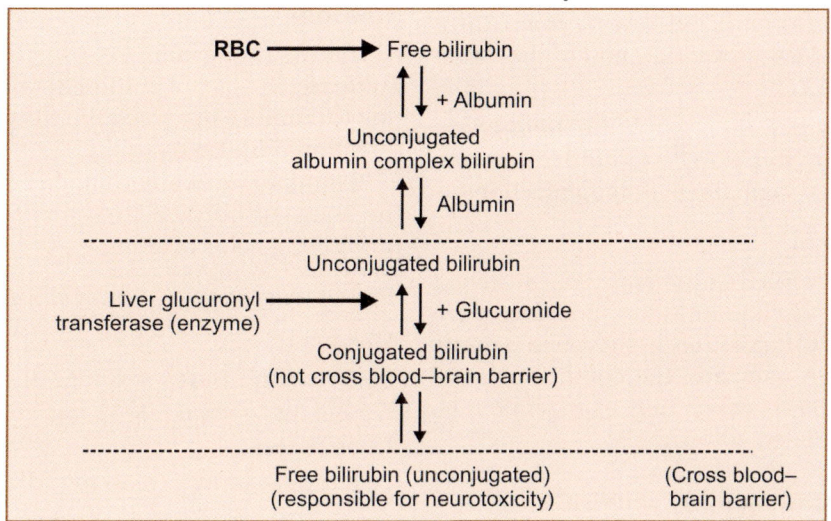

ii May damage or reduce the activity of enzymes
  a. Hypoxia
  b. Hypothermia
  c. Infections
  d. Thyroid deficiency
iii. May compete for or block the enzyme
  a. Drugs
  b. Other substances
iv. Leads to an absence or decreased amounts of the enzyme or reduction of bilirubin.
  a. Genital defect
  b. Prematurity.

PHYSIOLOGICAL JAUNDICE OF NEWBORN

Incidence

It is seen in 60% of term and 70% of preterm babies.

Definition

Physiological jaundice of newborn usually appears on 3rd day or 72 hours of age; maximum intensity is seen on 4th or 5th day and disappears by 7th day. The bilirubin level usually does not exceed 10 mg/dl.

Causes

i. It is due to breakdown of fetal red blood cells and production of bilirubin.
ii. Limitation in conjugation and excretion of bilirubin by liver due to deficiency of glucuronyl transferase.
iii. Due to lack of bacteria in the gut in early part of neonatal life, conjugated bilirubin entering the gut cannot be converted to urobilin. Instead it is deconjugated by β-glucuronidase and recirculated to the liver through enterohepatic circulation.

Features

There is no characteristic feature of physiological jaundice. In newborn, level of indirect bilirubin in umbilical cord is 1–3 mg/dl and rises at the rate of less than 5 mg/dl/24 hr.

This jaundice becomes visible on 2nd or 3rd day. The maximum intensity reaches on 5th–7th days and decreasing below 2 mg/dl between 5th and 7th days of life and disappears by the age of 8–14 days.

In premature infant rise is similar, little slower than term so maximum peak in between 4 and 7 days of life.

Diagnosis

Diagnosis depends on onset, maximum intensity and disappearance and exclusion of pathological causes.

Exaggerated in following circumstances

Prematurity, hypoxia, circulatory insufficiency, drugs, cephalhematoma, infections.

Management

This does not need any therapy but watched for severity. Adequate fluids and feeds are given to baby. Reassurance is given to parents about benign nature of the condition; associated conditions which may exaggerate this, should be treated accordingly.

PATHOLOGICAL JAUNDICE

Any of the following alert signs in neonatal jaundice when present it is assumed as pathological jaundice.

a. Clinical signs in first 24 hours of life.
b. Total serum bilirubin (TSB) increased by >5 mg/dl/day or 0.5 mg/dl/hr
c. TSB >15 mg/dl
d. Conjugated serum bilirubin >2 mg/dl.
e. Clinical jaundice presenting >2 weeks age in term and 3 weeks in preterm.

Appearing within 24 hours of age

1. Hemolytic disease of newborn, RH, ABO and minor group incompatibility.
2. Intrauterine infections—viral, bacterial, malaria.
3. G6PD deficiency.

Appearing after 24 hours of age

1. All of the above
2. Physiological
3. Polycythemia
4. Concealed hemorrhages
   a. Cephalhematoma
   b. Subarachnoid bleeding
   c. Intraventricular hemorrhage
5. Sepsis
6. Neonatal hepatitis
7. Metabolic disorders

Clinical Assessment of Jaundiced Newborn

Dermal staining may be used as a clinical guide to the level of jaundice staining of skin due to jaundice progresses in a cephalocaudal direction (Fig. 2.30).

Examine the newborn in day light, blanch the skin with digital pressure and note the underlying color of skin.

Part of body	Serum bilirubin	Zone
Head and neck	4–6 mg/dl	1
Neck to umbilicus	6–8 mg/dl	2
Umbilicus to knee	8–12 mg/dl	3
Knee to feet	12–14 mg/dl	4
Feet, upper limb	>15 mg/dl	5

Serum levels of total bilirubin are approximately estimated as follows.

Evaluation

- Examine usually every 12 hr during 3 to 5 days.
- Transcutaneous bilirubin (TcB)—used for screening.
- Total serum blirubin (TSB) estimation (Table 2.4).
  Babies needing phototherapy should be evaluated for:
  1. Hemoglobin, reticulocyte count, peripheral smear for evidence of hemolysis.
  2. Blood group—mother, baby
  3. G6PD deficiency
  4. Other sepsis screen.
- Thyroid function test
- Urine for reducing substances to identify galactosemia
- Specific enzyme/genetic studies for Crigler-Najjar, Gilbert and Sullivan genetic enzyme deficiencies.

Management of Pathological Jaundice

Management of neonatal pathological jaundice is directed towards reducing the level of bilirubin and preventing CNS toxicity.

- Prevention of hyperbilirubinemia by early and frequent feeding.

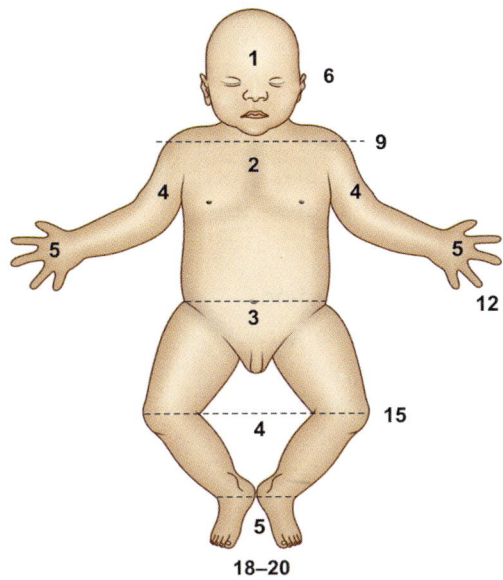

Fig. 2.30: Clinical assessment of neonatal jaundice.

Table 2.4: Guideline for phototherapy and exchange transfusion for hyperbilirubinemia cut off TSB mg/dl

Gestation (weeks)	Phototherapy	Exchange transfusion
<28	5–6	11–14
28–29	6–8	12–14
30–31	8–10	15–18
34	12–14	17–19

- Reduction of bilirubin this is achieved by:
  1. Phototherapy and/or
  2. Exchange transfusion

Preterm neonates: Guidelines to treat hyperbilirubinemia in preterm neonates gestational age <35 is as weeks follows (Table 2.5).

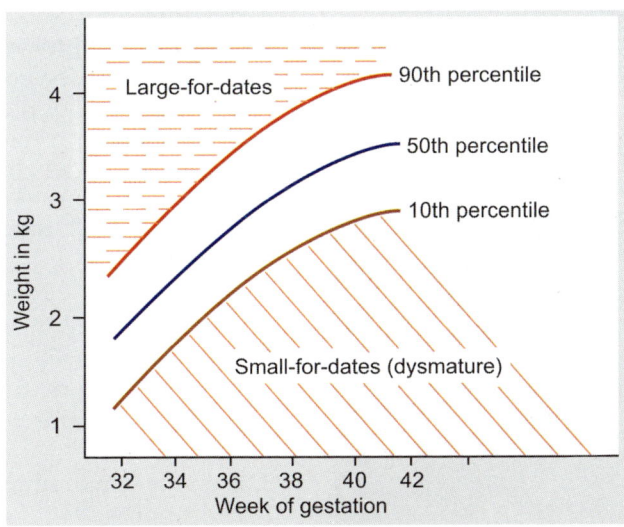

Fig. 2.31: Graph of weight and gestation showing large-for-dates and small-for-dates babies.

Table 2.5: Guideline to treat hyperbilirubinemia in preterm neonates

Birth weight (gm)	PT TSB (mg/dl) in healthy	PT TSB (mg/dl) in sick	BET TSB (mg/dl)
>1000	05–07	04–06	10–12
1000–1500	07–10	05–08	12–15
1500–2000	10–12	08–10	15–18
2001–2500	12–15	10–12	18–10

PT: Phototherapy; TSB: Total serum bilirubin; BET: Blood exchange transfusion

For 35 weeks or higher gestational age neonate

Guidelines for neonates >35 weeks gestational age are divided in three groups.

1. Infants at lower risk >38 weeks and well
2. Infants at medium risk >38 weeks + risk factors

   Or 35–37 weeks and well (no risk factor)
3. Infants at higher risk 35–37 weeks + risk factors.

Risk factors are isoimmune hemolytic disease G6PD deficiency, asphyxia, significant lethargy, temperature (instability), sepsis, acidosis, serum albumin <3.0 gm/dl.

Phototherapy (Tables 2.4 and 2.5)

This involves exposure of the naked baby to blue light/CFL/LED of wave length 460–490 nm.

Ideal irradiance of phototherapy (PT) with irradiance in blue green spectrum at least 20–30 $\mu w/cm^2/nm$.

Types of phototherapy light—phototherapy units are commercially available compact fluorescent lamp (CFL) in most commonly used device (Fig. 2.32).

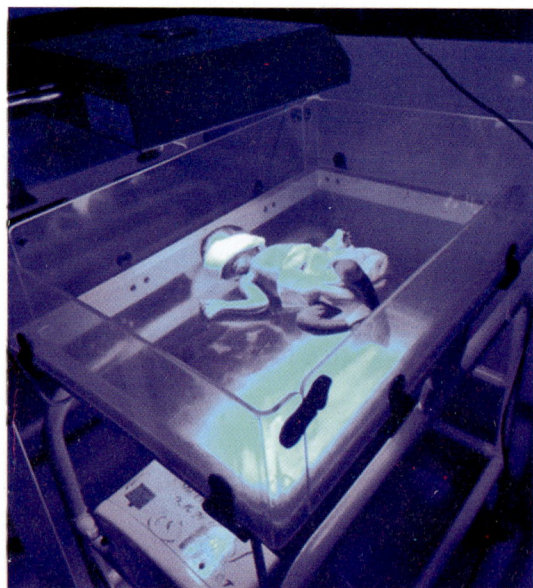

Fig. 2.32: Phototherapy unit.

Phototherapy has various types of light source that include fluorescent lamps of different colors (white, blue, green blue or tourquoise).

Other types of light source include light emitting diode (LED). Fiberoptic light source.

LED has long life and higher irradiance than CFL.

Mechanism of Action

It acts by converting insoluble (unconjugated) bilirubin into nontoxic soluble form isomers that is easily excreted in urine.

Method

1. Remove all the clothes of baby. External genitalia should be covered.
2. Cover the baby is eye with an eye patch.
3. Place the naked baby under the light in a cot or bassinet.
4. Keep the 25 to 45 cm distance between baby and light (or manufacturer recommendation). It is a noninvasive technique (an advantage of phototherapy).
5. Baby will appear bleached when under phototherapy so clinical assessment of jaundice is not reliable.
6. Check serum bilirubin every after 12 hours of stopping phototherapy. In hemolytic jaundice, rebound increases in serum bilirubin may occurs.
7. Ensure breastfeeding baby. Baby can be taken out for breastfeeding, remove eye shades for better mother infant interaction.
8. Monitor temperature of the baby every 2 to 4 hours.
9. Discontinue phototherapy once when two TSB values 12 hours apart fall by 2–3 mg% below current age specific cut off.
10. Prophylactic PT does not offer any clinical benefit.

Side effects of phototherapy

1. Increased insensible water loss.
2. Loose green stools.
3. Skin rash

4. Bronze baby syndrome occurs if baby has conjugated hyperbilirubinemia—discontinue phototherapy.
5. Hypo- or hyperthermia.

All these side effects are reversible.

Exchange Transfusion (Tables 2.4 and 2.5)

Indication: Double volume exchange transfusion (DVET) should be performed.
1. TSB levels reach to age specific cut-off level for exchange transfusion.
2. Signs of bilirubin encephalopathy are seen irrespective of TSB levels.
3. Indication at birth
   a. Cord blood bilirubin is 5 mg/dl or more.
   b. Cord Hb is 10 g/dl or less.

Conjugated Hyperbilirubinemia

This is rare in newborn period. Direct bilirubin level is >2 mg/dl.

It is never physiological. Causes may be extrahepatic biliary atresia (surgical cause), galactosemia, etc.

Breastfeeding jaundice: Breastfeed babies may have different type of physiological jaundice.

Appears between 24 and 72 hr of age, peaks by 5–15 days and disappear by third week of life. It may persist 2nd to 3rd months of life. It is due to inadequate breastfeeding. Ensure optimal and exclusive breastfeeding.

Breast milk jaundice: 2–4% of babies may have breast milk jaundice. Serum bilirubin 10 mg/dl at 3rd or 4th week of life. Baby may require phototherapy. Do not stop breastfeeding.

NEONATAL SEPTICEMIA

This is a clinical syndrome characterised by symptomatic systemic illness and bacteremia.

Etiology

Most common organisms are *E. coli* and group B Streptococcus (in 50–75% cases). *Staphylococcus aureus*, Enterococcus, Klebsiella, *Enterobacter* sp, *Pseudomonas aeruginosa*, *Proteus* sp, *Listeria monocytogenes* are other organisms causing it.

Predisposing Factors

May be febrile maternal illness, prolonged ruptured membrane, amnionitis, instrumentation, mouth to mouth breathing, umbilical sepsis, face mask.

Portal of entry in most cases is the umbilical vein. GIT and some other infections also cause septicemia.

Clinical Features

Baby who has been sucking normally gradually or suddenly becomes lethargic, inactive, unresponsive and refuses to suck. Often mother states that infant does not look well or feeds poorly.

There may be anorexia, loose motion; vomiting, lethargy, temperature instability, jaundice, respiratory distress, hepatomegaly, abdominal distension and pallor.

Hypothermia is more common and dangerous manifestation.

Meningitis may be associated with septicemia; convulsion may occur. Neck stiffness and bulging are absent in 70% cases.

High pitched cry, bulding fontanel, sign of shock, bleeding, renal failure, cyanosis or tachycardia also other manifestations.

Sclerema neonatorum manifests as diffuse hardening of subcutaneous tissue resulting in a light smooth skin that feels bound to the underlying structures of the body.

Diagnosis

1. Diagnosis of neonatal sepsis on clinical manifestations mostly.
2. Blood culture should be sent prior to starting antibiotics.
3. Sepsis screen should be performed.
   - Total leukocyte count (TLC)—below 5000/cu mm.
   - Absolute neutrophil count (ANC) less than 1800 per cu mm.

- Immature band cell + myelocyte + meta-myelocyte to total neutrophil ratio (ITR more than 20%). Because bore marrow pushes even the immature cells into circulation to fight infection.
- CRP (C-reactive protein)—value of >10 mg/dl is taken as positive.
- The micro-ESR elevated >15 mm.

4. *Lumbar puncture:* CSF should be examined within 30 minutes of drawing of the CSF because WBC and glucose falls rapidly with time.

Normal value of CSF

Cells	Preterm	Term
Leukocytes/mm^3	7	9
Polymorph (%)	61	57
Protein (mg/dl)	90	115
Glucose (mg/dl)	52	50

Sepsis is diagnosed when

WBC count	>8/mm^3 in term
	>10/mm^3 preterm
Protein	>120 mg/dl in term
	>170 mg/dl in preterm
Glucose	>20 mg/dl in term
	>24 mg/dl in preterm.

Treatment: Prompt treatment of neonatal sepsis consists of supportive care and antibiotics.

Supportive Treatment

i. Management of fluid and electrolyte balance, ventilatory assistance, fresh whole blood transfusion or exchange transfusion.
ii. Support of blood pressure with dopamine, dobutamine or steroids.
iii. Appropriate management of sepsis.
   - Maintain TABC.
   - Start oxygen maintain (SpO$_2$ 90–94%)
   - Assess peripheral circulation
   - Pulse rate

- Capillary refill time (CRT) normally >2–3 seconds.
- Skin color

If circulation is poor

IV normal saline or Ringer lactate 10 ml/kg over 5–10 minutes repeat it if no improvement, 1–2 times. If no improvement, dopamine or dobutamine is given.

Hypoglycemia should be treated with:
- IV 10% dextrose in a dose of 2 ml/kg stat
- Provide maintenance fluid with electrolyte and glucose.
- Potassium should be supplemented if normal urine flow is established.
- Consider exchange blood transfusion in sclerema.
- Administer vit K$_1$ mg IV/IM
- Avoid enteral feeds if hemodynamically compromised, give IV fluid. As soon as baby in stable give orogastric feeds.
- Blood transfusion—transfuse packed cells if baby has a low hematocrit (<35–40%).

Antibiotic Therapy: Antimicrobial therapy is an essential part of treatment of sepsis, blood sample for culture and sensitivity is taken but do not wait for the results and start antimicrobial therapy which covers the common causative bacteria.

Treatment after an etiologic agent is known depends on sensitivity report, give appropriate antibiotic.

Septicemia and pneumonia

First line:	Ampicillin or penicillin and gentamycin.
Second line:	Ampicillin or cloxacillin and amikacin
	Piperacillin + tazobactam and amikacin
Third line:	Cefotaxime and amikacin

Dose

Ampicillin 50 mg/kg/dose 12 hourly/8 hourly IV 7–10 days

Cloxacillin 50 mg/kg/dose 12 hourly/8 hourly IV 7–10 days and

Gentamicin 5 mg/kg/dose 24 hourly IV 7–10 days.

Duration: 7–10 days, IV route.

Monitoring: Monitoring should be done regularly.

Meningitis

First line drugs

Cefotaxime 50 mg/kg/dose 12 hourly IV 3 weeks

Amikacin 15 mg/kg/dose 24 hourly IV 3 weeks

Second line drugs

Meropenem 40 mg/kg/dose 8 hourly IV 3 weeks

Amikacin 15 mg/kg/dose 8 hourly IV 3 weeks

Change of antibiotics: If no improvement occurs after 48 hr of antibiotic treatment then change the antibiotic (second line).

Stop antibiotics: Asymptomatic neonates, blood culture is sterile.

Worsening of neonatal sepsis: When respiratory failure, unresponsive shock persistent and refractory convulsion, disseminated intravascular coagulation, baby requiring exchange transfusion.

Prevention of neonatal sepsis

- Safe delivery practice
- Meternal immunization for tetanus and treatment of maternal illness.
- Early and exclusive breastfeeds
- No prelacteal feeds
- Cord stump should be kept clean and dry
- Avoid overcrowding handling
- Maintain hygiene

CAPUT SUCCEDANEUM

This is a diffuse, nonfluctant, edematous swelling of soft tissue of scalp of newborn on the presenting part. This may extend across the midline and across suture lines. Edema disappears within few days of life. Sometime, it may be ecchymosis. No specific treatment is needed for this. If there is extensive ecchymosis phototherapy is indicated for hyperbilirubinemia. Rarely blood transfusion is required for shock due to hemorrhage. Moulding of head and overriding of parietal bones are generally associated with caput but it disappear during first week of life (Fig. 2.33).

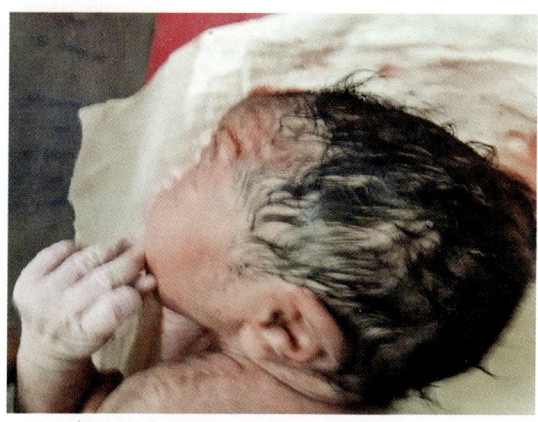

Fig. 2.33: Caput succedaneum.

CEPHALHEMATOMA

This is subperiosteal hemorrhage and collection of blood at the scalp of newborn following normal or complicated delivery.

This is always limited to one cranial bone, so does not cross suture line. Thus, it differs from caput. It has well developed margin (Figs 2.34 and 2.35).

Swelling is visible after several hours after birth. There may or may not be discoloration of scalp, sometimes underlying fracture of bone may be associated with it.

This is differentiated from menigocele in which positive crying impulse and associated, bone defect seen on roentgenographic examination. This is reabsorbed within 2 weeks to 3 months.

In few cases this remains for years and seen as cyst-like defect or widening of diploic space on radiological examination.

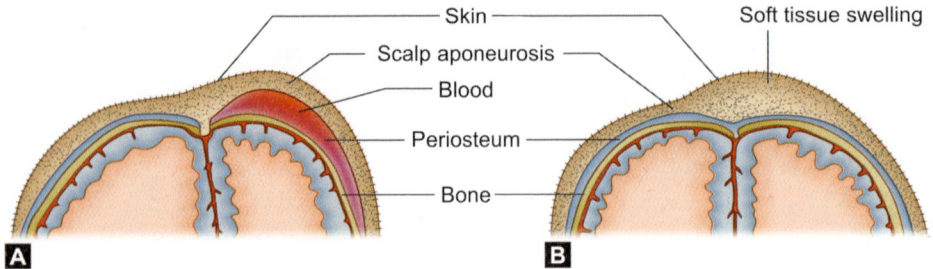

Skin — | — Soft tissue swelling
Scalp aponeurosis —
Blood —
Periosteum —
Bone —

A   **B**

Fig. 2.34: (A) Cephalhematoma; (B) Caput succedaneum.

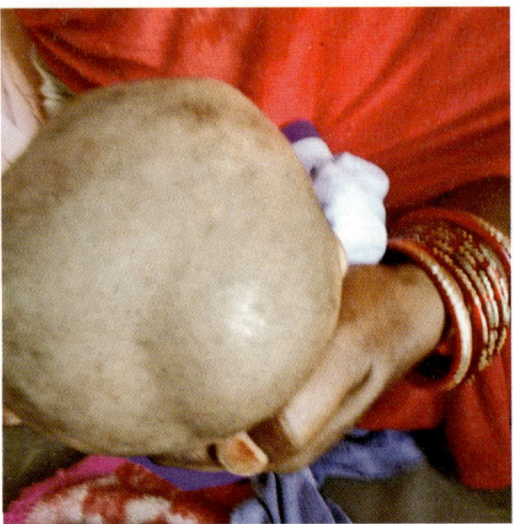

Fig. 2.35: Cephalhematoma.

This requires no treatment. Incision and drainage are contraindicated due to risk of introducing infection. Phototherapy is required for hyperbilirubinemia and blood transfusion for massive blood hemorrhage. Vitamin K 0.1 mg intramuscular given to correct coexisting coagulation defect.

PERINATAL MORTALITY

Death occurring during perinatal period is quite high in India. It includes stillbirth and death occurring in the first seven days of life.

Perinatal mortality rate is the number of stillbirths and first week deaths per 1000 total births (live and still).

Causes of perinatal mortality: Five common causes are:

i. Low birth weight babies
ii. Perinatal hypoxia and birth trauma
iii. Neonatal infections
iv. Congenital malformations
v. Rhesus isoimmunization

Other causes are

vi. High risk pregnancy
vii. Low socioeconomic group, maternal malnutrition, anemia and chronic illness of mother, elder mother.

High Risk Babies

i. Preterm baby
ii. Retarded fetal growth
iii. Post-term babies
iv. Twins
v. Jaundiced babies
vi. Rhesus incompatible
vii. Diabetic babies
viii. Congenital malformations
ix. Genetic defects of newborn

NEONATAL SEIZURES

Convulsions in newborn are always due to disorders of central nervous system or biochemical abnormality. In one-fourth cases no cause is identified. Incidence is 0.5%. The newborn babies do not manifest febrile convulsions.

Causes

1. Perinatal complications—birth asphyxia, intracranial injuries
2. Hypocalcemia

3. Infections—intrauterine infections, septicemia, meningitis
4. Hypoglycemia
5. Metabolic conditions
6. Development defects
7. Acute systemic illness
8. Narcotic addiction syndrome—in babies born to mothers addicted to heroin, morphine or alcohol.
9. Phenothiazine toxicity—use of large doses of these drugs for the management of eclampsia may lead to convulsions in newborn.
10. Local anesthetics—local injection of anesthetic into fetal scalp during paracervical block during delivery.
11. Hypomagnesemia
12. Pyridoxine dependency—prolonged maternal administration of vitamin B_6 during pregnancy may predispose to this condition.
13. Dyselectrolytemia (hypo- or hypernatremia).

Common causes

1. Hypoxic ischemic encephalopathy (about 50%)
2. Sepsis
3. Bacterial meningitis

Common types

Subtle—most common
- Repetitive blinking, eye deviation or staring.
- Repetitive movements of mouth or tongue.
- Purposeless movements of limbs as if baby is bicycling or swimming.

Clonic—repetitive movements of the limbs or face.

Tonic—continuous flexion and extension of limbs.

Myoclonic—sudden jerky movements of limbs.

Neonatal seizures should be differentiated from

1. Jitteriness—provoked by stimulus and abolished by restraining EEG normal.

2. Neonatal tetanus—involuntary contraction of muscles, trismus, opisthotonus, baby is conscious throughout often crying with pain.

Manifestations: Generalized tonic or clonic convulsions (as in grand mal epilepsy) are not seen in neonates. The manifestations are subtle and pleomorphic.

Manifest seizures are uncommon in preterm babies. Larger the baby, more powerful are the sizures. Seizures may be generalized twitching without jacksonian pattern or tonic or myoclonic type.

Diagnosis: Diagnosis depends on age of onset, positive family history and investigations of associated condition.

Blood

Blood glucose—low, serum calcium—low serum magnesium (low), serum electrolyte.

Sepsis Screening

Lumbar puncture—for diagnosis of meningitis.

Age of onset of convulsions

1st day	Birth asphyxia, intraventricular hemorrhage 'first day' hypocalcemia, inborn error of metabolism, narcotic withdrawal syndrome, pyridoxine dependency.
2nd day	Cerebral contusion, intracranial hemorrhage.
3rd day	Hypoglycemia.
4–7th day	Tetany, kernicterus, developmental malformations, meningitis.

Management

Step 1: Resuscitate the neonate if needed, place in thermoneural environment to prevent hypothermia, ensure patent airway, effective breathing and adequate circulation (TABC).
- Start oxygen
- Ensure IV assess, take blood sample for investigation.

Step 2: If blood sugar is less than 45 mg/dl correct hypoglycemia—10% dextrose–2 ml/kg followed by maintenance infusion 6–8 mg/kg/min.

Step 3: Estimate the calcium level, if less than 7 mg/dl or calcium level not available.

Give 10% calcium gluconate 2 ml/kg IV over of distilled water and then push.

If seizures persist after correction of hypoglycemia and hypocalcemia.

Step 4: Anticonvulsant drugs (ACD)

a. *First line acid drugs:* Phenobarbitone 20 mg/kg IV over 20 minutes. If baby has no further seizures, do not give maintenance.
b. *If seizures persist* after initial administration of phenobarbitone.
c. Administer further bolus of phenobarbitone 5 mg/kg/up to total of 40 mg/kg.
   If seizures are not controlled.
d. **Second line drugs:** Phenytoin or fosphenytoin 20 mg/kg IV over 20 minutes of 1 mg/kg/min. Assess after 30 minutes.
   Phenytoin only should be mixed with normal saline not with dextrose because it may precipitate in dextrose.
e. Once the seizures are *controlled*
f. Start a maintenance dose of phenobarbitone and phenytoin in dose of 3–4 mg/kg/day.
   Stop phenytoin once seizure free for 48 hr.
g. *If seizures persist*—lorazepam 0.05–0.10 mg/kg IV may be infused.
h. *If seizures persist*—consider referral to higher centre.

Maintenance

Once the seizures are controlled start a maintenance dose of phenobarbitone and phenytoin in dose of 3–4 mg/kg/day daily once a day.

Stop phenytoin once seizure free for 48 hr.
If seizures controlled maintain with phenobarbitone 3–4 mg/kg, stop when seizures free for 48 hr.

Specific Situations

1. In case of cerebral edema—dexamethasone and hypertonic mannitol are drugs of choice.
2. Infections—infections are treated with appropriate antibiotics.
3. Exchange transfusion is indicated for metabolic disorders, accidental injection of anesthetic to the fetus, kernicterus and in transplacental transfer of maternal chlorpropamide to the fetus.
4. Narcotic withdrawal syndrome—administration of phenobarbitone or chlorpromazine and attention to hydration.

Prognosis

About one-fourth of babies of neonatal convulsions die, if onset is before 24 hours of age. Perinatal hypoxia, birth injuries leading to intraventricular or subdural hemorrhage, meningitis are associated with grave prognosis and increased incidence of sequelae.

Hypocalcemia, narcotic withdrawal syndrome and subarachnoid hemorrhage associated with good prognosis.

NEONATAL SHOCK

Shock is defined as a clinical state of poor perfusion of the body tissues in which the body's demands of oxygen and nutrients are not met.

Identification

1. Tachycardia HR <160/min
2. Capillary refill time (CRT)

Apply gentle pressure by the tip of finger on central part of the body such as chest for 3–5 seconds. This results in blenching of the underlying surface. Lift the finger and observe how fast the blenched area refills and become pink.

Normal capillary refill time is <3 seconds. Prolonged CRT is sign of shock.

Other features are—poor peripheral pulses, pallor, rolling of skin, cold extremities.

Types of shock

- Hypovolemic—due to blood loss, fluid loss
- Cardiogenic—low cardiac output due to birth asphyxia, congenital heart disease, sepsis, etc.
- Obstructive—example coarctation of aorta, tension preumothorax, etc.
- Distributive—due to anaphylaxis
- Septic shock

Management

Supportive: Maintain TABC, give oxygen, treat hypoglycemia and hypothermia.

Specific

Fluid resuscitation: Infuse fluid bolus of 10 ml/kg of normal saline over 20–30 min assess the improvement by improvement in CRT and decrease in heart rate by at least 10 beats per minutes—if no improvement.

Bolus of 10 ml/kg of normal saline should be given.

Assess urine output and pulse volume over 4–6 hr for improvement.

Vasopressors

1. **Dopamine:** Dose 5–10 µg/kg/min. If no improvement increase by increments of 5 µg/kg every 20–30 minutes to a maximum 20 µg/kg/min
2. **Dobutamine:** Dose same as dopamine
3. **Hydrocortisone:** If baby dose not respond to vasopressor, give hydrocortisone 1 mg/kg/dose every 8–12 hourly for 2–3 days.

Unresponsive shock: Consider blood transfusion if Hb <12 gm% and refer to higher centre.

HYPOTHERMIA

Hypothermia is an important cause of neonatal mortality. It can be prevented by simple measures.

Heat loss: Heat loss may be due to:
1. *Evaporation:* After birth due to evaporation of amniotic fluid on surface of baby.
2. *Conduction:* Due to contact of baby with cold surface such as tray, etc.
3. *Convection:* Air current in which air replaces warm air around the baby, e.g. open window.
4. *Radiation:* Due to cold objects in vicinity walls.

Assessment of Hypothermia

Normal axillary temperature is 36.5–37.5ºC (97.7–99.5°F). Hypothermia say if temperature is below 36.5ºC.

Grading of hypothermia

Cold stress—36.4–36°C (97.5–96.8°F)

Moderate hypothermia—35.9–32.0°C (96.2–89.61ºF)

Severe hypothermia <32°C (89.6°F)

Temperature recording: Temperature in newborn should be recorded axillary temperature. It is as good as rectal and safer. It can be recorded by digital thermometer, thermometer probe attached over upper abdomen. Body's temperature can be assessed with human touch with reasonable precision.

Clinical Signs and Symptoms

Signs and symptoms are nonspecific, common signs and symptoms are lethargy, irritability poor feeding, and breathing difficulty (tachypnea, apnea).

Severe hypothermia may present with hypoglycemia, sclerema, DIC, internal bleeding.

Concept of warm chain: It is to prevent heat loss and promote heat gain. Warm chain in a set of 10 interlinked interventions carried out at birth of baby and later, which minimize the likely hood of hypothermia.

1. Warm delivery room (26°–28°C)
2. Warm resuscitation
3. Immediate drying
4. Skin to skin contact between baby and mother.
5. Breastfeeding
6. Postponing bathing and weighing

7. Appropriate clothing
8. Keeping mother and baby together
9. Warm transportation
10. Awareness—raising of health care pro-
    viders.

Prevention and Management

In the delivery room—room should be warm
(26–28°C) close the door, off the fans.
- Immediately dry the newborn with a sterile
  and warm towel.
- Heat source—radiant heat warmer and
  other sources of heat bulb, heater kept on
  before delivery.
- Use other warm towel to wrap the baby in
  two layers, use blanket to cover with
  clothing.
- Skin to skin contact (kangaroo mother care).
- Keep the baby with mother so her temperature will keep the baby warm.

Kangaroo Mother Care (KMC)

KMC is a technique used to keep the baby
warm the neonate in held skin to skin contact
with mother or any other adult caretaker.

Mother clothing—KMC works well with
a bloused and side gown, or shawl (*refer to
Fig. 2.26*).

Technique

Mother is advised to sit or recline well. Place
the baby between the breasts of the mother in
skin to skin contact in upright position, turn
the head of the baby to one side to prevent
airway obstruction. Slightly extended position
of the head facilitate eye contact to mother.

Abdomen of the baby should be in close
proximity to the epigastrium of the mother.
Mothers's breathing stimulate the baby so
reduces chances of apnea. The hips should
be flexed and bottom of the baby should be
supported in this way the baby clings to the
mother in frog like position.

Support the baby is bottom with sling or
binder.

Initiation: <1200 gm—may take two weeks
before KMC can be initiated.

1200–1800 gm—few days
>1800 gm—can be initiated immediately
after birth.

Duration: KMC should be provided for a duration of at least one hour or as long as possible.

Advantages

1. It gives thermal protection of neonates.
2. Increases milk production, it initiate breastfeeding, increase exclusive breastfeeding.
3. Reduces respiratory tract and nasocomial
   infections.
4. Improve emotional bonding and improve
   weight of the baby, reduces hospital stay.

Other heat sources

100 watt bulb, heater, warm blanket can be
used to prevent hypothermia.

Clothing of baby should be proper to
prevent hypothermia.

Management

Mild hypothermia (35.5°–36.4°C)

1. KMC
2. Warm the room using radiant heat warmer,
   or other heating devices.
3. Cover with warm clothes.
4. Keep the room warm and draught free.
5. Continue breastfeeding.
6. Monitor temperature every 30 minutes till
   it reaches 36.5°C then 3 hourly.
7. Wrap the baby well with cap.

Significant Hypothermia

1. Remove cold clothes from the baby, cover
   with warm clothes.
2. Place under radiant heat warmer or room
   heater or other devices to warm the baby.
3. KMC may be only option sometimes.

Monitor temperature every 15–30 min.

JITTERINESS

Jitteriness or coarse tremors are characterised
by movements in identical in all directions;
which is differentiated from clonic fits in

which rapid alternation of fast and slow phase of movements occur.

Many normal infants manifest jitteriness. Other causes are cerebral hyperexcitability, hypocalcemia, hypoglycemia, congenital thyrotoxicosis, infants of diabetic mother, narcotic withdrawal syndrome and drug toxicity.

Management includes identification of cause and treat accordingly. Tremors disappear spontaneously or following administration of phenobarbitone or chloral hydrate.

HEMORRHAGIC DISORDERS OF THE NEWBORN

Causes

Fetal hemorrhage: Twin to twin transfusion, fetomaternal hemorrhage, antepartum hemorrhage, administration of anticoagulant to mother, accidental incision of placenta during cesarean section.

Neonatal hemorrhage

i. Hemorrhagic disease of newborn.
   a. Low prothrombin level (transient) at birth due to deficiency of vitamin K.
   b. Transient deficiency of factors VII, IX and X.
ii. Thrombocytopenia or decreased production of platelets in bone marrow.
iii. Increased destruction of platelets by maternal antibodies.
iv. Idiopathic thrombocytopenic purpura.
v. Purpura of the mother or platelet incompatibility with isoimmunization.
vi. Local or traumatic causes.
   a. Umbilical cord bleeding due to slipped ligature or laceration of cord during delivery.
   b. Superficial injuries of the scalp, intracranial or visceral hemorrhage.
   c. Trauma due to catheters, tube, rectal thermometer.
   d. Cephalhematoma.
   e. Gastrointestinal bleeding due to swallowed maternal blood, acute peptic ulceration, perforation of gut, volvulus, necrotising enterocolitis.
   f. Subconjunctival hemorrhage due to increased venous pressure during passage in birth canal during delivery.
   g. Retinal hemorrhage—may be normal. But may be associated with increased viscosity of blood and polycythemia.
vii. Hepatic insufficiency due to anoxia, hepatitis, immaturity or metabolic disorders.

Deficiency of vit K incidence is higher in breastfed babies due to low content of its breast milk and in prolong administration of antibiotic, which eliminates intestinal flora resulting in vit K deficiency.

Clinical Features

Most commonly bleeding appears in the gastrointestinal tract either as malena or hematemesis. The vomited blood is bright red. There may be dark tarry stool.

Less often bleeding manifests as intracranial hemorrhage, hematuria, umbilical bleeding or vaginal bleeding.

Acute hemorrhagic pneumonia manifests as rapid pallor and blood stained froth in the mouth.

Intraventricular hemorrhage manifests as deterioration in respiratory and circulatory functions, e.g. inability to suck well and swallow, poor ineffective cry, twiching or convulsions, intermittent cyanosis, bulging fontanelle, rigidity of limbs, squint, nystagmus and local paralysis.

When blood or malena is sole manifestation during first 48 hours, the possibility of maternal swallowed blood is excluded by Apt and Downey test.

The sign of acute blood loss such as pallor, rapid breathing, rising heart rate and falling blood pressure are seen, if blood loss is excessive. Infant may die in few hours or after 2–3 days. Premature babies are at risk due to increased vascular permeability and irritability to effectively utilize vitamin K for the synthesis of coagulation factor.

Management

i. In all cases vitamin K is given 2 mg Intramuscularly or intravenously.

ii. Blood transfusion—if blood loss exceeds 20% of his volume.

- Fresh blood transfusion—for thrombocytopenia or deficiency of clotting factor is present.
- Platelet transfusion—for thrombocytopenia
- Fresh plasma transfusion—for cases where deficiency of clotting factor does not respond to administration of vitamin K.

iii. Administration of antibiotic, supportive therapy for shock, acidosis, treatment and control of hypothermia are other adjuvent measures.

iv. Exchange transfusion and corticosteroids are indicated in platelet isoimmunization.

v. If bleeding is due to rupture of vessels (e.g. in velamentous insertion of cord or in placenta previa), identify the bleeding vessel and ligate.

vi. Manage the cause after investigation.

HEMOLYTIC DISEASE OF NEWBORN

Hemolytic disease of newborn is caused by incompatability between mother's blood group and that of the baby. When fetal RBC crosses and reaches in maternal circulation, they produces antibodies in the mother. If antibodies cross the placenta and enter in babies circulation, they cause hemolysis of RBC resulting anemia, jaundice and other features of hemolysis.

Two types of incompatibilities are seen:

i. Rh incompatibility

ii. ABO incompatibility

Rh HEMOLYTIC DISEASE

Rhesus factor is an antigen present in the majority of human red cells (85% in the white but very low or nil in Chinese and Japanese). This antigen was also found on red cells of rhesus monkey. Injection of red cells of rhesus monkey into rabit produce antibody (called agglutinin).

The persons whose red cells could be agglutinated with rabbit antiserum were classified as "rhesus positive" and those in which agglutination did not occur were called "rhesus negative".

Genetic Constitution

An individual caries the six main rhesus genes on two chromosomes (gene pairs), three of which are dominant C, D and H and three of their alleles (alternative forms at particular locus) the c, d and e which are recessive genes. Each chromosome contains a group of three genes. The arrangement is as follows:

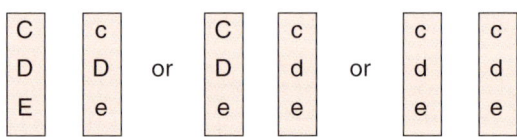

D is most powerful antigen and antibodies formed by it are also most powerful. If an

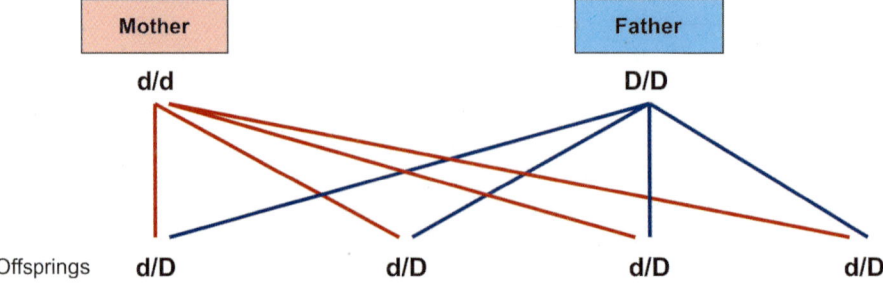

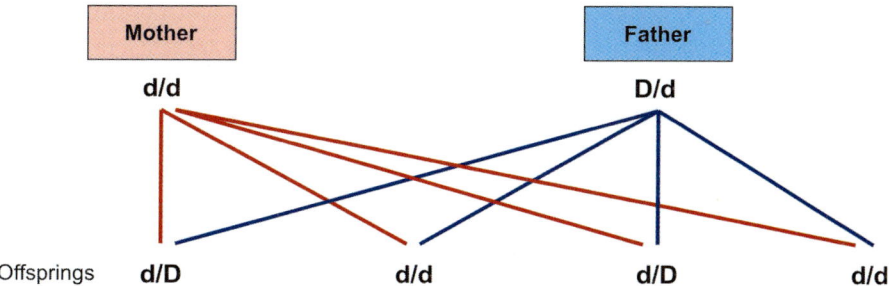

individual possessing D in either chromosome is called 'rhesus positive' when' D' locus is occupied by 'd' recessive gene in both chromosomes of the individual then it is called "Rh negative". 'd' is very weak antigen and, therefore, its antibodies are also very weak. If an individual contains D antigen in both genes (as cDe/CDE) it is called homozygous while if individual contains dominant gene D in one and recessive gene d in other chromosome (as CDE/cde) is called heterozygous.

Transmission

i. A homozygous rhesus positive man (D/D) married to rhesus negative women. D is transmitted to all of his offspring and all the babies will be affected.

ii. If father is heterozygous rhesus positive and mother is rhesus negative then 50% chances of being rhesus positive and 50% chances of rhesus negative.

Rhesus Sensitization and Immunization

Contrary to ABO group the serum of Rh positive or Rh negative individual does not possess any natural Rh antibody (agglutinin) except under following circumstances:

i. When blood transfusion of Rh positive donor is given to Rh negative individual. It will stimulate antibody formation and recipient shows severe transfusion reaction.

ii. By the presence of Rh positive fetus in Rh mother, some of the baby's Rh positive red cells cross over into maternal circulation where they act as foreign antigen. Rhesus isoimmunization occurs in two stages:

1. Sensitization
2. Isoimmunization

1. *Sensitization:* Mother is usually sensitized at the time of delivery because most of the transplacental hemorrhage occur during delivery. RBCs of Rh positive fetus evoke antibody response in maternal antibody system. So, first infant usually escapes rhesus hemolytic process.

Primary sensitization during pregnancy is unusual possibly because mother is more resistant to sensitization during pregnancy and they provide weak antigen during this time.

Sensitization also occurs at the time of abortion because transplacental hemorrhage may occur.

2. *Isoimmunization:* The sensitized maternal red cells are stimulated in second pregnancy to produce antibody against Rh antigen to destroy the antigen. The maternal Rh antibody passes through the placenta to enter the fetal circulation and causes hemolysis of Rh positive fetal cells by causing antigen antibody reaction resulting in anemia, jaundice and other features.

Sensitization of mother is cumulative so disease tends to become more and more severe with successive pregnancies.

This antibody formation is permanent and differs from antibody formation against bacterial antigen which is temporary.

Magnitude of fetomaternal bleeding: Entry of Rh positive fetal cells into maternal circulation through transplacental hemorrhage can be detected by Kleihaur-Betka technique which can identify fetal RBC by virtue of fetal hemoglobin (HbF) in contrast to adult hemoglobin (HBA). Fetal cell countmore than five or more in 50 low power fields is termed 'significant'. It shows that about 0.25 ml of fetal blood entered the mother circulation.

Clinical Features

Many Rh negative mothers do not get isoimmunized. There is a wide range of clinical manifestations. Clinical picture is characterized by increasing severity of the disease with each subsequent pregnancy. Severe disease is likely to result when there is coexisting ABO incompatibility.

Major clinical manifestations of the disease are on fetus as follows:
  i. Hemolytic anemia
  ii. Icterus gravis neonatorum (grave jaundice)
  iii. Hydrops fetalis

Hemolytic anemia: Anemia may be mild. In severe form there may be profound anemia resulting fetal death. Generalized pallor or pale lemon color of the skin may be apparent between the third and fourth days. Hemoglobin is low. Hepatosplenomegaly is noticed.

Icterus gravis neonatorum (grave jaundice)— The severe form of jaundice is rarely detected at birth since serum bilirubin from the hemolyzed red blood cells of the fetus is excreted through the placenta into maternal circulation. After birth liver of newborn is unable to detoxicate the extent of bilirubin and, therefore, jaundice develops within 24 hours of birth and rapidly increases in intensity.

The amniotic fluid and umbilical cord may be faintly or markedly stained yellow. A deeply jaundiced baby is most likely to develop kernicterus.

Hydrops fetus: This is the most serious manifestations of rhesus incompatibility. Baby at birth is pale, grossly edematous with enlarged abdomen due to fetal ascites. The infant is often preterm and may die *in utero* or shortly after birth from severe anemia and congestive cardiac failure.

Placenta is greatly enlarged, pale in color and edematous and water may ooze from it. Weight is more (normal 1/8 of baby's weight).

Radiologically fetus assumes a frog-like attitude with a big hallo around the skull.

Diagnosis

  i. *Rh typing:* Rh typing of mother and infant shows that mother is Rh negative and infant is Rh positive. Her husband's Rh typing should also be done.
  ii. *Direct Coombs' test:* Direct Coombs' test should be done on cord red blood cells. If test is positive means infant is affected with rhesus isoimmunization.
  iii. Rh antibody titre of mother is high (tested in 32–38 weeks of pregnancy in primigravida and 30th week in multipara). Rising titre is subsequent pregnancies suggest isoimmunization.
  iv. Amniotic fluid spectrophotometric scanning—amniotic fluid is taken by amniocentesis at 28–29th week of pregnancy and fluid is examined photometric method for bilirubin. It gives idea about severity of the disease and serves a guide about need of intrauterine transfusion or optimum time for termination of pregnancy.
  v. *Genotyping:* Genotyping of father is done to determine whether father is homozygous (D/D) or heterozygous (D/d).
  vi. Blood examination of baby for serum bilirubin reticulocytosis, anemia, anti-Rh agglutinins and hypoglycemia.

Prevention: Anti-D Gammaglobulin

Method of administration: If mother is Rh negative and fetus is Rh positive 200–400 micrograms of anti-D gammaglobulin are given to mother intramuscularly within 48 hours of delivery. Since abortion also involves risk of transplacental hemorrhage and so maternal sensitization. Rh negative mother should be given an intramuscular injection of Rh immunoglobulin.

Rh immunoglobulin should be given on first pregnancy so protection is offered to the next Rh positive pregnancy. When the mother is already sensitized and the serum of mother contains Rh antibody. It has no role.

If mother is Rh negative and fetus is Rh negative there is no need to treat with anti-gammaglobulin.

Purpose: The purpose of injection of anti-D immunoglobulin is to prevent Rh sensitization. Anti-D immunoglobulin blocks the D antigen on the surface of the red cells and, therefore, there is no antibody stimulation on entry into maternal circulation (Fig. 2.36).

1. Intrauterine blood transfusion (fetal intraperitoneal)

   Indications
   i. In severely affected fetus
   ii. When intrauterine fetal death is apprehended
   iii. History of stillbirths or hydrops in previous pregnancies.

   Method: Group O rhesus negative packed cells are injected into peritoneal cavity of the fetus before the 32 weeks of pregnancy. 80 ml of red cells injected at 28–30 weeks and 100 ml after this time. The packed cells enters the fetal circulation by lymphatics or through thoraric duct is an ill stood mechanism.

2. Premature termination of pregnancy is indicated at 34th week when hemolytic disease is anticipated from high titre of Rh antibodies.

3. Management of labour—uterus should be handled gently at 3rd stage of labour to prevent severe fetomaternal hemorrhage. Clamp the umbilical cord properly after birth so to avoid additional loading of fetal circulation.

Treatment

a. Exchange transfusion is done within 6 hours of birth as soon as possible preferably with Rh negative and ABO compatible blood, in event of non-availability of Rh negative blood, Rh positive blood may be given. But mother's blood should never be given because it contains antibody.

   Exchange transfusion prevents CCF and kernicterus has reduced death rate about 3% in infants.

b. Phenobarbitone for hemolytic disease reduces need for exchange transfusion.

c. Digitalization for CCF, diuretics and thoracocentesis and paracentesis for massive fluid in serous cavities and other measures.

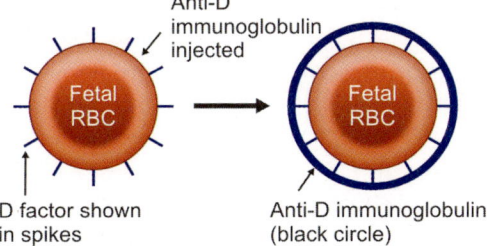

Fig. 2.36: Anti-D immunoglobulin blocks the D antigen on the surface of red cells therefore there is no antibody stimulation when it enters into the maternal circulation.

ABO HEMOLYTIC DISEASE

Contrary to Rh hemolytic disease it is generally mild. If mother's group is O and infant's group is A or B. She develops anti-A or anti-B antibodies in her blood.

Clinical manifestations include jaundice, anemia, hepatosplenomegaly. Jaundice is delayed up to 48–72 hours.

No specific treatment is needed in majority. Exchange transfusion is indicated if serum bilirubin exceeds 20 mg%.

RESPIRATORY DISTRESS IN THE NEWBORN

Respiratory difficulties are the most common cause of morbidity in newborn. It may be due to:
a. Depression of respiratory centre in the brain
b. Interference with pulmonary ventilation (include hyaline membrane disease)
c. Congestive cardiac failure.

RESPIRATORY DISTRESS

Respiratory distress in the newborn is common problem accounts for significant morbidity and mortality.

Definition: Breathing difficulty or respiratory distress is characterized by any one of the following.
• Respiratory rate >60 breaths per minutes.
• Severe chest indrawing
• Grunting
• Apnea (not breathing)
• Gasping.

Causes of Respiratory Distress in Newborn

Respiratory system: Prenatal or postnatal aspiration, intrauterine pneumonia, postnatal pneumonia, hyaline membrane disease, massive pulmonary hemorrhage, pneumothorax, transient tachypnea, Wilson milky syndrome, pleural effusion, congenital malformation of upper respiratory passages. Esophageal atresia with tracheoesophageal fistula; diaphragmatic hernia, pulmonary agenesis, lobar emphysema, pulmonary lymphangiectesis, cysts and tumors.

Cardiovascular system: Cardiac failure, cardiomyopathies, myocarditis, arrhythmias.

Central nervous system: Central nervous system, trauma, asphyxia, diaphragmatic paralysis, paralysis of intercostal muscles.

Hematological causes: Anemia, polycythemia.

Metabolic disorder: Variable.

Metabolic causes: Hypoglycemia, hypothermia, metabolic acidosis, inborn error of metabolism.

Abdominal causes: Omphalocele, gastroschisis, ascites, diaphragmatic hernia, drugs that depress CNS.

Common causes: Aspiration, infection, hyaline membrane disease, massive pulmonary hemorrhage, pneumothorax and congenital malformations.

Common Causes

Preterm baby
• Respiratory distress syndrome (RDS/HMD)
• Congenital pneumonia
• Miscellaneous—hypothermia, hypoglycemia.

Term baby
• Transient tachypnea of newborn (TTNB)
• Meconium aspiration
• Pneumonia
• Asphyxia

Surgical causes
• Diaphragmatic hernia
• Tracheoesophageal fistula
• B/C choanal atresia

Other causes
Cardiac—congenital heart disease
Metabolic—acidosis, inborn error of metabolism.

RESPIRATORY DISTRESS SYNDROME (RDS)
(HYALINE MEMBRANE DISEASE: HMD)

The term describes a characteristic neonatal respiratory distress which is predominantly seen in small preterm at birth but which may also be observed in babies of diabetic mother, babies delivered by cesarean section or in babies where mother suffered from anoxia or severe fall of blood pressure.

Idiopathic respiratory distress syndrome or hyaline membrane disease (HMD) is one of the causes of ventilatory disturbance.

Incidence: 8 per 1000 live births.

Etiopathogenesis: These factors contribute to the pathogenesis of hyaline membrane disease.

i. The deficiency of surfactant in the pulmonary alveoli.

ii. The alveoli are small, inflate with difficulty and do not remain air filled between inspiration.

iii. The chest case is weak and compliant. Surfactant (saturated lecithins) reduces the surface tension at alveoli thus preventing their collapse at the end of expiration when the alveoli are reduced. It is produced by type II alveolar lining cells in lungs. Synthesis of surfactant start at 20 weeks fetal life. Over 90% of surfactant is produced after 35 weeks of gestation.

The surfactant (surface active material) is deficient in preterm babies born before 37 weeks of gestation thus do not prevent alveoli to collapse. So, these alveoli are not properly ventilated resulting in reduced oxygenation of blood.

The hypoxemia causes pulmonary vasoconstriction resulting shunting of blood from pulmonary to system side across the patent ductus arteriosus. Thus, further reduces the pulmonary blood flow.

Reduced blood flow is lungs causes epithelial necrosis, which results effusion of proteinacious fluid containing cellular debris and components of infants serum into alveoli and terminal bronchioles. This material lining the alveoli forms a membrane which again interfere with ventilation. Due to peculiar staining property of the membrane give the name hyaline membrane disease.

If newborn survives for 3–4 days, the surfactant production in the alveoli becomes normal and the pulmonary function starts improving rapidly.

Maternal diabetes mellitus delays maturation of fetal lungs. Infants delivered by emergency cesarean section also predispose to develop hyaline membrane disease due to greater chances of perinatal hypoxia.

Damage to alveolar cells due to birth asphyxia, acidosis, hypothermia, antepartum hemorrhage and shock may suppress surfactant synthesis.

The alveolar diameter and ducts and respiratory bronchioles are significantly smaller in the preterm than term so requires greater force to inflate them and a relatively larger transpulmonary pressure at the end of expiration to keep them away from deflating.

Thus, in preterm babies small chest units and compliant and weak chest wall lead to atelectasis, rapid rate of respiration, increased airway resistance.

Clinical Features

The signs of hyaline membrane disease usually appear within minutes of birth. Sometimes symptoms may not be recognized for several hours. The babies are hypotonic and inactive and develop rapid breathing with progressively increasing respiratory distress. The breathing is entirely diaphragmatic type. The lower sternum may become permanently in drawn with hyperventilated upper chest. In very ill babies respiration may be depressed.

Characteristically tachypnea, grunting respiration, flaring of alae nasae, retraction of ribs and sternum, intercostal and subcostal retractions and duskiness are usual presentations.

Cyanosis increases gradually often unresponsive to oxygen and caused by pulmonary vasoconstriction reduces pulmonary blood flow and right to left-shunting of unoxygenated blood continues.

Extremities become pale and edematous due to poor peripheral circulation. Visceral circulation also becomes poor resulting oliguria and anuria. Abdomen becomes distended with diminished bowel sounds. On auscultation breath sounds are reduced, fine rales are heard.

Investigations

A. During antenatal period

i. *Lecithin sphingomyelin ratio in amniotic fluid:* A ratio more than two indicates full maturation and 1.5 to 1.99 borderline maturation. Ratio 1–1.44 develop mild form of HMD and ratio less than 1 is always associated with severe RDS.

ii. *Bubble stability test:* The amniotic fluid shaken within alcohol. Production of stable bubbles suggest good maturation of surfactant.

B. During postnatal period

i. *Gastric aspirate shake test:* Add 1 ml of absolute alcohol in 0.5 ml of gastric aspirate. Shake vigorously for 15 seconds. If the bubbles cover less than one-third of liquid surface there is increased chances of respiratory distress.

ii. *X-ray chest:* X-ray chest shows ground glass opacity of both lungs and air bronchogram effect.

Treatment

Oxygen therapy

Saturation of oxygen should be directed with pulse oximeter. Saturation below 90% should be treated with oxygen supplementation. Oxygen is a drug and should only be used if the baby has hypoxia as it is harmful to eyes, brain and lungs.

Administration of oxygen—oxygen may be administered with the help of:

1. Nasal prongs—appropriate size prongs which fit the neonate well should be used. Adjust flow of oxygen (0.5–2.0 L/min) to achieve target saturation.

2. Head box—place a head box over baby's head so that baby's head stays within the head box, even when baby moves (Fig. 2.37).

Adjust flow of oxygen (3–5 L/min). It achieves desired oxygen saturation.

Continuous positive airway pressure (CPAP)

It is a technique for maintaining end expiratory airway pressure greater than atmospheric pressure.

CPAP in non-invasive modality of support where a continuous distending pressure (5–7 cm of water) applied at nostril level to keep alveoli open in spontaneously breathing neonate.

CPAP may be applied nasal prongs or nasopharyngeal tube.

Mechanical Ventilation

May be indicated if hypercapnea or acidosis develops.

Exogenous surfactant

Since exogenous surfactant deficiency is the cause of RDS exogenous surfactant is administered through intratracheal route.

It is given to treat moderate and severe RDS. It is also given all neonates less 28 weeks of gestation prophylactically (even RSD present or not)

It deceases duration and level of ventilation support.

Ensure baby is intubated, give surfactant and extubated to CPAP.

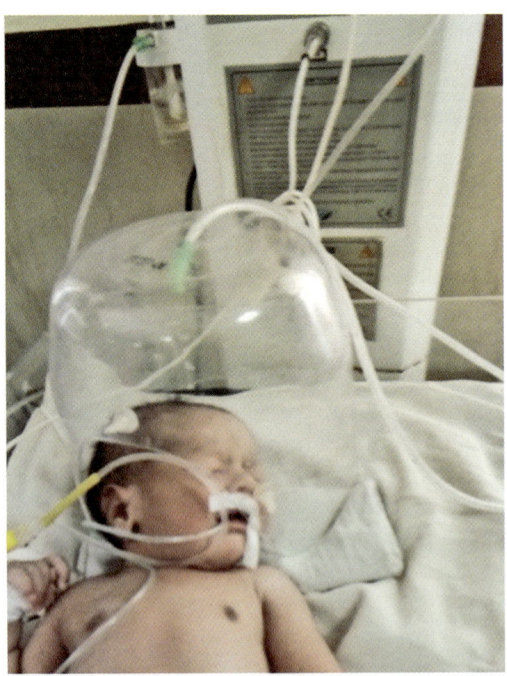

Fig. 2.37: Oxygen head box.

Prevention: Steroids should be administered intramuscularly to all mother in the preterm labor (<35 weeks) during antenatal period to prevent RDS.

Dexamethasone 6 mg two times for 2 days or betamethasone 12 mg once daily for 2 days.

Complications

Acute complications: Pneumothorax, emphysema, intraventricular hemorrhage, sepsis, and right to left shunt across a patent PDA.

Chronic complications
1. Bronchopulmonary dysplasia
2. Retinopathy of prematurity

Supportive
1. Maintain normal body temperature.
2. Expressed breast milk by gavage feeding may be given in mild to moderate RDS.
3. Give IV fluids if baby does not accept breastfeed or has severe respiratory distress.
4. Maintain blood glucose if low, treat hypoglycemia.
5. If baby has apnea stimulate by rubbing the back or flicking the sole provide positive pressure ventilation with bag and mask.
6. Mild breathing distress—oxygen is only needed.
7. Monitor the baby's response to oxygen.
8. Antibiotics. Take blood sample for sepsis screen. Start antibiotics IV ampicillin and gentamicin, if sepsis screen in negative stop antibiotics after 48 hr. If sepsis screen is positive but culture is negative, baby shows clinical improvement gives antibiotics for 5–7 days.
   If culture is positive for gram-positive cocci give antibiotics for 7–10 days and for gram-negative for 10–14 days.
9. After improvement give breast milk by orogastric tube then allow breastfeeding or by expressed mother milk using cup and spoon or paladay.
a. **Antibiotics:** Antibiotics are given only in presence of infections.

b. **Correction of acidosis:** Intravenous fluid especially 1.2% sodium bicarbonate in 5–10% dextrose in water is given to treat acidosis.

c. **Feeding:** Nasogastric feeding is employed. Avoid over feeding. In very ill babies glucose, bicarbonate, fluid and electrolytes can be administered through catheter inserted in umbilical cord.

d. **Nursing:** Proper nursing to maintain proper temperature and respiration.

Prognosis: Prognosis is bad. If child survives 2–5 days, he may suffer from neurological, pulmonary and ophthalmic sequelae.

Prevention: One or two doses of 6 mg of betamethasone acetate is given to pregnant mother intramuscularly whose lecithin in amniotic fluid shows lung immaturity and who is likely to deliver with in 24–72 hours or whose labour is delayed 24–72 hours or more.

MECONIUM ASPIRATION SYNDROME (MAS)

Meconium is first stools consist of material in the fetal gut water, mucopolysaccharides, desquamated skin and gastrointestinal mucosal epithelium, vernix, bile salts and amniotic fluid.

Definition: MAS is an acute respiratory disorder caused by aspiration of meconium into the airways of the fetus or neonate.

Pathophysiology: Meconium is often passed as a result of distress hypoxemia in the fetus at term. Meconium staining of amniotic fluid occurs in 10–14% of pregnancies.

Aspirated meconium can block the large and small airways *in utero.*

It causes atelectasis and emphysema, fetus becomes hypoxic and develops gasping or deep respiration movements or may occur at time of birth. It also induces chemical pneumonitis.

Clinical Features

Symptoms of respiratory distress develops within 6 hours of birth and develop 24–48 hours. Severe cases develop respiratory failure, sign of hypoxemia and cyanosis.

Evaluation

X-ray chest—bilateral hetergenous opacities, diffuse patchy area of atalectesis and parenchymal infiltrates alternating with hyper inflation pneumothorax, pneumatocele may occur.

Management

1. Good supportive care includes prevention of hypothermia, hypoglycemia, maintenance of calcium level, etc.
2. Oxygenation and mechanical ventilation.
3. Prevention is of paramount importance, suctioning of the trachea via endotracheal tube just after birth is necessary.

Complications

PPHN, bacterial pneumonia, long-term reactive airway disease.

HYPOGLYCEMIA

Hypoglycemia is said to be present when glucose falls under 30 mg% in term and 20 mg% in preterm babies.

Clinical symptoms are convulsions, tremors, cyanosis and apneic spells. Treatment consists of administration of 10% solution of glucose by intravenous route. Steroids are given for short period.

NEONATAL TETANY

Newborn on cow's milk formula suffers from tetany. It manifests as convulsion, jitteriness, laryngeal spasm, tremors, muscular twitching and carpopedal spasm. The baby remains symptomless between attacks. On investigation serum calcium is reduced almost always below 8%. Serum phosphate is high. Treatment is administration of 5–10 ml of 10% calcium gluconate by intravenous route followed by oral administration of calcium for maintenance.

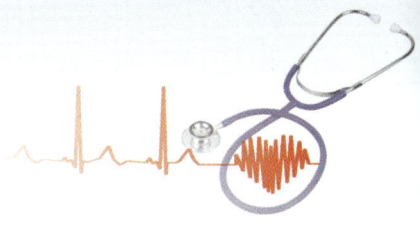

Growth and Development

3

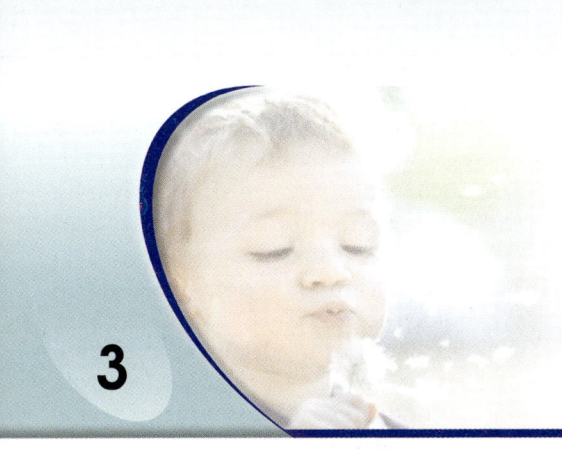

Growth and development are essential features of life of a child and both the terms are interrelated.

Growth

Growth is a measure of physical maturation signifies an increase in mass of tissue. This can be measured in term of centimeters and kilograms.

Development

It is a measure of functional or physiological maturation. It denotes accomplishment of mental emotional and social adaptation abilities.

Contrary to adult growth is an essential feature of life of a child.

Human newborn has the slowest rate of growth and development among mammals.

Rules of Development

1. The development is a continuous process from conception to maturity, and
2. Proceeds in a cephalocaudal direction. Development depends upon the maturation or myelination of nervous system. When myelination is complete the skill is rapidly learnt by individual as soon as opportunity is given.
3. The sequence of development is same in all children but the rate of development varies from child to child.

4. Certain primitive reflexes have to be lost before relevant milestones are attained.
5. During the process of development generalized mass activity is replaced by specific individual responses. For example, the infant expresses pleasure by massive general response of vigorous kicking of arms and legs, rapid respiration and guttural sounds during early period. While an elder child expresses pleasure with a smile only.

Girls mature faster than boys and adolescence is earliar in them by 2 years. Skeletal maturation is faster in girls than boys resulting shorter height in girls than boys.

Factors affecting growth and developement

i. **Genetic factor:** Hereditary factors usually decide physical shape and size, e.g. tall parents have tall children and so on.

ii. **Prenatal factors and maternal factors**
   1. *Maternal malnutrition*: Maternal malnutrition specially deficiency of macro- and micronutrients have adverse effect on birth weight and child development.
   2. *Exposure to drugs and toxins:* Certain drugs, e.g. antiepileptic drugs, alcohol abuse and environmental toxins affect adversely.
   3. *Maternal disease:* Adverse factors are:
      • Hypertension, hypothyroidism, malnutrition and fetoplacental insufficiency.

- Acquired infections, e.g. syphilis, rubella, toxoplasmosis, etc.
- Exposure to free radicals.

Neonatal risk factors: Adverse factors are:
- IUGR
- Prematurity
- Perinatal asphyxia

Postnatal factors: Risk factors are:
- Severe calories deficiency
- Deficiency of vitamins A, B_{12}, D, E, riboflavin
- Iron deficiency
- Iodine deficiency
- Infectious diseases—diarrhea, malaria
- Environmental factor
- Acquired insult to brain—trauma, infections
- Socioeconomic
- Emotional
- Chronic illness
- Lack of stimulation—social and emotional deprivation and lack of interaction and stimulation effects adversely.
- Violence and abuse—domestic and community effects adversely
- Maternal depression effects negatively.

Protective factors
- *Breastfeeding*: Breastfeeding has promotive effects on development.
- *Maternal education*: Education of mother is a protective factors and reduce mortality and promote development.

iii. **Nutritional:** Dietary deficiency in protein and calories results in retarded growth, while overnutrition causes obesity. Undernutrition affects weight than length.

iv. **Environmental:** Physical surrounding such as lack of sunshine and poor hygiene effects growth. Emotional factors, e.g. at home, school may affect growth.

Adverse condition during prenatal and postnatal period, e.g. mother illness affects adversely child growth.

v. **Socioeconomic:** Poverty affects adversly in the development of growth and development.

vi. **Emotional:** Growth is better in child in which affection and love is given. Anxiety, lack of support, love, emotional influences body by neurochemical regulation of growth hormone.

vii. **Chronic illness:** Chronic diseases affect the body; chronic renal, cardiac or metabolic disorders result retardation in growth. While high level of growth hormone results in gigantism.

viii. **Growth potential:** If smaller is child in term of gestation. He will be smaller in further years. If longer at birth longer will be in subsequent years.

ix. **Prenatal or intrauterine growth:** Intra-uterine growth retardation, endometritis, maternal infection, rubella, diabetes affect the fetus and newborn.

x. **Postnatal growth pattern:** Growth pattern of all body tissue is not similar in any age; following pattern which it is expressed by various curves.

a. *General type:* Body as a whole, external dimensions of various organs of body including bone and muscles. There are two periods of rapid general growth—infancy and adolescence.

b. *Genital type:* It includes growth of testes, ovary, epididymis, uterine tube, prostate, prostatic urethra, seminal vesicles.

c. Genital growth is most rapid during adolescence. Before it, almost stationary.

d. *Neural type* (brain and its parts, optic apparatus, spinal cord). It continues rapidly during the first few years of life and then approaches the adult size.

e. *Lymphoid type:* Thymus, lymph glands, intestinal lymphoid masses. Lymphoid

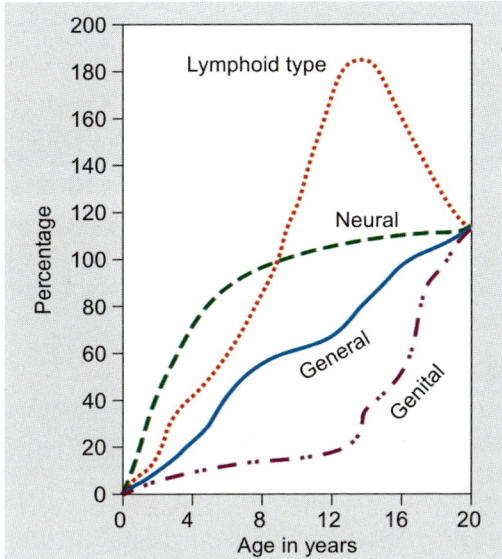

Fig. 3.1: Pattern of growth.

growth is rapid in infancy and highly accelerated during period of child-hood (Fig. 3.1).

Laws of Growth

a. Growth and development of children is a continuous process and orderly.
b. Every individual has its own growth pattern but general pattern of growth is predictable.
c. Different tissue of the body grow at the different rates, e.g. brain, lymphoid, etc.

Assessment of Growth

Physical growth is assessed by:
  i. *Body measurement:* Weight, length, head circumference.
  ii. Velocity of physical growth.

Weight

Weight of child is taken without clothes; best in lever type of scale. Spring type of scale is less accurate (Table 3.2).

At birth 7 lbs, at 6 months twice of birth weight, at 12 months thrice of birth weight, 2 years four times of birth weight (Table 3.4).

Height (Length)

Length is recorded in case of babies up to 2 years in infantometer or stadiometer and height by standing (Table 3.3).

If height is below 3rd percentile (dwarfism) and if height is above 97th percentile (gigantism).

Head Circumference

Head circumference which also reflects growth of brain, is measured by cross tape technique (Table 3.5).

Chest Circumference

It is measured by tape at the level of nipple midway between inspiration and expiration, when child is in recumbent position.

At birth head is larger than chest circumference; after 1 year chest becomes larger than head.

Velocity of Growth

Comparison of child's height and weight with standard norms helps in assessing present situation of growth whether normal or not.

Weight: Mostly newborn babies lose weight during first few days. Term babies lose up to 5% of birth weight and regain by the age of 7 days. Malnourished small-for-dates babies when fed adequately do not lose any weight. Preterm babies may lose 10 to 15 percent of birth weight and regain up to second week.

During first year of life average daily weight gain is 30 gm is first quarter, 20 gm in second quarter and 10 gm in third quarter.

At birth weight (7 lbs) becomes double at 6 months, triple at 1 year and four times at 2 years age.

During period of 4 to 12 years average yearly weight gain is about 2 kg per year. It is less in comparison to previous period; so mostly parents are worried unnecessarily about the weight gain and appetite during this phase. *Height:* Height velocity during first year is 25 cm, second year 12.5 cm, third year 7.5–10 cm and subsequently 5.0–7.5 cm per year. *Head circumference:* Growth velocity of head circumference is 2 cm per month for first 3 months then 2 cm every 3 months for further months till first year of age (8 cm during first six months).

1–3 years of age head growth is 2 cm per year and subsequently it is only 1 cm per year up to the age of 5–6 year.

Head size does not increase during school age significantly.

Eruption of Teeth

Different teeth erupt at different times. Temporary or milk teeth or deciduous teeth are 20. Delayed dentition may be familiar, malnutrition or due to vit D deficiency. Permanent teeth are 32 and they erupt in different order.

Temporary Teeth

Age	Teeth eruption
At birth	Nil
6–7 months to 10 months	First central and lateral incisors
1¼ years	First molar
1¼–1¾ years	Cuspids
2–3 years	Second molar

Permanent Teeth

Age	Teeth eruption
6 years	First molar
8 years	Central and lateral incisors
9 years	Bicuspids (anterior)
10 years	Bicuspids (posterior)
11–12 years	Canines
12–1 3 years	Second molar
17–25 years	Third molar

Number of Teeth

$$\text{Temporary } \frac{edcba \mid abcde}{edcba \mid abcde} = 20$$

$$\text{Permanent } \frac{87654321 \quad 12345678}{87654321 \quad 12345678} = 32$$

Dentition is not reliable criteria for assessment of growth. Teeth may be present at birth. Non-eruption of teeth is a feature of ectodermal dysplasia.

Ossification Centers

At birth five ossification centers present—at tibia (knee lateral)—two; at tarsal bones (ankle lateral)—three

Up to the age of 6 years take X-ray of wrist. On general No. of ossification centers in wrist = Age in years +1 (e.g. at 1 year age, have 2 ossification centers and at 2 years age, have 3 ossification centres).

At the age of 6 months, two ossification centers are present at wrist.

Domains of development: For assessment of development, domains are:
1. Gross motor development
2. Fine motor skill development
3. Personal and social development and general understanding
4. Language
5. Vision and hearing

ASSESSMENT OF DEVELOPMENT

Motor Development (Gross)

It involves control of the child over his body which is observed in following positions:
a. **Ventral suspension:** Baby is lifted up from prone position. Examiner is supporting the chest or abdomen of the baby with palm of his hand. See whether head drops down or controls above the horizontal plane (Fig. 3.2).
b. **Supine position:** The infant is placed in the supine position and is gently pulled by the arms to a sitting position, observe the movement of his head and curvature of spine. Note head lag or head control (Figs 3.3 to 3.5).

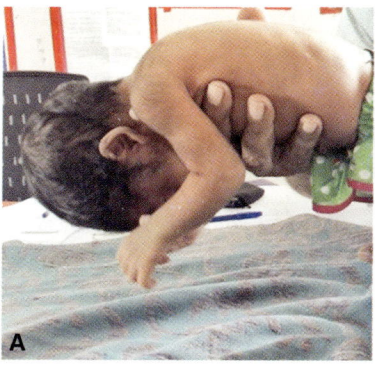 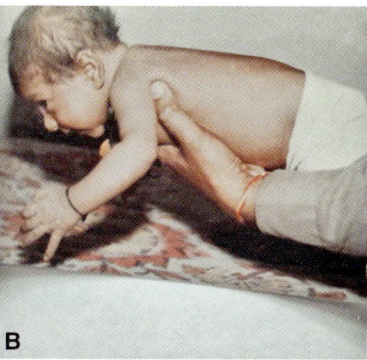 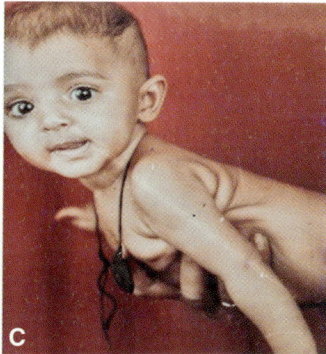

Fig. 3.2A to C: (A) Ventral suspension head hangs completely; (B) Head maintained in same position as rest of body; (C) Head maintained beyond the plane of the rest of the body.

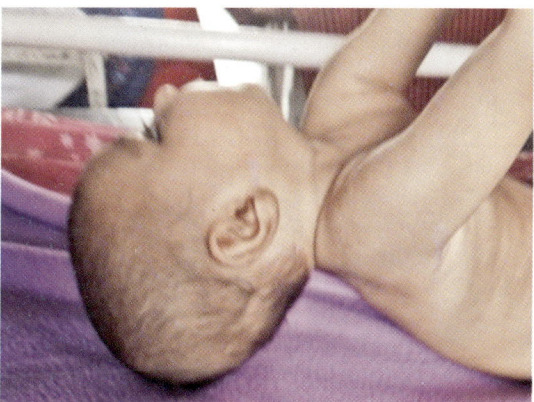

Fig. 3.3: Traction response. Complete head lag.

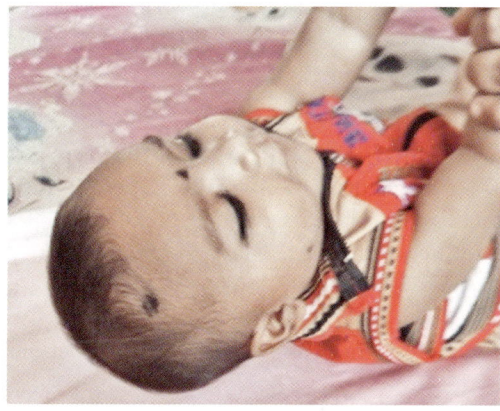

Fig. 3.5: Traction response. No head lag (12 weeks).

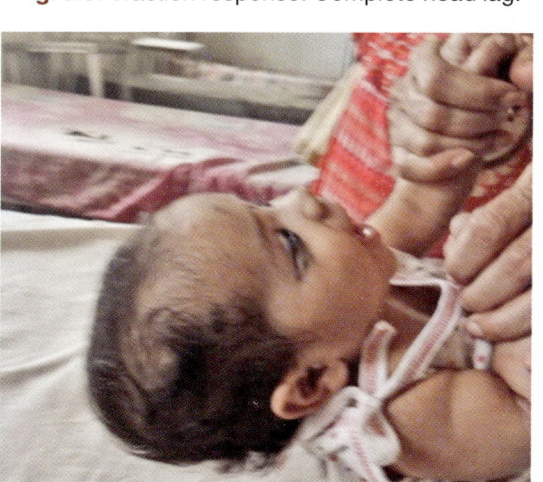

Fig. 3.4: Traction response. Head is maintained at plane of body.

c. **Prone position:** Observe the baby while baby is lying in the prone position.

   At few days after the birth head can be turned to one side, at the 1 month baby lifts the chin up momentarily in midline.

d. **Sitting position**: Look about the control on sitting position, sitting with support or without support. He can turn himself from supine to sitting position.

e. **Standing and walking:** See early stepping movements when his feet are placed on the surface of the table (9 months), standing with support or standing without support, walking (Fig. 3.9).

f. **Climbing stairs:** At the age of 2 years he can climb up to stairs.

Fine Motor and Adaptive Development

It is tested as follows.

Hand Eye Coordination

At the age of 4 months and infant try to grasp the red rattle, ring, etc. dangling infront of him. Initially he may overshoot but he get it to his mouth.

Eye Coordination

A lighter pen torch or red ring tied to a string is brought infront ot the infant and kept at 20 cm distance. Infant can regard it (4 weeks).

He can follow the object moved side to side by unsteady excursion of eyes (6 weeks).

He can follow the object with steady movement of the eyes and also converge and focus his eyes (2–3 months).

Social and Personal Development

Social smile: He smiles when the examiner tries to speak to him or smiles to him without touching him by 2 months.

Language

Hearing: At 1 month—turn his head towards sound of a bell or rattle.

Sound: By 9 months—he can produce words 'da da' 'ma ma'.

Understanding: Respond to appropriate verbal request, e.g. 'where is papa'.

True speech: Up to age of 1 year he can use three words.

Vision and Hearing

Vision: Check the vision by moving object 8–10 inches in front of eye. See fixation of eyes on care taker's face.

Hearing: Sound is produced 1 and ½ feet away the ear and see the response as turning of head one side and then downward when sound is produced below the ear.

Normal Developmental Milestones
(weeks-wise)

Neonatal period (first 4 weeks)	
Prone	Lies in flexed attitude, turn head from side to side, head hangs on ventral suspension.
Supine	Generally flexed and little stiff. Complete head lag.
Visual	May fixate face or light in line of vision.
Reflex	Grasp reflex active.
Social	Visual preference to human face.

At 4 weeks	
Prone	Head momentarily lifted up to the plane of rest of body on ventral suspension.
Supine	Head lags on pulling to sitting position (Fig. 3.3).
Visual	Watches mother when she specks, follow object up to 90°, quiten on sound of bell.
Social	Beginning to smile on response to examiner voice and smile.

8 weeks	
Prone	Head maintained in the same plane as rest of the body on ventral suspension and momentarily lifted beyond this (Fig. 3.2B).
Supine	Head lags on pulling to sitting position (Fig. 3.3).
Visual	Follows moving objects.
Social	Smile on social contact, listen to voice (Fig. 3.11).

12 weeks	
Prone	Lifts head and chest; head above plane of body on ventral suspension (Fig. 3.2C).
Supine	Hold rattle (toy) place in hands.
Sitting	Head held up when supported in a sitting position but it tends to bob forward.
Reflex	Makes defence movements.
Social	Sustained social contact, turn head toward sound.

16 weeks	
Prone	Lifts head and chest—plane efface is about 90° to bed, arms are stretched out in full extension.
Supine	Touches and grasps objects and brings them to mouth.

Sitting	Sitting with support. No head leg on pulling to sitting position.
Standing	When erect pushes with feet.
Social	Laughs loudly, may show displeasure if contact broken, exited at sight of food and seeing a toy.

28 weeks

Prone	Rolls over.
Supine	Lifts head.
Sitting	Sits with support of pelvis (Fig. 3.6).
Standing	May support most of the weight, bounces anteriorly.
Adaptive	Reaches out for and grasp object, transfer objects from hand to hand.
Language	Monosyllables like ba, da, ma are produced.
Social	Prefers mother, enjoys mirror.

40 weeks

Sitting	Sits up without support (Fig. 3.7).
Standing	Pulls to standing position.
Motor	Creeps or crawls.
Adaptive	Grasp object with thumb and forefingers.
Language	Repititive consonant sounds (mama, dada).
Social	Responds to sound of name, wave 'bye' 'bye'.

52 weeks (1 year)

Motor	Walks with one hand held, walks on holding on to furniture (Fig. 3.8).
Adaptive	Picks up pellets, releases object to other person on request.
Language	Few words besides 'mama', 'dada' sakes head for No.
Social	Plays simple ball games, makes postural adjustment to dressing.

15 months

Motor	Walks alone, crawls up stairs (Fig. 3.9).
Adaptive	Makes tower of 2 cubes.
Language	Follow simple commands, tells mother what he wants, name familiar object (ball).
Social	Feeds self, kisses parents.

18 months

Motor	Runs stiffly, sits on small chairs with one hand held.
Adaptive	Piles 3 cubes, dump pellets from bottle.
Language	10 words average, name picture.
Social	Feeds self, may complain when wet or soiled (domestic mimicry, Fig. 3.10)

24 months

Motor	Runs well, walk up and down stairs, open door, climbs furniture.
Adaptive	Tower of 6 cubes, scribbling.
Language	Puts 3 words together (subject, verb, object). Repeat what is said uses the word 'I', 'me', 'you'.

30 months

Motor	Jumps.
Adaptive	Tower of 8 cubes, make vertical and horizontal strokes.
Social	Helps put things away, pretends in play.

36 months

Motor	Rides tricle, stands momentarily on one feet.
Adaptive	Tower of 9 cubes, copies a circle, initiate a cross.
Language	Knows age and sex, repeat number.
Social	Plays simple games, helps in dressing, unbutton clothing, put on shoes, washes hands.

48 months

Motor	Throws ball overhead.
Adaptive	Copies cross and square, draw a man.
Language	Tells a story.
Social	Plays with several children, goes to toilet alone.

60 months

Motor	Skips.
Adaptive	Draw triangle form copy, name heavier for 2 weights.
Language	Name 4 colors, counts to pennies correctly.
Social	Dresses and undresses, ask question about meaning of words.

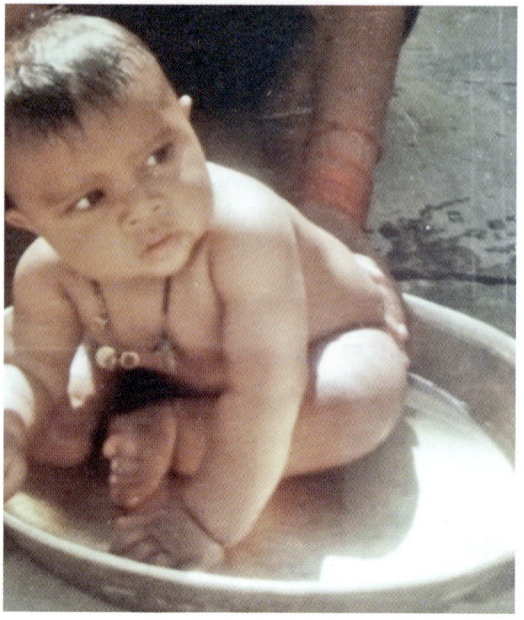

Fig. 3.6: Sitting with support of both hands.

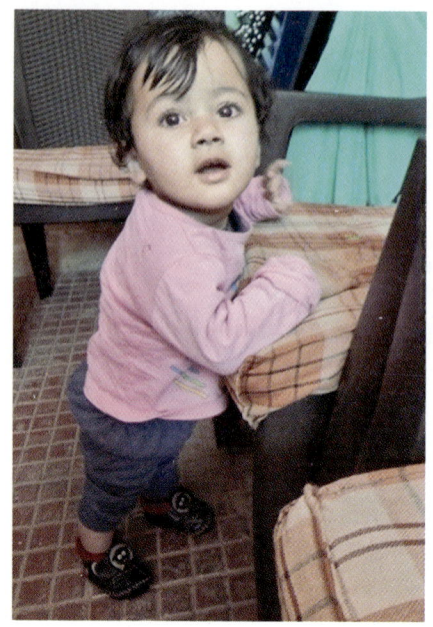

Fig. 3.8: Standing with support.

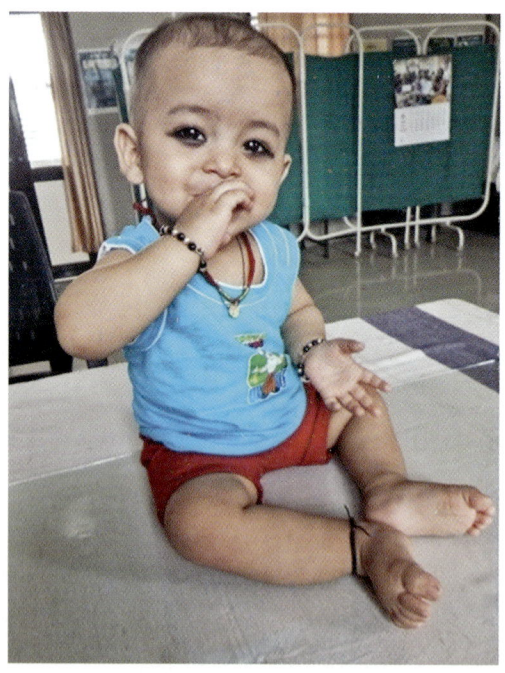

Fig. 3.7: Sitting without support.

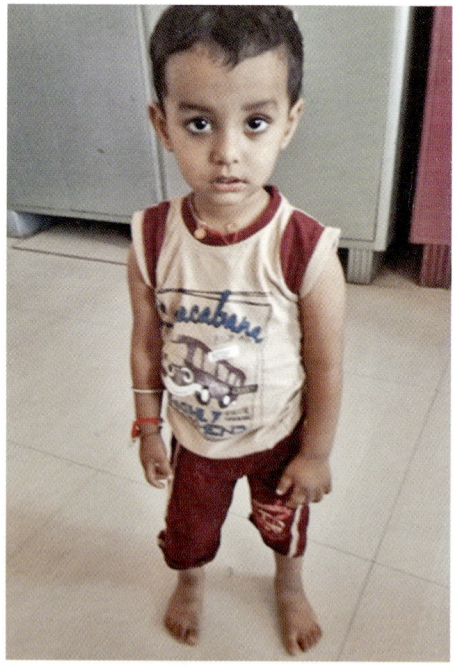

Fig. 3.9: Standing without support.

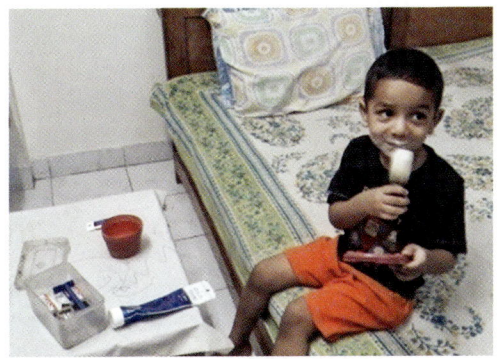

Fig. 3.10: Domestic mimicry.

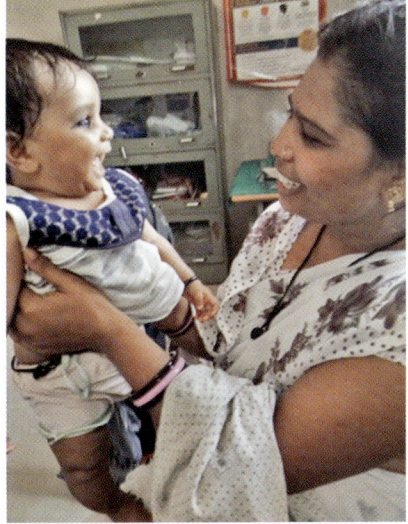

Fig. 3.11: Social smile.

There may be great variation and wide range in a child development.

General evaluation of milestones is as follows

Social smile (4–6 weeks), holds rattle (12 weeks), turn his head (12 weeks), first able to go for rattle (20 weeks), begins to roll from his front to his back (24 weeks), from back to his front (28 weeks). Begins to take an object one hand to another (26 weeks) sits with support (28 weeks), sits without support (32 weeks), stands holding furniture (36 weeks), crawl on abdomen (40 weeks), walk holding furniture (48 weeks), walk with one-hand held (52 weeks), walk without help (13 months), creeps upstairs (15–18 months), joins two or three words in sentence (21–24 months), takes some clothes off (24 months), dresses self (3–4 years).

Developmental Milestones

Infant and children change as per age, some infants and children reach milestone early another later. Reaching milestones early or later generally do not indicate whether an infant of children will be advanced or delayed later in life.

Developmental milestones

Milestones during newborn to 1 month.

Physical
- Infants keep their hand clenched in fists most of the time.
- Develop basic reflexes sucking, swallowing, grasping, blinking and starling.
- Eyes are not coordinated and appear as cross.
- Cannot organize their hands and eyes to work together.

Congnitive
- Watch an object about 12–15 inches away specially if it is moving slowly from one side of their field of vision to the other.
- Investigate their own hands and fingers.
- Prefer their own mother's voice.
- Distinguish smells and taste, prefer sweet tasting liquids and will recoil from unpleasant smells.

Language
- Communicate mostly by crying or some-times by making other noises.
- Prefer certain sounds, for examples, they may settle or become still where they hear familiar voices.
- Turn in the direction of familiar voice.

Social and emotional development
- Sleep an average 17 and 19 hours a day as a series of short sleeping periods
- Enjoy being held and rocked.

2 months to less than 4 months

Gross motor	Moves both arms, and both legs, freely and equally when awake.
Raises head	Occasionally
Fine motor	Keeps his hand open and relaxed
Hearing	Responds sound
Speech	Vocalizes by cooking specially after feeding
Vision	eye contact

Cognition and socialization: Social smile

4 months to less than 6 months

Gross motor	Holds head straight while sitting or when head on shoulder.
Fine motor	Reaches and tries to grasps an object grasp of the object is in the ulnar side of palm.
Hearing	When spoken to responds by looking directly at speaker's face
Speech	Lough aloud
Vision	Follows an object

Cognition and stabilization: Sucks on hands.

6 months to less than 9 months

- *Gross motor*: Roll over or turn over in either direction
- *Fine motor:* Grasps a small object by using his whole hand
- *Hearing:* Locate source of sound
- *Speech*: Child utters consonant sounds like 'P', 'b', 'm'
- *Vision*: Child watches TV without lifting his/her head
- *Cognition and socialization*
- Child stretches his arms to be picked up by the parents, child looks for a spoon or toy that has dropped.

9 months to less than 12 months

Gross motor: Can sit without support. Transfer object from hand to hand.

Hearing: Respond to his/her name.

Speech: Babbling example, 'ba', 'da', 'do', 'ma', 'mo'.

Vision: Avoid bumping into objects.

Congition and socialization: Child enjoys playing hide and seek (peek-a-boo).

12 months to less than 15 months

Gross motor: Reciprocal crawling on hands and knees.

Fine motor: Child picks up small objects using thumb and index finger.

Hearing: Child stops activity in response to 'No'.

Speech: Child says one meaningful word clearly like 'mama', 'dada'.

15 months to less than 18 months

Gross motor: Child walks alone.

Fine motor: Child put small thing into a container, points to object.

Hearing: Follow simple one step direction 'sit down', give me the ball'.

Speech: Child says at least two words other than mama or *dada like—dog, cat.*

Cognition and socialization: Child manipulates or explores boy with his fingers like poking, pulling the toy.

Imitate action like 'bye-bye', 'clap', 'kiss'.

- Cries when a stranger picks him up.
- Child searches for completely hidden objects.

Developmental Assessment

Assessment of development is essential to diagnose developmental delay, which is present in about 10% of child. Speech impairment, hyperactivity and emotional disturbances are often not detected by parent unit the age of 3–4 years. Learning disabilities are detected at school going age. Early identification and proper learning help in better outcome. Various types of developmental screening tests have been suggested.

Developmental Screening

Assessment of development of child requires repeated observation at periodic intervals. It helps in making only intervention and to identify disability.

Common screening tests used in India are described below.

Revised Denver development screening test (DDST) or Denver

It assesses child development in four domains:
A. Gross motor
B. Fine motor adaptive
C. Language
D. Personal social behavior

These are presented as age norms in the form of growth curves.

Phatak Baroda screening test: It is developed by Dr Pramila Phatak, used up to 30 months of age, best system, diagnostic tools are commercially available.

Trivendrum development screening chart: Used to assess child development up to 2 years of age. Simple test, can be done by health worker in 5 min.

Clinical adaptive test and clinical linguistic and auditory milestone scale (AT/clams): It is used in 0–36 months of age useful to identify mental retardation.

Good enough—Harris drawing test: It is done with the help of pencil or pen, child in asked to draw a man. Performance is compared with norms. It is useful to determine child's intelligence roughly.

SHORT STATURE

Definition: Short stature is defined as height or length is below the 3rd percentile or less than –2SD from the mean, he or she is considered to be short stature (Fig. 3.12).

General Concepts

Growth velocity: Children grow 2 inch per year (5 cm per year) between 3 years of age and puberty. Children who have a growth velocity less than 5 cm per year is considered to have pathological growth disorder.

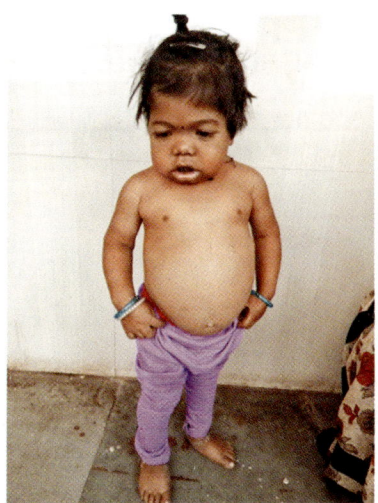

Fig. 3.12: 13-year-old dwarf.

If child height is third percentile (less than –3SD) below the mean but growth velocity is normal, he or she is considered normal variant short stature.

Midparental height (MPH): Take height of mother and father and estimate targeted midparental height (MPH) as follows.

$$\text{Male (MPH)} = \frac{\text{Father's height} + (\text{mother's height} + 5 \text{ inches})}{2}$$

For example

$$\begin{aligned}
\text{Boy} &= \frac{69 + 60 + 5}{2} = \frac{129 + 5}{2} \\
&= \frac{134}{2} = 67 \text{ inches} \\
&= 67 = 5 \text{ feet 7 inches} \\
&\pm 4 \text{ inches or } \pm 2\text{SD}
\end{aligned}$$

$$\text{Female (MPH)} = \frac{\text{Father's height} - 5 \text{ inches} + \text{mother's height}}{2}$$

For example

$$\begin{aligned}
\text{Girls} &= \frac{(69 - 5) + 60}{2} = \frac{64 + 60}{2} = \frac{124}{2} \\
&= 62 = 5 \text{ feet 2 inch} \\
&\pm 4 \text{ inches or } \pm 2\text{SD}
\end{aligned}$$

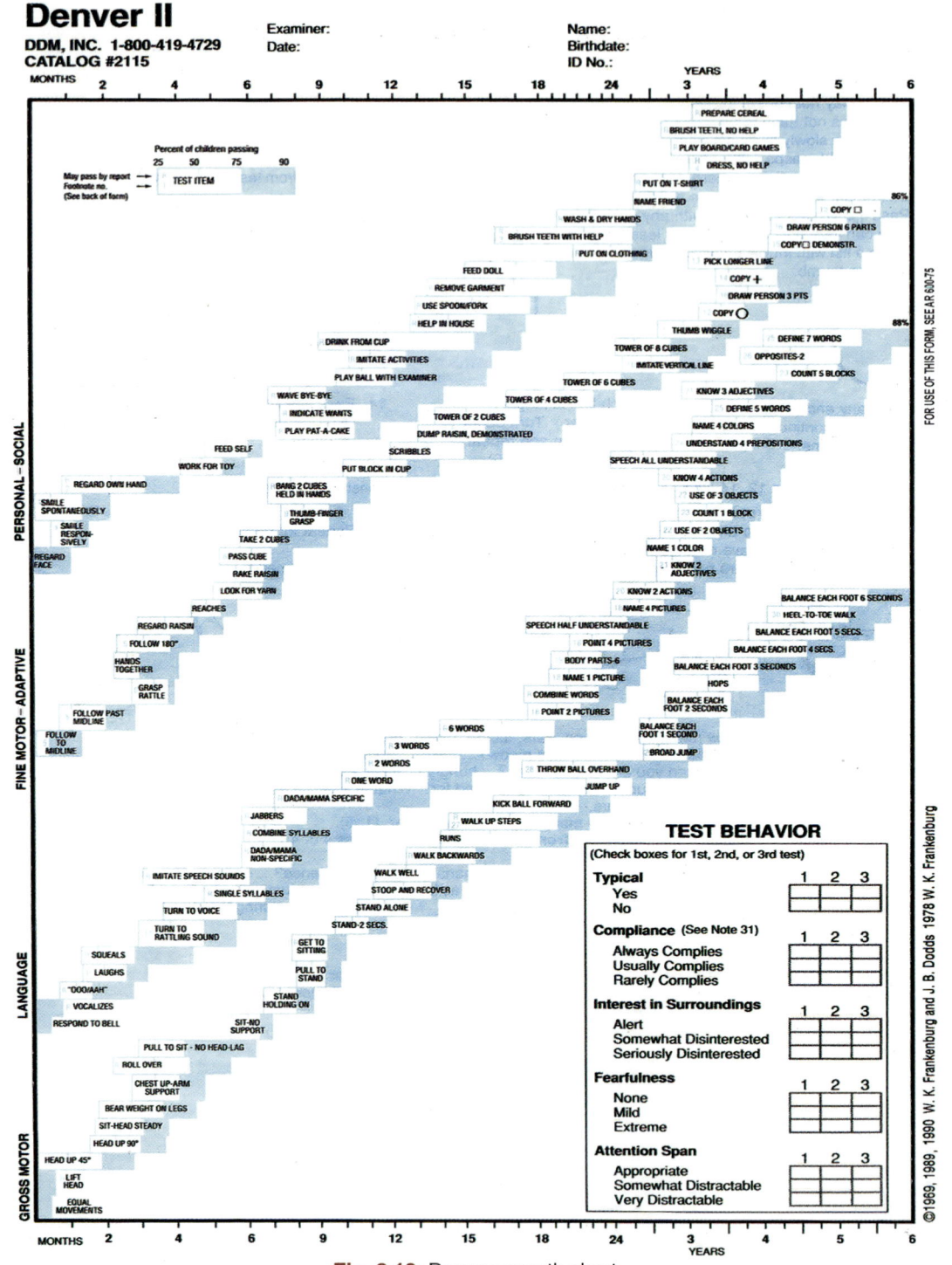

Fig. 3.13: Denver growth chart.

- So, most children when they have completed main growth are within ± 2SD, or 4 inches of their MPH. It is a normal variant short stature.
- If there is difference in growth percentile and targeted MPH. It is pathological.

PROPORTIONATE SHORT STATURE

CATEGORIZATION

A. Normal variant—short stature (page 94)
1. Familial short stature
2. Constitutional growth delay
B. Pathological
1. Proportionate—U/L ratio normal
2. Disproportionate—U/L ratio abnormal

Prenatal causes	Postnatal causes
1. Intrauterine growth retardation	1. Malnutrition (nutritional)
2. Intrauterine infection	2. Cyanotic heart disease
3. Genetic and chromosomal (renal, cardiopulmonary, malabsorption, chronic, infection, anemia)	3. Chronic visceral disease
4. Endocrine disease	
5. Psychosocial (emotional deprivation)	

A. Pathological Short Stature

It is defined as children whose height is below –3SD of the mean with abnormal growth velocity, growth velocity less than 2 inches or 5 cm per feet. It may be of two types.

1. Proportionate

Short stature with a normal upper and lower segment ratio (U/L). Onset may be prenatal or postnatal of such cases.

a. Prenatal onset
   i. Environmental exposures—*in utero* exposure to tobacco or alcohol.
   ii. Chromosomal disorders (e.g. Down syndrome)
   iii. Genetic disorders (e.g. Russel silver syndrome)
   iv. Viral infection in early pregnancy (rubella, cytomegalovirus)
   vi. IUGR

b. Postnatal onset
   i. Malnutrition
   ii. Social–emotional deprivation, neglect
   iii. Chronic systemic disease of body.

   GIT, cardiac disease, renal disease, lung disease, endocrinopathies (hypothyroidism, growth hormone deficiency, drugs—cortisone long-term use).

1. GIT diseases—inflammatory bowel disease, malabsorption syndromes, lactose intolerance, cystic fibrosis, coeliac disease, cow milk allergy.
2. Cardiac diseases—cyanotic congenital heart disease.
3. Renal deseases—renal failure, renal tuberculosis, pyelonephritis.
4. Chronic lung deseases—cystic fibrosis, asthma, empyema.
5. Endocrinopathies:
   - Hypothyroidism
   - Growth hormone deficiency
   - Cortisol excess
6. Chronic infections—tuberculosis, malaria, leishmaniasis, syphilis, causes of failure to thrive.

2. Disproportionate Short Stature

With short limbs
1. Achondroplegia
2. Hypochondroplegia
3. Chondrodysplasia punctata
4. Chondroectodermal dysplasia
5. Diastrophic dysplasia

6. Metaphysial chondrodysplasia
7. Deformities due to rickets and osteogenesis imperfecta

With short trunk

1. Spondyloepiphyseal dysplasia
2. Mucopolysaccharidosis
3. Mucolepidosis
   • Caries spine
   • Hemivertebrae

B. Normal Variant Short Stature

These are of two types:

a. *Familial (or genetic) short stature*—short stature with a short MPH. Normal growth velocity. Normal bone age, normal onset of puberty or earlier.

b. *Constitutional growth delay short stature*—height is –2SD below the mean with history of delayed puberty in either or both parents, delayed bone age and late onset of puberty and a minimum growth of 5 cm per year. Human gonadotropins and growth hormones after puberty are within normal range.

It requires no treatment. Parents should be reassured.

Evaluation of a Case of Short Stature

History

1. Perinatal history—assess intrauterine growth retardation (IUGR) or prematurity, hypoglycemia, prolonged jaundice.

   Cryptorchidism, micropallus is suggestive of hypopituitarism.
2. Chronic disease—assess such as renal failure, CNS disease, severe respiratory disease, sickle cell anemia, GIT disease.
3. Drugs—long-term use of steroids, stimulants.
4. Family history of parenteral growth and pubertal history.
5. Social history—related to emotional deprivation.

6. History of systemic disease—as per cause.
7. Dental history—delayed teeth eruption suggest delayed bone growth.

Physical Examination

1. Length—measure accurately
2. Measure upper segment to lower segment ratio (U/L).
   a. Lower segment : Pubic symphysis to the heel
   b. Upper segment : Total height minus lower segment
      • U/L   : Normal value
        At birth   : 1.7
        3 years of age : 1.3
        >7 years of age : 1.0
      • Abnormal U/L ratio suggest disproportionate short stature
3. *Systemic and general examination*: Any sign related to disease, e.g. thyroid, genetic disease, etc.

Investigations

I. Laboratory investigation

A. 1. Complete blood count (CBC)
   2. Erythrocyte sedimentation rate (ESR)
   3. T_3, T_4, TSH estimation
   4. Serum electrolyte calcium and phosphorus
   5. Serum creatinine and bicarbonate

B. Insulin growth factor 1 (IGF-1)—for growth hormone

C. Chromosome analysis in girls to evaluate Turner syndrome.

II. Radiographic studies

a. Bone age determination—AP film of left hand and wrist to assess epiphysis and compare with age.
b. CT scan
c. AP and lateral skull radiograph—to assess pituitary gland.

ENDOCRINE DISORDERS RESULTING SHORT STATURE

1. *Hypothyroidism:* Common cause of short stature. Patient blood investigation shows increased TSH, low T_4 and positive anti-thyroid peroxidase antibodies.
2. *Growth hormone deficiency:* Clinical features—prolonged neonatal jaundice, cherubic facies, obesity, microphallus, cryptorchidism and midline defect (e.g. cleft palate). Growth velocity is low (<5 cm per year). Diagnosis is established by estimation of growth hormone and during sleep or after provocative test. It is less than 10 ng/ml.
   a. Imaging studies
      1. Delayed bone age
      2. MRI—CNS lesion
   b. Lab studies
      1. Low IGF-1 levels
      2. Growth hormone stimulation testing shows poor response.
      Management
      Daily injection of growth hormone until a bone age—above 13–14 years of age in girls, 15–16 years of age in boys is achieved.
3. Hypercortisolism—history of prolonged use of cortisone with clinical features poor growth, increasing weight gain, purpuric marks on skin, and delayed bone age. Moon facies.
4. Cushing syndrome—excessive secretion of corticosteroids from adrenals.
5. Turner syndrome—female patient with poor growth velocity, lack of puberty, chromosome either missed or its part is missed.
6. Diabetes mellitus—juvenile diabetes mellitus is associated with significant growth retardation.

BODY MASS INDEX (BMI)

It is defined as children's weight in kilograms divided by square of his or her height in metres.

$$BMI = \frac{\text{Weight in kilogram}}{(\text{Height in metres})^2} = \frac{kg}{m^2}$$

Such as weight in 70 kg, height in 1.75 meters

$$BMI = \frac{70}{(1.75)^2} = 22.9$$

Contrary to adult BMI of children changes according to age and sex. It is called BMI for particular age and sex (Table 3.1).

Importance of BMI for Age

1. As per survey report many children of school going age are undernourished. Children 5–10 years, age group 60% of them who have BMI more than 95% suffers from hypertension, high cholesterol or other problems.
2. It gives level of fat of the body. Low or high BMI suggests malnutrition or obesity.
3. BMI changes from childhood to adolescence age and sex wise.

Classification

- Underweight or malnourished—BMI <−2SD, overweight—BMI in between +1SD and <+2SD
- Obesity—BMI >+2SD or 95 percentile for age and sex.

ADOLESCENCE

Adolescence is a stage of transition from childhood to adulthood.

Period: It is 10–19 years age. This is divided into 3 phases.
1. *Early:* 10–13 years age
2. *Mid:* 14–16 years age
3. *Late:* 17–19 years age

Puberty is early half of adolescence.

Adolescence is a period of life in which rapid change in physical, sexual, congnition and psychology occurs.

1. *Changes in growth*—it is a time of substantial physical growth and maturation. The average period of growth spurt is 2–3 years.

Table 3.1: Body mass index for the age

	Girls				Boys	
−3SD	Median	3SD	Age (year)	−3S D	Median	3SD
11.8	15.2	21.3	5.01 (61 month)	12.1	15.3	20.2
11.7	15.3	22.1	6	12.1	15.3	20.2
11.8	15.4	22.3	7	12.3	15.5	21.6
11.9	15.7	24.8	8	12.4	15.7	22.7
12.1	16.1	26.5	9	12.6	16	24.3
12.4	16.6	28.4	10	12.8	16.4	26.1
12.7	17.2	30.2	11	13.1	16.9	28
13.2	18	31.9	12	13.4	17.5	30
13.6	18.8	33.4	13	13.8	18.2	31.7
15.4	19.6	34.7	14	14.3	19	33.1
14.4	20.2	35.5	15	17.7	19.8	34.1
14.6	20.7	36.1	16	15.1	20.5	34.8
14.7	21	29.3	17	15.4	21.1	35.2
14.7	21.3	29.5	18	15.7	21.7	35.4
14.7	21.4	36.2	19	15.9	22.2	35.5

Nearly 50% of the ideal adult body weight and 25% of final adult height are gained during the pubertal spurt.

Growth spurt occurs 18–24 months earlier in female than the male.

2. Development of genitalia and secondary sexual characters.

   Endocrinologic changes: Factor responsible for initiation of puberty is unknown.

   Adrenarche: The onset of androgen steroidogenesis occurs 2 years before the maturation of hypothalamic pituitary gonadal axis.

   • *True puberty:* It occurs when gonadotropins such as LH, FSH and gonadal sex steroid oestrogen and testosterone increases.

Physical aspects due to hormonal changes

Hypothalamus: Pituitary gonadal axis activate and leads to production of gonadotropin, luteinizing hormone (LH), follicle stimulating hormone (FSH), sex steroids, oestrogen and testosterone.

• Gonadal sex steroids—secondary sexual character
   1. Breast development
   2. Increase in penile and testicular size
   3. Menarche
• Adrenal androgens—sexual hair, acne.

Onset and Sequences of Puberty

Changes in males

1. *Testicular enlargement:* Begins between ages of 11 and 12 years. It is a first sign of puberty.
2. *Facial and axillary hairs:* It occurs about 2 years after the growth of pubic hairs.

Stages (5 stages)

1. Prepubertal, no pubic hairs have, prepubertal testes.
2. Testes larger, sparse, long hair at penile base.
3. Testes further enlarged, penis length enlarged, darker, coarser and curl hair.
4. Darkening of scrotal skin, penis length and width increased, glans develops, coarse and curly pubic hair extending over symphysis pubis.
5. Testes and penis adult size and shape. Adult type pubic hair that spreads to medial surface of thighs.

GIRLS

- Breast development between 8 and 13 years of age
- Appearance of pubic hair
- Menarche (10–16 years of age)
- Sweet and fresh face
- Increase in height and weight
- Breast development.
- Nipples become hard
- Hair on axilla and genitals
- Maturity of genitals
- White discharge per vagina
- Menstruation starts.

5 Stages

1. Prepubertal, no terminal hair at external genitalia.
2. Appearance of breast bud, sparse straight hair along the labia.
3. Generalized breast enlargement extending beyond the areola, pigmented pubic hair begin to curl.
4. Nipple and areola form a second mount over the breast, hair increases, spread over the entire mons.
5. Mature and adult type of breast nipple projects and areola recedes.

Puberty in female begins with the development of breast buds at the mean age 9.5 years (*thelarche*).

Menarche—occurence of first menstrual cycle, occurs at the mean age of 12.5 years and occurs about 2–3 years of the thelarche.

Psychosocial development

Early (10–13 years of age): Early shift to independence from parent with declining interest in family activities, beginning with conflict with parents and behavior changes.

Middle (14–17 years of age)
- Increased conflict with parents
- Diminished preoccupation with pubertal changes
- Intense peer group involvement
- Increased abstract thinking
- Lack of impulse control with risk taking behaviors.

Late (17–19 years of age)
- Development of self-distinct from parent. Adolescents are better able to take and more likely to seek advice from parents.
- Being comfortable with own body image.
- Well developed abstract through process with fewer risk taking behaviors. Adolescents are able to articulate future educational and vocational goals.

Problems faced by adolescence

1. Nutrition and eating disorders
2. Mental health problems—anxiety, suicide, depression, juvenile delinquency, self-esteem.
3. Sleep disturbances—increased sleep is required at this period. Disturbance in sleep may lead to poor academic performance, day time drowsing, depression, anxiety.
4. Infections—they are exposed to TB, HIV, STD, skin and parasitic infection.
5. Genital infection and STD—vaginal discharge, candidiasis, gonorrhea, chlamydia, pelvic inflammatory diseases are common lifestyle diseases in obesity.

ATTENTION DEFICIT HYPERACTIVITY DISORDER

Attention deficit hyperactivity disorder (ADHD) is one of the common chronic problems affecting school age children and have poor family and peer relations. Without effective treatment, such children may develop long-term handicaps. It is more common in boys than girls.

Clinical Features

It is characterised by hyperactivity, impulsiveness and inattention in appropriate to age.

Three classes of ADHD are:
Class I: All three symptoms
Class II: Hyperactivity and impulsiveness
Class III: Inattention

Laboratory Studies

Laboratory studies have limited role investigations are carried out to rule out other causes

Table 3.2: Median weight, height and head circumference

Age	Weight (kg)		Height (cm)		Head circumference (cm)	
	Boys	Girls	Boys	Girls	Boys	Girls
0	3.3	3.2	49.1	49.1	34.5	33.9
3 m	6.4	5.8	59.8	59.8	40.5	39.5
6 m	7.9	7.3	65.7	65.7	45.0	42.2
9 m	8.9	8.2	70.1	70.1	45.4	43.0
1 yr	9.6	8.9	74.0	71.4	46.1	44.9
2 yr	12.2	11.5	86.4	86.4	48.3	47.2
3 yr	14.3	13.9	95.1	95.1	49.5	48.5
4 yr	16.3	16.1	107.0	102.7	50.2	49.3
5 yr	18.3	18.2	109.4	109.4	50.7	49.9
6 yr	20.5	22.2	116.4	115.1		
7 yr	22.9	22.4	121.7	120.8		
8 yr	25.4	25.0	127.3	126.6		
9 yr	28.1	28.2	134.3	138.4		
10 yr	31.2	31.9	142.7	145.0		
11 yr			149.1	150.7		
12 yr			162.8	156.9		
13 yr			133.1	156.9		
14 yr			163.2	159.8		
15 yr			186.5	161.7		
16 yr			172.9	162.5		
17 yr			175.2	162.9		
18 yr			176.1	163.1		
19 yr			176.3	163.2		

of hyperactivity such as lead toxicity, iron deficiency anemia, thyrotoxicosis.

Epidemiology and Etiology

1. ADHD is more common in boys than girls
2. The cause is unknown:
   a. Genetic factors: About 30–50% of affected children show genetic factors.
   b. Abnormality is neuromuscular, especially dopamine and norepinephrine also leads to such symptoms.

Clinical Features

1. Symptoms are usually in school going children before age of 7 years of age.
2. Symptoms are more in one environment (e.g. school, home)
3. Symptoms of inattentions such as not being able to focus during classroom instruction given, difficult with organization and forget fullness.
4. Symptoms of hyperactivity such as fidgeting, acting as if driven by a motor, excessive talking and difficulty remaining seated well in the classroom.
5. Symptoms of impulsivity such as blurting out answer before as question is completed.
6. Impairment in function in school and social environment.

Management: Management includes behavior and drug therapy.

1. *Behavior therapy:* Parents should be advised to stay calm as much as can and avoid confrontation. Instruct the parents with one

Table 3.3: Length for age (cm)

Boys				Girls		
Mean	−3SD	+3SD	Age	Mean	−3S D	+3SD
49.1	43.6	54.7	0	49.1	43.6	54.7
59.8	53.5	66.1	3 m	59.8	53.5	66.1
65.7	58.9	74.2	6 m	65.7	58.9	72.5
70.1	62.9	77.4	9 m	70.1	62.9	77.4
74.0	66.9	81.7	1 yr	71.4	66.3	81.7
86.4	76.7	96.1	2 yr	86.4	76.7	96.1
95.1	83.6	106.5	3 yr	95.1	83.6	105.6
107.0	89.8	115.7	4 yr	102.7	89.8	115.7
109.4	95.2	123.7	5 yr	109.4	95.2	123.7
116.4	101.2	131.3	6 yr	115.1	99.8	130.5
121.7	105.9	137.6	7 yr	120.8	104.4	137.2
127.3	110.3	144.2	8 yr	126.6	189.2	143.9
134.3	115.9	152.7	9 yr	138.6	114.2	150.8
137.8	118.7	156.9	10 yr	138.6	119.4	157.8
142.7	122.9	163.3	11 yr	145.0	125.1	164.9
149.1	127.4	170.3	12 yr	150.7	130.7	171.2
162.8	133.2	177.6	13 yr	156.9	133.6	177.2
163.2	140.1	186.3	14 yr	159.8	139.0	180.6
168.5	145.1	191.9	15 yr	161.7	141.0	182.3
172.9	149.6	196.2	16 yr	162.5	142.0	182.9
175.2	152.7	198.1	17 yr	162.9	142.8	182.9
176.1	153.7	198.4	18 yr	163.1	143.2	182.9
176.5	154.6	198.6	19 yr	163.2	143.5	182.9

thing to do at a time. Good works should be rewarded time to time. Study periods should be brief.

In school child should sit in first line with timely schedule.

2. *Drugs:* Drugs which stimulate frontal lobe of brain are choice of drug.
   a. Stimulants (methylphenidate, dextroamphetamine and fremoline)
   Start with low doses and given in morning their use is associated with variation in mood, state, motor tics, and abuse potential.

b. Atomoxetine is a non-stimulant that is approved for use in ADHD as the second line treatment.

These drugs give statistically significant and comparable improvements in the symptoms.

c. Tricyclic antidepressants (TCA) are used if above drugs failed. Clonidine, antipsychotic drugs, e.g. thioridazine, resperidone, fluxetine are used. But they have serious side effects than stimulants.

Prognosis is assessed time to time.

Table 3.4: Weight-for-age (kg)

Boys				Girls		
Median	−3SD	+3SD	Age	Median	−3SD	+3SD
3.3	2.1	5.0	0 (Birth)	3.2	2.0	4.8
7.0	4.4	9.0	3 m	5.8	4.0	8.5
7.9	5.7	10.9	6 m	7.3	5.1	10.6
8.9	6.4	12.3	9 m	8.2	5.8	12.0
9.6	6.9	13.3	1 yr	8.9	6.3	13.1
12.2	8.6	17.1	2 yr	11.5	8.1	17.0
14.3	10.0	20.7	3 yr	13.9	9.6	9.6
16.3	11.2	24.2	4 yr	16.1	10.9	25.2
18.3	12.4	27.9	5 yr	18.2	12.1	29.2
20.5	14.1	31.5	6 yr	22.2	13.5	33.4
22.9	15.7	36.1	7 yr	22.4	14.8	38.3
25.9	17.5	42.5	8 yr	25.5	16.6	45.2
28.1	18.8	48.2	9 yr	28.2	18.1	51.1
31.2	20.4	56.4	10 yr	31.9	20.3	59.2

Table 3.5: Head circumference (cm)

Boys				Girls		
Median	−3SD	+3SD	Age	Median	−3SD	+3SD
33.9	33.3	37.4	0 (Birth)	34.5	30.7	38.3
39.5	35.8	43.3	3 m	40.5	37.0	44.1
42.2	38.3	46.1	6 m	45.0	41.1	48.8
43.0	39.8	47.8	9 m	45.4	41.2	48.8
44.9	40.8	49.0	1 yr	46.1	42.2	48.8
47.2	43.0	51.4	2 yr	48.3	42.2	49.9
48.5	44.3	52.7	3 yr	49.5	45.2	53.8
45.1	49.3	53.6	4 yr	50.2	45.8	54.7
49.9	45.7	54.2	5 yr	50.7	46.3	55.2

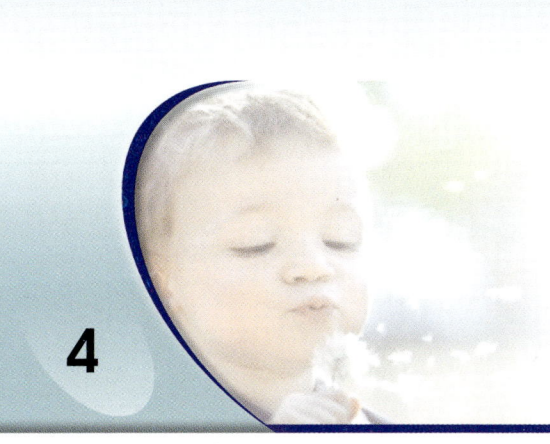

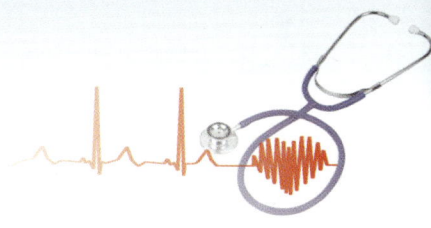

4

Nutritional Requirements

Sufficient and balanced diet is 'must' for proper growth and development of the child. Growth is fast during first five years of age. During this period nutrition has great importance. Nutrition is basic determinant of resistance against infection.

Water

Child requires more water than adult. As per body weight it is given in Table 4.1.

Calories

Calories are measurement of energy. An infant needs 100–120 calories per kg of body weight daily. At one year infant requires 1000 calories per day. Requirement is calculated for further age by increasing 100 calories for one year age. At one year age requirement (1000 calories),

e.g. 5-year child needs 1000 + 400 = 1400 calories per day.

In balanced diet calories must drive 50% from carbohydrate, 35% from protein and 15% from fat.

Daily requirement of protein and calories is given Table 4.2.

Proteins

Proteins are essential for growth and balance of body. Amino acids are essential for growth and development of body. Milk and nonvegetarian diet are rich in amino acids; so they are better than vegetarian diet. Lysine is deficient in cereals and methionine is deficient in pulses; so mixture of pulses and cereals known as 'khichdi' is a good combination.

Fats

Fats are rich source of energy. Fat-soluble vitamins are also dissolve in it. Linoleic acid

Table 4.1: Daily requirement of water

Age	Water requirement (ml/kg)
Newborn first 3 days	80–100
3–10 days	125–150
10 days–3 months	140–150
10 days–3 months	140–160
3–12 months	150
1–3 years	125
4–6 years	100
7–9 years	75
10–12 years and afterward	50

Table 4.2: Daily requirement of protein and calories

Age	Calories (k. claories)	Proteins required in grams
Birth to 6 months	600	11
6 months to 1 year	800	13
1–3 years	1200	18
4–6 years	1500	22
7–9 years	2800	33
10–12 years	2100	41

Table 4.3: Daily requirement of vitamins and minerals

Vitamins and minerals	Daily requirement
Vitamin A	1500–5000 IU
Vitamin B$_1$ (thiamine)	0.5–1.5 mg
Vitamin B$_2$ (riboflavin)	0.6–2.5 mg
Niacin	8–20 mg
Vitamin B$_6$ (pyridoxine)	0.4–1.4 mg
Vitamin B$_{12}$ (cyanocobalamin)	1–15 µg
Folic acid	25–100 µg
Vitamin C	35–60 mg
Vitamin D	400 IU
Calcium	0.6–1.4 gm
Phosphorus	0.5–1.4 gm
Iron	15–18 mg

is essential for body. In deficiency of it, dryness of skin occurs.

Vitamins and Minerals

These are essential for metabolic activities of the body (Table 4.3).

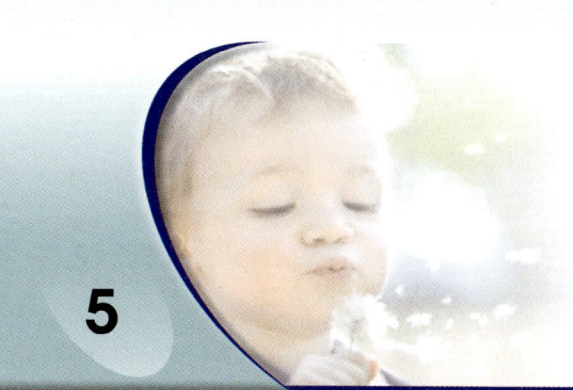

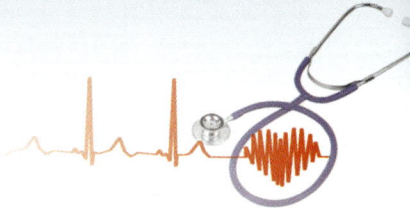

5

Infant Feeding

Nutrition has great importance for infants. Milk is basic food for infants. Act of feeding meet nutritional as well as emotional and psychological needs of the infants.

Breast milk is best for the infant and breast-feeding should be encouraged.

Milk Secretion

Anatomy of breast

Inside the breast alveoli which are very small sacs made of milk secretory cells. Around the alveoli are smooth muscle cells which contract and squeeze out the milk.

Small tubes or ducts carry milk from the alveoli to the outside of the nipple. Beneath the alveoli the ducts become wide and form lactiferous sinuses, where milk collects in preparation for a feed. The ducts become narrow again as it passes through the nipple.

The secretory alveoli and ducts are surrounded by supportive tissue and fat which gives the breast its shape (Fig. 5.1).

Physiology of milk secretion

Prolactin reflex: When the baby sucks at the breast impulses go from the nipple to the brain. In response the anterior pituitary gland secretes prolactin hormone. Prolactin goes in the blood to the breast and makes the milk secreting cells produce milk.

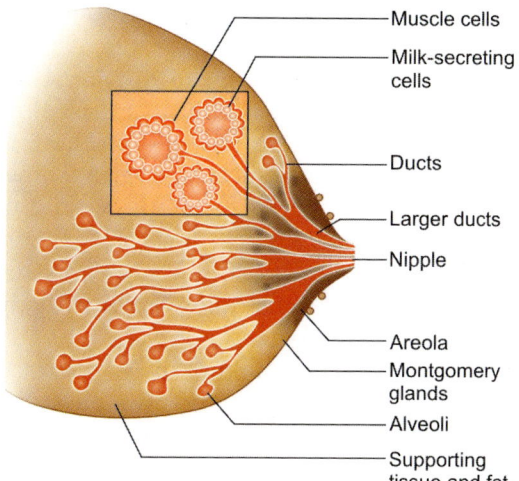

Fig. 5.1: Anatomy of breast.

Most of the prolactin is in the blood milk is in about 30 minutes after the feed so it makes the breast to produce milk for the next feed. For this feed the baby takes the milk which is already in the breast.

It tells us if her baby suckles more, her breast make more milk. So, more suckling make more milk, as in case of twin babies.

If baby suckles less, the breast make less milk. If a baby stops suckling, the breasts soon stop making milk.

More prolactin is produced in night and makes a mother feel relaxed and sometime sleepy. Prolactin and suckling itself by stimulating the release of endorphin suppress ovulation so breastfeeding can help of delay a new pregnancy. Breastfeeding in night is important for this.

Oxytocin reflex: When baby suckles sensory impulses go from the nipple to the brain. In response to this posterior part of pituitary secretes the hormone oxytocin. Oxytocin goes to the blood and make the muscle cells around the alveoli to contract.

This makes the milk (which has collected in the alveoli) flow along the ducts to the lactiferous sinuses.

This is oxytocin reflex or milk ejection reflex.

Oxytocin produced more quickly than prolactin. It makes the milk in breast flow for this feed. Oxytocin can start working in 3–10 minutes before a suckles, when a mother learns to expect a feed or simply crying or playing with the baby.

The oxytocin reflex sometimes called let down reflex. The same reflex can be brought out by synthetic oxytocin.

Oxytocin makes a mother's uterus contracts after delivery. This helps to reduce bleeding.

Good feeling, for example, pleased with her baby or thinking lovely of him and feeling confident that her milk is best for him, can help the oxytocin reflex to work and her milk to flow. Sensations such as touching or seeing her baby or hearing him cry can help the reflex.

If a mother is separated from her baby in between feeds her oxytocin reflex may not work easily. But bad feeling, such as pain worry or doubt, she has not enough milk can hinder the reflex and stop her milk flowing. When infect the breasts are producing milk but it is not flowing out.

Inhibitors of breast milk: There are substances which can reduce or inhibit milk production.

If one breast stops making while the other breast continues to make milk although oxytocin and prolactin go equally to both breasts.

If a lot of milk is left in the breast, the inhibitors stop the cells from secreting any more.

BREASTFEEDING

Breastfeeding is natural. Exclusive breastfeeding term denotes it a baby has no other food or drinks except breast milk.

Advantages of Breastfeeding

1. *Nutrients in human milk*

Carbohydrate: The sugar lactose is the main carbohydrate in milk. Starch is very important nutrient for older children and adults but young babies cannot digest starch easily.

Breast milk contains more lactose than other milk.

Protein: Quality and quantity
1. There is less casein in human milk in comparison to cow's milk and it forms softer curds which are easier to digest.
2. Human milk contain much of the whey protein consists of anti-infective properties against infection.
3. The anti-infective proteins in human milk includes lactoferrin, which binds iron and prevents the growth of bacteria which need iron and lysozymes (which kills bacteria) as well as antibodies (immunoglobulin, mostly IgA) which protects from infections.
4. It contains bifidus factor which promotes growth of lactobacillus, inhibits the growth of harmful bacteria and give breastfed babies stool their yogurt smell.
5. Research has shown that the breast milk also contains antiviral and anti-parasitical factors.
6. Artificially fed babies may develop intolerance to protein from animal. Babies who are fed animal milk or formula may develop allergies such as eczema and possibly asthma.

7. Human milk contains alpha lactalbumin while animal milk contains beta lactalbumin and lacks the amino acid cystine, and formula milk lacks taurine which is needed for brain growth.

Fat

1. Human milk contains essential fatty acids which are needed for growth of eye and brain of the baby. While cow milk or formula does not contain.
2. *Lipase:* At birth a baby's gut has not developed all the enzymes which are needed to digest milk fat. The lipase in breast milk helps to complete digestion of the fat in the gut.

Vitamins: Human milk contains vit A and vit C more than cow milk. Cow milk contains plenty of vit B but goat milk lacks vit B, folic acid and cause anemia.

Iron: Only about 10% of iron of cow milk is absorbed in gut but about 50% of the iron from breast milk is absorbed, so it protects iron deficiency anemia until at least 6 months of age and after longer.

2. Protection against infection

1. Breast milk contains white blood cells and a number of anti-infective factors which help to protects a baby against infections.
2. Breast milk also contains antibodies against infections which mother has had in past. When a mother becomes infected white cells becomes active and makes antibodies IgA to protect her. Some of the antibodies go to the breast and make antibodies which are secreted in her breast milk to protect her baby this is called enteromammary circulation.
   - Growth of mumps, influenza, vaccinia and Japanese encephalitis virus can be inhibited by substance in human milk.
   - *Protection against diarrhea and respiratory infection.*

Artificially fed babies get diarrhea more often partly because artificial feeds lack anti-infective factors and partly artificially feeds are often contaminated with harmful bacteria. Breast milk is not contaminated.

- Breast milk contains anti-poliomyelitis titre. Which protects from poliomyelitis.
- Bile salts lipase kills Giardia and *Entamoeba histolylica.*
- Breast milk also protects ear infections and meningitis.
- Cost of artificial milk especially in poor is a disadvantage for artificially feeding. But beast milk is free.
- Breast milk is readily available can be given at any time.
- Breast milk is at desired room temperature for the baby.
- Incidence of breast cancer is less in mother who is breastfeeding to her baby.
- *Pschychological benefits:* It forms close, loving relationship which makes mother feel deeply satisfied emotionally. This is called *bonding.*
- Colostrums has anti-infective properties, protects children from infections.

Variation in composition of breast milk

Colostrum: It is a special breast milk produced in the first few days after the delivery.

It is thicker and yellow or clear in color. Over the few days colostrum changes into mature milk.

1. Colostrum has more antibodies and other anti-infective proteins than mature milk, more WBC, more protein. Antibodies provide first immunization against the disease that body meets after delivery.
2. Colostrum has mild purgative effect which helps to clear the baby gut meconium. This clear bilirubin from the gut and helps to prevent jaundice.
3. Colostrum contains epidermal growth factors, helps to develop immature villi of

intestine of the baby afterbirth. This helps to prevent the baby from developing allergies and intolerance to other food.

4. It contains more vit A, so reduce severity of infections.
5. It contains more vit K which prevents bleeding in the newborn.
6. Antibodies in colostrum probably help to prevent allergies by coating the intestinal mucosa.

Foremilk: It is a bluish milk that is produced early in a feed contains protein, lactose, other nutrients and water.

Hind milk: It is white milk that is produced later in feed which contains more fat than foremilk.

Quantity

600–900 ml milk up to 6 months and many mother's can produce 400 ml of milk a day during the period of 6 months and 100–150 ml during second year.

Various positions for breastfeeding a baby

- Underarm position
- Using the opposite arm
- Mother in lying down position.

Key points in position

1. Baby's head and body should be straight.
2. Baby's face should face mother's breast.
3. Baby's body should be close to her body so she should support the baby's whole body.

Mother how to support her breast

She should put her fingers below her breast. First finger used to support the breast. Thumb is placed above the areola, helping to shape the breast.

Attachment of the body

Good attachment is essential for successful breastfeeding. Ask the mother to express a little milk on her nipple and touch the body's lips with her nipple. Wait until baby's mouth

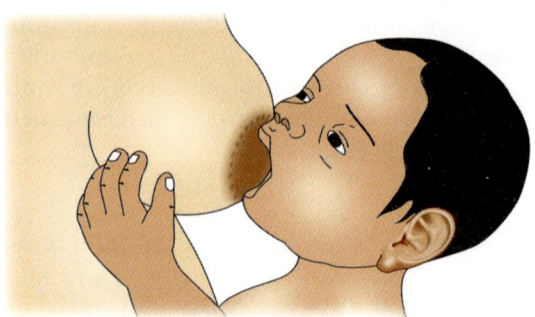

Fig. 5.2: Good attachment.

is opening wide and tongue is down and forward (Fig. 5.2).

Move the baby quickly onto her breast aligners the nipple towards the baby's nipple so his lower lip well below nipple.

Key points of good attachment

1. More areola is visible above the baby's mouth than below it.
2. Baby's mouth is wide open.
3. Baby's lower lip is turned outwards. So, he is reaching with the tongue under the lactiferous sinuses to press out the milk.
4. Baby's chin is touching the breast.
5. Cheeks are gulped out.

Problems of poor attachment

- Pain or damage to nipple.
- Poor milk supply so baby is not satisfied, poor weight gain
- Breast engorgement because milk is not removed.
- Poor attachment is seen mostly if baby is also has bottle feeding.

This protects the breast from the harmful effects of being to full. It is needed if a baby stops breastfeeding for some reason.

If breast milk is removed by suckling or expression, the inhibitors are also removed. Then the breast makes more milk.

So, if baby stops suckling from one breast that breast stops making milk, or a baby suckles more from one breast, that breast make more milk.

So, if a baby cannot suckle, the breast milk must be removed by expression to enable production to continue.

Exclusive breastfeeding means only breast milk should be given to the baby up to age of 6 months. Do not give ghutti, water, gripes, honey, animal or powdered milk. Never use bottles or pacifier. Bottle feeding is always at risk of contamination of milk which may cause diarrhea.

- Burping
- Oral pills that may be used and a contraceptive device may interfere with milk secretion.
- Size of breast has no correlation with secretion of milk.
- Babies who are less than about 30–32 weeks of gestational age need to fed expressed milk by nasogastric tube or by cup or spoon.
- In sick babies—expressed milk in a cup can be given.

Baby born after cesarean section: It is usually possible for a mother to breastfeed within 4 hours of cesarean section as she regained consciousness.

Early breastfeeding: Oral feeding is possible as soon as a baby is born. The first feed should be given within 2–3 hours after delivery to prevent hypoglycemia (early breastfeeding).

CONTRAINDICATIONS

Mother

1. Acute illness of mother—septicemia, nephritis, eclampsia, profuse hemorrhage, active tuberculosis, typhoid fever, malaria.
2. Chronic poor nutrition, debility, severe neurosis.

Temporary cesation of nursing is required

If mother requires diagnostic radiopharmaceuticals, chloramphenicol, metronidazole, sulfonamides or anthraquinone derivative laxative: Breastfeeding is not contraindicated in the following situations:

a. Resumption of menstruation
b. Pregnancy
c. Hemolytic disease of newborn

Schedule of breastfeeding

Initiate breastfeeding on putting baby immediately but not later than 2 hours after the delivery. Colostrum is good for the body and should not be discarded. Afterward put baby to breast whenever the baby demands through crying.

In time schedule feeds are given at particular time interval. But ultimate aim is that baby should be hungry at the time of feeding.

Adequacy of breast milk supply

Adequacy is assessed as follows:

a. Baby sleeps 2–4 hours after feed.
b. Baby gains weight satisfactorily. 'Test feed' means weigh the baby before and after feed. It is satisfactory method because it causes anxiety in mother thus reduces let down reflex and milk supply.
c. *The wetness test:* If breast fed baby who is not given other fluids urinate at least six times in 24 hours then it is almost certainly taking enough breast milk.

Average production of milk is 600–700 ml/day which is adequate for 5–6 months of life.

Basic method of breastfeeding

a. While breastfeeding mother should hold the baby firmly with the head resting on the upper arm and she should support the breast with the other hand. She should touch the mouth of baby with the nipple and allow to suck.
b. The baby need not be covered during feeding.
c. The child should be fed alternating on both breasts.
d. Act of feeding should be followed by 'burping' to 'kick out' swallowed air. For it, hold the baby on mother shoulder or making him sit in mother's lap and put

Table 5.1: Composition of human, cow, buffalo and goat milk

Component	Human	Cow	Buffalo	Goat
Protein (gm%)	1.0	3.5	4.2	4.4
Fat (gm%)	5.0	3.5–7	7.5	4.1
Calories (100 ml)	60	50–100	80–120	70
Water %	88	87	83	87
Lactose %	7.0	5.5	4.8	4.9
Ironmg%	0.1	0.2	0.2	0.2
Vit A (IU/100 ml)	170–670	140–280	80	80
Vit C (mg%)	2–6	1–4	1–4	1–4

or rub his back so that swallowed air comes out.

e. Mother should be encouraged for breast-feeding because psychological inadequate bonding between the mother and baby increase out put of milk. Milk diet also should be adequate during lactation period for adequate supply of milk.

Complementary Feeding

Extra feeds of water and artificial milk may be required in some babies whose appetite is greater or breast milk is inadequate.

Supplementary Feeding

It is artificial feeding where artificial feed is given instead of breastfeeding. It is also called artificial feeding.

ARTIFICIAL FEEDING

Artificial feeding means infant feeding by means other than breastfeeding and involves the use of human milk substitute such as liquid

Table 5.2: Amount of milk and frequency of feeding

Age	Amount/kg/day	Frequency/day
Birth to 1 month	50–75 ml	6–7
1–2 months	75–100 ml	6–7
2–4 months	100–125 ml	5–6
4–6 months	150–175 ml	5
6 months onward	175–200 ml	4–5

milk of cow's, buffalo, etc. or dried milk which are commercially available.

Indications

1. When mother's milk is insufficient or contraindicated due to any reason.
2. After death of mother.
3. When mother cannot give proper time, e.g. service class mother, due to industrialization or any other reason.
4. When lactose intolerance is due to mother's milk.

Types of Milk

Cow, goat or buffalo milk are given. Cow milk is best. Fat content is high in buffalo milk (Table 5.1). When needed buffalo milk can be given after removal of cream. Milk should not be diluted. Diluted milk causes malnutrition due to insufficient nutrients. Milk should be boiled before feeding. Commercially available food can be advised for economically well to do person but instruction should be followed properly. In all, it is essential to prevent contamination.

Method (Table 5.2)

Milk can be given by feeding bottle, droper, or spoon and cup. Spoon and cup is better because it can be cleaned easily. Wide mouth straight bottle is better than boat-shaped bottle because it can be cleaned easily. Use of bottles should be discouraged because they are difficult to clean. Unhygienic feed may lead to infection.

The rubber teats with flanged basis are hygienically superior to the plain and finger-like teats. The hole at teat can be made with red hot needle. Its size should allow 12–15 drops/minute of milk. When bottle is kept upside down so baby can suck and swallow better without choking.

Milk is kept in bottle or in cup what is needed at a time. During feeding bottle should be held is such a way that only milk is allowed not the air. Child should be burped after feeding.

Addition of Vitamins and Minerals

Artificially fed babies should receive vit A, vit C, and iron supplementation. They are deficient in it.

WEANING

Mother's milk is inadequate for requirement after 4 months age of infant. Introduction of semisolid in the diet of infant is termed weaning.

In India, in many community it is called 'Ann Prasan', a traditional ritual.

Time

If mother milk is sufficient then it can be initiated about 6 months of age. But in India, it should be started from 3 months of age and completed up to 1 year of age. At that age child should be taking almost the adult diet.

How

i. During initial phase apart from mother's milk, bananas, ragi, mashed potatoes, rice, etc. are given.

ii. It is not essential to give particular food. Food depends on liking of child and economic status of family. Food must be fresh and out of contamination.

It is given by cup and spoon if child takes with his own hand, let them do.

Commercially available food can also be given but not encouraged. Fish, eggs should be introduced later on due to probable risk of allergy of protein.

Time of nutritional stress: Weaning is the time of nutritional stress for infant because he has to balance with different types of bacteria and parasites in food. At the same time emotional deprivation from withdrawl of mother's milk. Deficiency of vit A, kwashiorkor and malnutrition begins during this period mainly because insufficient cooked food may give rise to deficient digestion during this period. So, in words of Dr C. Gopalan, most happiest period of child's life is up to 6 months when he is dependent on mother's milk.

iii. Weaning is done from common food items which the family is already using. Carefully taken out from the family food without spicy.

COMMON FEEDING PROBLEMS

Regurgitation

Child vomits or regurgitate just after feeding. It is due to swallowed air in milk child grow and gain weight properly. Burping after feeding is required.

Constipation

For constipation glucose should be mixed with water should be given or honey is given. Milk of magnesia 1–2 teaspoonful may be given.

Failure of Lactation

It is common in primipara and due to fear, anxiety and lack of self confidence. It is increased when lactation is not established in first few days. She should be encouraged and sympathetic attitude toward her helps to combat this problem.

INFANTILE COLIC

It is excessive crying of baby due to abdominal colic common below 3 months of age.

Features

Baby cries for few to many hours. During this time face is flushed, abdomen distended, he draws legs to abdomen, soles are cold. Attacks are common at evening or late hours of the day.

It is due to swallowed air during feed, over feeding or high carbohydrate content in food.

Abdominal colic is due to 'gas' and relieved when it is passed out by mouth or rectally.

Attacks are repeated.

Treatment

1. Hold the child erect and put on bed prone.
2. Suppository per rectal or enema also gives relief due to passage of gas.
3. Sedation is less useful in long lasting attack.
4. No use of carminative before feeding.
5. Burping is essential after feeding.

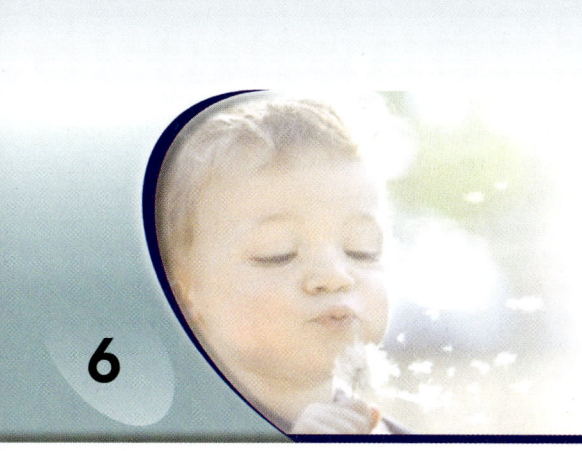

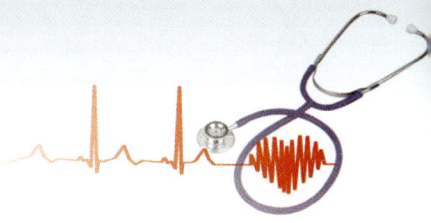

6

Immunization

Immunity is the protective ability of human body to tolerate the presence of material indigenous to the body (set) and to identity and eliminate foreign (non self) material.

Immunity provides protection from infectious diseases. It is generally very specific to a single organism or a group of closely related organism.

There are two basic mechanisms for acquiring immunity.

1. Active
2. Passive

Active immunity: It can be natural following an infection and can last a lifelong or following immunization.

It is a stimulation of immune system to produce antigen specific humoral (antibody) and cellular immunity. It lasts for many years, often a lifetime.

Active immunity is acquired

a. When one survives infection from the disease causing organism to which body responds by memory cells. Upon reexposure to the same antigen these memory cells begin to replicate and produce antibodies very rapidly which re-establish protection.
b. Another way to produce active immunity is by vaccination. Vaccine produce same antibodies but they do not subject the recipient to the disease.

Herd immunity

It is a type of immunity that occurs when the vaccination of a portion of the population (or herd) provides to unprotected individuals.

Passive immunity: When antibody produced by one human or animal is transferred to another. It degenerates over time, e.g. antibodies from mother protect the child from certain diseases for up to a year.

How immunization works?

A vaccine contains components similar to the infecting organism so immune system works same to both. Successful vaccination produces lifelong memory lymphocytes that respond more quickly and microbes are destroyed quickly. Protection may not be complete but the severity of illness reduced.

When vaccine is given first time, it stimulates the immune system known as primary. Immune system responds to antigen by producing antibodies and immune cells. Initially immunoglobulin M (IgM) antibody is produced in small amount. After few days immune system begins to make immunoglobulin (IgG) antibody which is more specific to microbes and last long than IgM.

Subsequent administration of same vaccine stimulates the subsequent response which is faster than primary and IgG is produced predominantly rather than IgM, which provide long lasting protection.

GENERAL CONSIDERATION ABOUT IMMUNIZATION

1. Interval between doses should not be less than one month.
2. Doses of all vaccines are as indicated. Polio drops are given orally (2 drops), check the label of the vial before use.
3. Older children may be given primary immunization on demand
4. Primary immunization of each child should be completed within 1 year of age.
5. Vaccines are effective if full coarse of the potent vaccine is given at the right time.
6. Measles vaccine is not given before 9 months of age because antibodies received from mother still protects the child from mother interact and will not allow the vaccine to work in the infants body.
7. Sterilization of syringes and needles and maintenance of cold chain are two essentials for best result of immunization.
8. Measles and BCG are freeze dried vaccine should be constituted with diluents before use.
   - Vaccine is administered with AD syringe (auto-disabled syringe). Syringe is locked after once use second time cannot be used (Fig. 6.1).
   - *Open vial policy.* When vaccine vial is opened and some vaccine is used at the place of immunization, remaining vial with vaccine is returned and kept in ice lined refrigerator. This remaining vaccine is used afterward for immunization this is called open vial policy.

Vaccines under open vial policy are OPV, pentavalent, IPV, DPT, TT, PCV.

But BCG, measles, rotavirus vaccine vials once opened can be used up to 4 hours after opening. Afterward discarded. For these vaccines open vial policy is not applicable.

Adverse events following immunization (AEFI) After vaccination, few children develop some untoward side effects due to vaccine. There effects are called AEFI.

Completely immunized child. Child who has received all the schedule vaccine up to 2 years of age.
- **Fully immunized child (FIC):** When child has received pentavalent or DPT (3 doses) and hepatitis B (3 doses), OPV (3 doses) and measles vaccine (one dose) up to 1 year age. He is called fully immunized child.

COLD CHAIN

The pieces of equipment and persons that keep vaccine cold from manufacturer to the expectant mother and the child are together called the 'cold chain'.

Storage and Transportation

All the vaccines must be kept between +2°C and +8°C during storage and transportation.

Heat, sunlight, and freezing can damage potency of vaccine permanently. Heat or freezing cannot make it potent again.

The vaccine must be collected quickly from the airport by the state stores. Transported to regional stores and from there to district stores in +2°C to +8°C.

ILR (ice lined refrigerator) and deep freezer are used for storage.

ILR (Ice Lined Refrigerator) (Fig. 6.2)

All vaccines are stored in ILR.

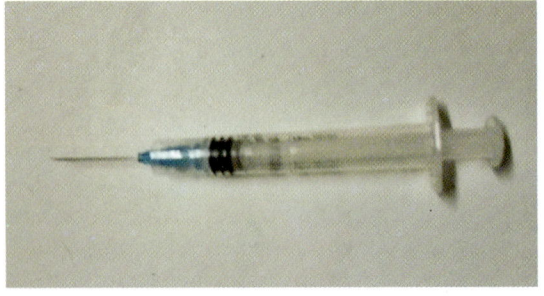

Fig. 6.1: AD syringe.

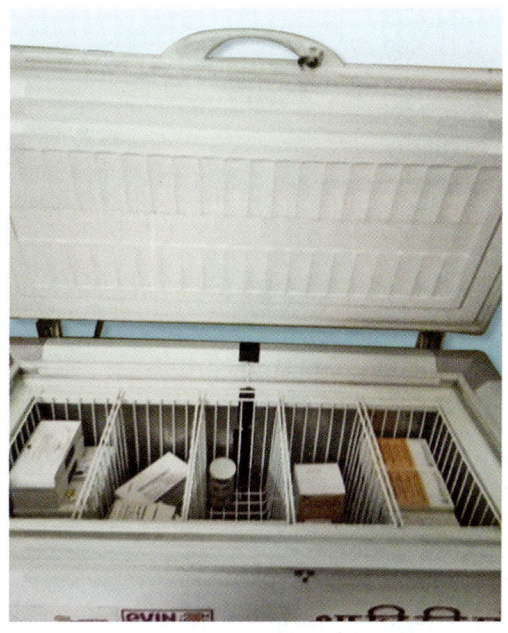

Fig. 6.2: ILR—internal view.

The bottom of these types of refrigerator is coldest place. DPT, DT, TT should not be kept directly on the floor of ILR as they can freeze and get damaged. Keep these vaccine in baskets provided with ILR.

There is no freezer compartment of ILRs. You cannot freeze ice packs or ice refrigerator because the risk of cold chain failure is far less in an ILR because safe temperature range maintained even with an electricity supply of 8 hours in 24 hours cycle.

Deep Freezer

Used for polio or measles vaccine storage in special situation such as in pulse polio, mop up round and freezing the ice packs.

Conventional Refrigerator

These are used less these days for storing vaccine. Correct arrangement is as follows:
a. Keep measles and poliovaccine on top self near the freezer.
b. Keep DPT, TT, DT, BCG on the middle self.

c. Keep diluent for measles and BCG in the refrigerator near the freezer but not is freezer because ampule will break.
d. Keep plastic bottle of water or ice packs on the lower self to keep the refrigerator maintain the low temperature in case of electricity failure.

Vaccine Carrier

Cold vaccines from refrigerator is kept in vaccine carrier in which vaccine is kept between frozen ice packs and vaccine is transported. Temperature is maintained for 48 hours (Fig. 6.3).

Day Carrier

Vaccines are transported from taking at PHC level to place of immunization in day carrier for vaccination session. It can keep vaccine cold for 6–8 hours. Ice packs are kept in sides of carrier, vaccine in between them.

Icepacks

These are flat plastic bottles filled with water. The ice packs are prepared by keeping them

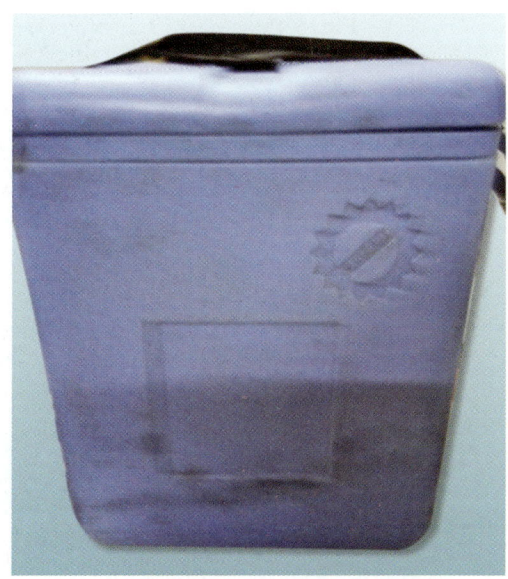

Fig. 6.3: Vaccine carrier.

in the deep freezer or in the freezer compartment or in ordinary refrigerator. They are used for lining the walls of vaccine carrier to keep them cold. It has depressions to keep the vaccine vials during session of immunization after its removal from vaccine or day carrier (Fig. 6.4).

Devices which indicate temperature of vaccine is below zero degree are also commercially available (*Tracker*) (Fig. 6.6).

• **Vaccine vial monitor (VVM):** Every vaccine vial have vaccine vial monitor at its surface. It is in the form of as shown in Figs 6.5 and 6.7.

When temperature of vial goes up, color of vaccine vial monitor changes.

Usable

Stage 1   Color is white
Stage 2   Color is slight faint

Not usable

Stage 3   Color is same as surrounding
Stage 4   Color is dark than surrounding

• Vaccine with VVM stage 1 and 2 is used for vaccination. Stages 3 and 4 are discarded and not used.

Heat sensitive vaccines: These are vaccines which lose their efficacy when exposed to high temperature—BCG, measles, OPV, rotavirus.

Cold sensitive vaccines: These are vaccines which lose their efficacy when exposed to low temperature.

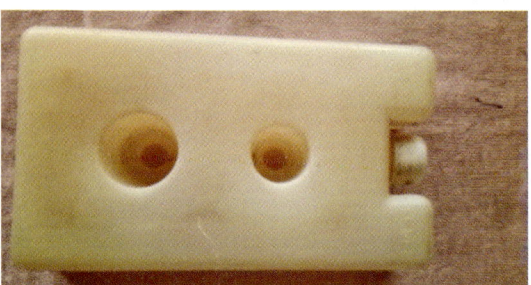

Fig. 6.4: Ice pack.

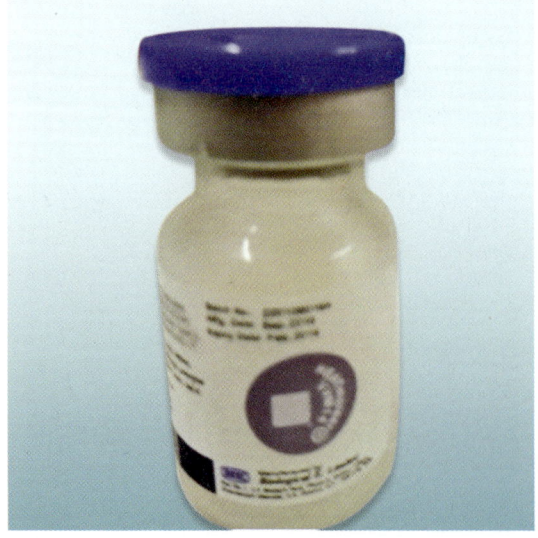

Fig. 6.5: Vaccine vial with vaccine vial monitor.

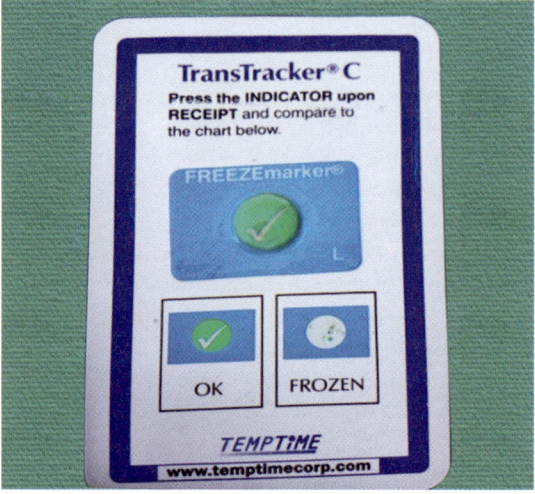

Fig. 6.6: Tracker.

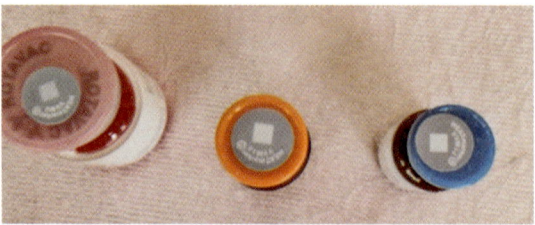

Fig. 6.7: VVM at cap of vaccine vial.

Pentavalent, tetanus toxoid, IPV, hepatitis B, PCV.

Measles and OPV can be stored in deep freezer up to district store in special situation, e.g. pulse polio, measles mass immunization.

Reverse cold chain: In some situation, e.g. AEFI due to vaccine, vaccine sample at the session site is transported in cold chain from session site to manufacturer for investigation of vaccine sample. Thus is called reverse cold chain.

Contraindications for immunization

a. During high fever.
b. Patient with history of convulsions or epilepsy.

BCG VACCINATION

Bacillus of Calmette-Guerin is an live attenuated vaccine. It produces controlled primary tuberculosis infection and protects against tuberculosis.

Vaccine

Freeze dried, heat stable best stored at +2°C to +8°C.

Age

Soon after birth as early as possible.

Site

The standard site is the middle of deltoid over left upper arm given intradermally (Table 6.1).

Method

Reconstitute the vaccine after dissolving in diluent. 0.1 ml or in case of newborn 0.05 ml is given intradermally with special BCG syringe. There will be clear, flat topped swelling in skin. The swollen skin may look pale with very small pits (like on orange peel). If skin does not swell it means you have injected under the skin by mistake, stop injecting and correct the position of the needle, give remainder of the dose but not more. If you already have given the whole dose under the skin consider the child injected and do not repeat the injection.

Reaction following vaccination

After 2–3 weeks of vaccination a papule appears at the injection site which increases in size. At about 4 weeks, it subsides or develops into ulcer which heals in about 3 months time.

In case of acclerated reaction, ulcer develops after 2–3 days of vaccination and lasting about 3 weeks. It is suggestive of tuberculin positive reaction.

Contraindication

No, except tuberculin (Mantoux test) positive in which there is no need to give. But in routine practice does not favour to do tuberculin test before BCG vaccination.

Complications

  i. Accelerated reaction in tuberculin sensitive.
 ii. Ulcer at site with bacterial infection.
iii. Abcess formation.
 iv. Regional lymphadenitis.
  v. Keloid formation over the site of vaccination.

POLIO VACCINATION

Oral polio vaccine (Sabin) is live attenuated vaccine containing all the three strains of polio virus (Lansing, Leon and Brunhide). Reinfection with wild virus prevented.

Salk vaccine is administered parenterally and does not interfere spread of wild virus infection.

Vaccine

Vaccine is best stored at 2°–8°C.

Age

0 (zero) dose is given just after birth before discharge from hospital. After that 3 doses are given at monthly interval starting from 6 weeks. A booster is given at age of 16–24 months of age or 1 year after 3rd dose.

Dose

Two drops of polio vaccine given directly into mouth of the child. This should be followed by feeding of some water to ensure administration.

In routine practice DPT and polio is given simultaneously.

Immunity Production

On entry in the gut strains of OPV multiply, which leads to production of antibodies like IgG, IgM and IgA. IgA gives local immunity while IgG, IgM give systemic immunity which protects central nervous system.

Contraindications

i. Child suffering from diarrhea
ii. Acute illness.

Complication

No complication.

DPT VACCINATION

Triple vaccine (DPT) protects against diphtheria, pertussis (whooping cough) and tetanus. Vaccine is best stored at 2°–10°C.

Age and Dose

3 doses of DPT are given after 6 weeks of age at monthly interval. A booster is given after 1 year of 3rd dose.

Dose is 0.5 ml given best on lateral aspect of thigh. After the age of 5 years pertussis component is not given due to risk of severe reaction. DT is given during this period.

Contraindications

i. Acute febrile illness
ii. History of convulsive disorders
iii. Polio epidemic.

Complications

i. Fever and febrile convulsions
ii. Local abscess at the site

iii. Collapse (hypovolemic, hypotonic shock) 1–3 hours after injection. Recovers in 1–2 hours.
iv. Allergic rash in skin.
v. Encephalitis.
vi. Provocation of polio during epidemic of disease.

MEASLES VACCINATION

Measles vaccine is a live attenuated vaccine (Schwartz's vaccine). It protects against measles.

Age

Given at the age of 9 months. Second dose given at 16–24 months of age.

Dose and Administration

Reconstitute the vaccine after dissolving in diluent (pyrogen-free distilled water). Inject 0.5 ml of freshly prepared vaccine into outer aspect of child's upper arm (right) subcutaneously. For it, pinch up the skin with your fingers push the needle into pinched up skin, not straight but sloping. Do not push the needle far in. Withdraw the plunger to check the blood, if not, press the plunger of syringe and inject the vaccine. Use reconstituted vaccine for 4 hours only. It can also be given intradermaly, intramuscularly.

Complications

Measles vaccine is very safe if reconstituted vaccine is used within 4 hours. One sterilized syringe and needle is used for injection. Complications are:

i. Malaise fever
ii. Rash 4–10 days after vaccination
iii. Convulsions
iv. Encephalitis

All deaths following measles vaccine reported are attributed to incorrect handling of the vaccine and not following the compromise on aseptic precautions.

TOXIC SHOCK SYNDROME (TSS)

It is a syndrome of symptoms followed by administration of contaminated measles vaccine. Contamination may occur due to the use of unsterile syringes and needles used to draw out the vaccine from the vials of reuse of measles vials more than one session on the same or frequent days. TSS occurs when the vaccine is contaminated with *Staphylococcus aureus.*

Symptoms are severe watery diarrhea, vomiting and high fever within few hours of measles vaccine administration. Disease progresses to hypotensive, hypovolemic shock within 48 hours, case fatality is high.

Treatment is IV fluids, antibiotics, steroids and antipyretics as well as symptomatic supportive therapy. If there is no improvement dopamine and steroids are given. Patient is shifted to ICU if above measures fail.

MUMPS VACCINATION

It is also live attenuated vaccine. Probations is 95%. It is supplied in powder form and used after reconstitution. The dose is 317 TCID (tissue culture infection doses) which should administered subcutaneously by jet.

RUBELLA VACCINATION

It is live attenuated viral vaccine protects against congenital rubella syndrome given to girls 1 year to age of puberty and to susceptible women of child bearing age. Not given in pregnant women and given only when conception is unlikely for subsequent 2 months.

PENTAVALENT VACCINE

Pentavalent is a vaccine which contains five antigen—diphtheria, pertussis, tetanus, hepatitis B and influenza type B.

Dose, route and schedule: As per national immunization schedule vaccination of pentavalent vaccine should be started for any child aged more than 1 month.

First dose—6 weeks age, second dose—10 weeks, third dose—14 weeks age. Total 3 doses. There is no booster.

Dose: 0.5 ml intramuscular at anterolateral aspect of left thigh.

If a child has received at least one dose of pentavalent vaccine before 1 year age then the child should be given further doses at 4 weeks interval.

Child who has initiated with DPT/hepatitis B vaccine will continue to receive subsequent doses of DPT/hepatitis B and not pentavalent vaccine.

Side effects

1. Redness, swelling and pain at the site of injection given.
2. Fever, vomiting, irritability, loss of appetite.

Contraindications

1. Severe allergic reaction to pentavalent vaccine
2. Age below 6 weeks
3. Child suffering from severe or moderate acute illness.

INACTIVATED POLIO VACCINE (IPV)

Inactivated polio vaccine is produced from wild type of poliovirus strains of each serotype that have been inactivated (killed) with formalin.

Dose and administration: If one dose of IPV is used, it should be given at 14 weeks of age because this is the age when maternal antibodies have diminished and immunogenicity is significantly higher.

It is administered intramuscular or subcutaneous routes. In national immunization program 0.5 ml of this vaccine is given intramuscular on anterolateral aspect of right thigh. It is given at 14 weeks of age along 3rd dose of pentavalent vaccine.

Various studies suggested that two doses of 0.1 ml of IPV are about equal to single dose of 0.5 ml of intramuscular do. So, *fractional IPV (f IPV)* doses at two intervals are called *fractional IPV (f IPV).* This reduces cost of vaccination and reduces burden of manufacturing. Fractional IPV is given subcutaneously on right arm.

IPV gives protection against poliomyelitis by forming very good humoral antibody. From April 2016 trivalent oral polio vaccine (P1, P2, P3) is replaced by bivalent OPV (P1, P3) because P2 strain was responsible for vaccine derived poliomyelitis (VDP). Since poliomyelitis due to P2 strain is not reported for many years so there was no need of trivalent vaccine and there was risk of VPP cases.

So, introduction of IPV in immunization produces immunity against all 3 strains and there is no risk of polio either.

IPV is to be given in addition to the existing oral polio vaccine in order to boost population immunity.

Side effects are less serious:
- Redness, pain, swelling or a lump where vaccine is injected.
- Low fever
- Joint pain, body aches
- Drowsiness
- Vomiting

ROTAVIRUS VACCINE

Rotavirus vaccine is a live vaccine used to protect against rotavirus infections. These viruses are the leading cause of severe diarrhea among young children. The vaccine prevents 15 to 34% of severe diarrhea is developing world and 37 to 96% of severe diarrhea in developed world.

Dose and schedule: Three doses of rotavirus vaccine are given before one year of age.

First dose at 6 weeks of age, second dose at 10 weeks of age, and third dose at 14 weeks of age.

Five drops of vaccine are given *orally*.

Side effects. It is safe vaccine, a few side effects are:

Mild transient symptoms

1. Irritability, mild or temporary diarrhea or vomiting after getting a dose of rotavirus vaccine.
2. Gastroenteritis mostly after 1st dose.
3. *Serious problems:* Intussusception in occasional case.

PNEUMOCOCCAL CONJUGATE VACCINE

Pneumococcal conjugate vaccine (PCV) is a vaccine which prevents pneumonia caused by *Streptococcus pneumoniae.*

Types: Pnemococcal conjugate vaccine (absorbed) (PCV 10 vaccine) contains 10 serotypes and PCV 13 vaccine contain 13 serotypes.

PCV 10—serotypes 1, 4, 5, 6B, 7f, 9v, 14, 18C, 19F, 23F

PCT 13—all serotypes in PCV 10 and serotypes 3, 6A, 19A

Table 6.1: Vaccine–dose, route and site of administration

Vaccine	Dose	Route of administration	Site
BCG	0.1 ml	Intradermal	Left shoulder
OPV	2 drops	Oral	
Hep B	0.5 ml	Intramuscular	Anterolateral aspect of thigh (left)
Pentavalent	0.5 ml	Intramuscular	Anterolateral aspect of thigh (left)
DPT	0.5 ml	Intramuscular	Anterolateral aspect of thigh (left)
IPV	0.5 ml	Intramuscular	Anterolateral aspect of thigh (right)
Rotavirus vaccine	5 drops	Oral	
Measles vaccine	0.5 ml	Subcutaneous	Posterior aspect of right arm
TT	0.5 ml	Intramuscular	Arm or anterolateral aspect of thigh
FIPV	0.1 ml	Subcutaneous	Right arm
PCV	0.5 ml	Intramuscular	Anterolateral aspect of right thigh

Table 6.2: Immunization time table (IAP)

Age	Vaccine
Birth	BCG, OPV 0, Hep-B1
6 weeks	DTwP-1, IPV1, Hep-B2, Hib 1, rotavirus 1, PCV1
10 weeks	DTwP-2, IPV2, Hib 2, rotavirus 2, PCV2
14 weeks	DTwP-2, IPV3, Hib 3, rotavirus 3, PCV3
6 months	OPV 1, Hep-B3
9 months	OPV 2, MMR-1
9–12 months	Typhoid conjugate vaccine
12 months	Hep-A1
15 months	MMR2, varicella 1, PCV booster
16–18 months	DTwP B1, DTaP B1, IPV B1, Hib B1
18 months	Hep-A2
2 years	Typhoid booster
4–6 years	DTwPB2, DTaPB2, OPV3, varicella 2, typhoid booster
10–12 years	T dap/Td, HPV

IAP recommended vaccine for routine use

Table 6.3: Immunization schedule (UIP)

Age	Vaccine
At Birth	BCG, OPV Zero dose, Hep-B-birth dose
6 weeks	OPV-1, Pentavalent 1, Rota 1, fIPV-1, PCV-1
10 weeks	OPV-2, Pentavalent 2, Rota 2,
14 weeks	OPV-3, Pentavalent 3, Rota 3, fIPV-2, PCV-2
9 months	Measles 1/MR-1, Vit A, JE-1*, PCV-B
16–24 month	DPT first booster dose, OPV booster dose, measles 2/MR-2, JE-2 age
5–6 years (up to 7 years of age)	DPT second booster dose
10 years	TT
16 years	TT

*JE in 231 endemic district

Storage: PCV is freeze sensitive vaccine. It should be stored at temperature ranging between +2°C and +8°C in ice lined refrigerator (ILR).

Schedule: PCV in the UIP is recommended for infants (up to 1 year of age).

Three doses, 2 primary doses and 1 booster is given.

- PCV1 first dose—at 6 weeks of age.
- PCV2 second dose—at 14 weeks of age.
- PCVb booster—at 9 months of age.

If the doses are delayed within the first year of life. Delayed doses must be separated by a minimum interval of 2 months.

Route, site and dosage: PCV vaccine should be given at anterolateral aspect of right thigh intramuscular with autodisable syringe (AD syringe) (Table 6.1).

Dose: 0.5 ml

Efficacy: Efficacy is more than 80%.

Coadministration: PCV can be coadministered with UIP vaccines.

Contraindication: It is a safe vaccine.

1. Children with severe allergic reaction to a prior dose or to pentavalent vaccine.
2. Children with severe illness.

Side effects: Irritability, crying, swelling and tenderness at injection site, transient fever >39°C (102°F).

Open vial policy: Open vial policy is applicable to PCV 13.

Age limit for vaccination

1. BCG can be given up to 1 year of age.
2. DPT can be given up to 5–6 years of age (not beyond 1 year of age).
3. Pentavalent vaccine should be given under 1 year of age.
4. Measles vaccine can be given up to 5 years of age.
5. JE vaccine can be given up to 15 years of age.
6. IPV vaccine should be given at 14 weeks of age. Along with pentavalent vaccine in delayed cases, IPV can be given maximum up to 1 year of age.
7. Rotavirus vaccine can be given up to 1 year of age. Afterward no need because child acquired immunity up to age due to natural infection.
8. PCV can be given up to 1 year of age.

COMBINED MMR VACCINATION

It is combined vaccine of measles, mumps and rubella.

INFLUENZA VACCINATION

It is killed virus given in dose 0.2 ml by subcutaneous route.

TYPHOID VACCINATION

It protects against typhoid fever given as intramuscular injection just after school entry.

Vaccination against hepatitis B (Tables 6.1 and 6.2)

IAP recommended vaccine for high risk children:

1. Influenza vaccine—after 6 months
2. Meningococcal vaccine—after 4–6 months
3. Japanense encephalitis vaccine—after 12 months of age
4. Cholera vaccine—after 12 months of age
5. Rabies vaccine—any age
6. Yellow fever vaccine—after 2–3 years of age
7. Pneumococcal polysaccharide vaccine (PPSV 23)—after 2 years of age.

High Risk Category Children

HIV infection, chronic cardiac, pulmonary, hematologic, renal, liver disease, children on long-term steroid, immunosuppressive or radiation therapy, diabetes mellitus, cerebrospinal fluid leak, cochlear implant, malignancies, functional or anatomic asplenia, hyposplenia. During disease out breaks, laboratory workers, travelers, children having pets in home. With higher threats of being bitten by dogs.

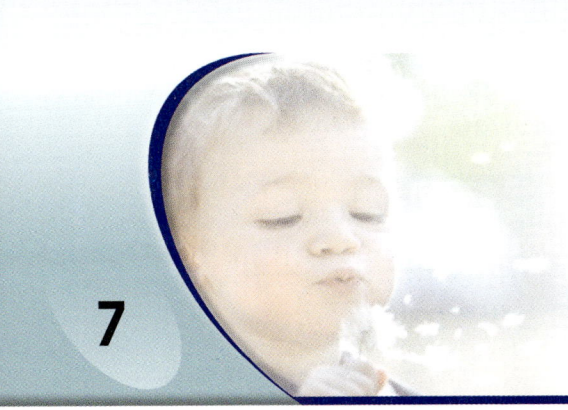
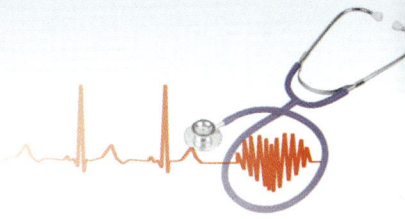

7

Nutritional Disorders

MALNUTRITION
(PROTEIN ENERGY MALNUTRITION)

Definition

Malnutrition is a clinical condition due to complete or incomplete deficiency or excess of food or constituents of food.

In our country malnutrition means under-nutrition. 25% of total disease in children comprise to this group. It is an important cause of morbidity and predispose to other disease.

Old name of protein calorie malnutrition is now better termed protein energy mal-nutrition.

Magnitude of the Problem

Prevalence of malnutrition is extremely widespread in our community. Very few cases of severe malnutrition are brought to medical centres. The major part of which is hidden and out of our knowledge which show *'malnu-trition Iceberg'* because of lack of awareness.

Protein Calorie Malnutrition (Protein Energy Malnutrition)

In every type of malnutrition there is mixed deficiency of both protein and calories. Marasmus and kwashiorkor both conditions result, from protein and calories deficiency. But marasmus results mainly due to calorie deficiency and kwashiorkor results from mainly protein deficiency.

EVALUATION AND PATHOGENESIS

There are two theories about pathogenesis of malnutrition.

1. **Classical theory:** According to this theory kwashiorkor is due to mainly protein deficiency and marasmus is due to calorie deficiency. But both are deficient in both conditions.
2. **Newer theory of free radicals:** Free oxygen radicals are normally buffered by proteins and neutralized by antioxidants such as vitamins A, C and E and selenium. In malnourished child deficiency of these nutrients in presence of infection or aflatoxin may damage liver cells giving rise to kwashiorkor.

FACTORS CAUSING MALNUTRITION

Causes

I. Deficiency of food intake

i. Due to poverty—poor person cannot purchase sufficient diet.
ii. Incomplete diet due to ignorance—such as thinking that commercially available food is good; urban, educated women discontinue breastfeeding.

iii. Defective feeding habits, e.g. dilution of milk, starvation, during infectious disease, etc. prolonged breastfeeding.

iv. Inadequate intake due to emotional deprivation.

v. Inadequate intake due to false beliefs and habits—particular food is hot or cold wrong customs, beliefs.

vi. Insufficient intake due to diseases in the body
   • Cleft palate, stomatitis, hypertrophic pyloric stenosis
   • Infections—causing anorexia.

vii. A large families—mother remains busy in care of large families so few children remain neglected.

viii. Inadequate distribution of food in family. Women and preschool children often receive less food than economically active male adult.

ix. Defective digestion—infections of gastrointestinal tract, liver diseases.

II. Defective digestion

Infection of gastrointestinal tract, liver diseases.

III. Defective absorption

Digested food is not absorbed from the gut and components of food are not reached in the blood. Thus, producing state of malnutrition, e.g. Giardia infection, lactose intolerance, milk allergy, diarrhea, vomiting, worm infestation.

IV. Absorption is adequate but metabolism is defective

For example, in infection, liver diseases, tuberculosis, diabetes.

V. Assimilation of nutrients is improper

Low birth weight, mental retardation, renal disease.

VI. Increased demand of nutrients during stress, disease, administration of antibiotics, catabolic or anabolic drugs.

Assessment of Nutritional Status

Nutritional status can be assessed in following ways:
   i. *History of dietary intake:* Cereals, vegetarian diet, pulses, fruits, eggs, etc. and assess daily consumption of proteins, calories, fat and roughly vitamins and minerals.
   ii. Clinical examination of signs of malnutrition and deficiency of vitamins and minerals (e.g. hair changes, xerosis).
   iii. Anthropometric measurements: Weight, height, skin fold thickness, mild arm circumference, chest and head circumference ratio, calf and foot length ratio, subcutaneous fat.
   iv. Biochemical tests, e.g. Hb level, serum proteins, amino acid level in blood and urine, hydroxy proteins excretion in urine, urinary and creatinine ratio, serum transferrin, etc.

Why common in children?

The state of malnutrition is common in children because they are growing and children must consume enough nitrogenous food to maintain a positive nitrogen balance while adult need only maintain nitrogen equilibrium.

Malnutrition worsen infection and infection worsen malnutrition

Malnutrition worsen infection

   i. Nutrition is basic determinant of resistance against infection. Resistance of human against organism is adversely effected due to reduced antibody formation due to lack of protein.
   ii. Skin and mucous membrane continuity is effected so it does not offer effective physical barrier against infection.

The period of infectivity is prolonged because increased duration of replication and shedding of pathogens. Recovery is delayed and infection is more severe.

Infection worsen malnutrition, due to:
1. Reduced appetite or food is not given by parents due to false belief.
2. Defective absorption and digestion of food.
3. Loss of electrolytes, protein, e.g. in diarrhea, in hookworm infestation.
4. Increased protein demand due to increased catabolism during infection.
5. Protein is lost due to tissue breakdown and in exudates.

Classification

Types of malnutrition:
1. **Stunting—low height for age:** It is an indicator of chronic malnutrition, results of long duration, food deprivation and/or chronic disease.
2. **Wasting—low weight for height:** It is an indicator of acute malnutrition, result of more recent food defect or illness.
3. **Underweight—low weight for age:** It is a combined indicator of both acute and chronic malnutrition, under weight may be classified into two:
   a. Moderate malnutrition—if weight is less than –2SD
   b. Severe acute malnutrition—if weight is less than –3SD (SAM).

Indicators of growth: SD score, length for age, weight for age, weight for length/height.

SD score	Length for age	Weight for age	Weight for length/height
O median	Normal	Normal	Normal
Below –1SD	Normal	Normal	Normal
Below –2SD	Stunting	Low weight	Wasting
Below –3SD stunting	Severe	Severe low weight	Severe
	cSAM	wasting	

In wasting weight for length is less. In stunting weight-for-age is less but weight-for-height may be low, normal or more because length is less.

WHO Classification

The latest classification of children (under 5 years of age) with severe malnutrition divides them into two categories based presence of pitting of nutritional basis
a. Edematous
b. Non-edematous

Presence of edema in used as independent tool to screen cases of malnutrition as it has strong association with mortality.

Kwashiorkor represents the more worst form of edematous malnutrition when striking clinical features such as the skin (flaky paint dermatosis/crazy pavement sign) and hair changes are present.

IAP guideline for grading malnutrition

As for IAP guideline weight for length/height for sex is taken.

Weight grade

Median normal
Less than –1SD mild malnutrition
Less than –2SD moderate malnutrition
Less than –3SD severe malnutrition (severe acute malnutrition—SAM)

CLINICAL CLASSIFICATION

1. Marasmus
2. Kwashiorkor
3. Marasmic kwashiorkor

NUTRITIONAL MARASMUS

This state of malnutrition is common in infancy and below 3 years of age.

How Marasmus Occurs?

Mother's milk is adequate for the infant only up to about 6 months of age. In case of lactation failure it is insufficient even up to 6 months. Artificial feeding by milk of cow, buffalo is done to compensate it. If it diluted then nutritional constituents are insufficient in it. Chances of contamination are also more resulting infections: Infection causes loss of appetite and infant receive inadequate nutrition resulting loss of weight gradually and gradually. Thus, producing clinical stage of marasmus.

Clinical Features

a. Child is usually infant and below 3 years of age. Early features are irritability, hunger and craves for food. Child is alert initially, later on becomes apathetic.
b. Loss of weight occurs. Usually body weight is less than 60% of expected weight-for-age. Low BMI.
c. There is gradual loss of subcutaneous fat from the different parts of the body. Muscles become atrophic. Marasmus is classified according to loss of subcutaneous fat as follows:

Grade I: Loss of subcutaneous fat in axilla and abdomen and gluteal region.
Grade II: Loss of subcutaneous fat in axilla, groin, abdomen and gluteal region.
Grade III: Loss of subcutaneous fat in axilla, groin, abdomen, gluteal region, chest and spine.
Grade IV: Loss of subcutaneous fat in axilla, groin, abdomen, gluteal region, chest, spine and even buccal region.

Buccal pad of fat is depleted at last because higher portion of fatty acids are stored there (Fig. 7.1).
It gives child 'skin and bone appearance'. Diminished buccal pad of fat gives him 'old man appearance.'

d. Eyes are sunken and lose their lusture.
e. Body has subnormal temperature and pallor over face and pulse remain slow because basal metabolic rate is low.

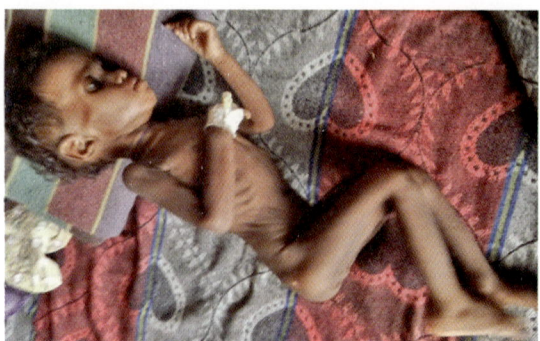

Fig. 7.1: Marasmus.

f. Infections are frequent afterward recovery is delayed.
g. Edema is absent from body. Signs of vitamins and minerals deficiency are seen.
h. Mood changes (mental changes) are absent.
i. Constipation is frequent but diarrhea may occur.
j. Skin is dry inelastic and prone to infection. Loose folds of skin are prominent at gluteal region on inner side.
k. Abdomen is distended due to wasting, hypotonia of muscles and gaseous distension.
  i. Mid arm circumference reduced.
  ii. Clinical features of the disease causing malnutrition.
  iii. Biochemical changes
l. Anemia is mild to moderate.
m. Serum protein slightly reduced.

Essential features of marasmus (minimum diagnostic criteria)
  i. Growth retardation as evidence by loss of weight, height.
  ii. Skin and bone appearance due to loss of subcutaneous fat.
  iii. Edema absent.

Non-essential features (variable)
  i. Hair changes absent.
  ii. Dermatosis absent.
  iii. Hungry instead of anorexia.
  iv. Mineral and vitamin's deficiency.

KWASHIORKOR

'Kwashiorkor' is a clinical syndrome that results from a severe deficiency of 'proteins and inadequate calorie intake' (Fig. 7.2).

The word kwashiorkor was originally given by Cicely Williams (1930), which means 'red boy' because of characteristic pigmentary changes in skin. But the better interpretation of term means 'deposed child' due to arrival of another child.

Etiology and History

After the age of 6 months, mother milk is insufficient to infant and weaning food is introduced. If due to poverty and due to another reason food intake is inadequate; in this time child requires first class protein which is not available in his food. Apart from this it is common age for respiratory tract infection and diarrhea which causes loss of weight.

If child suffers from infections, e.g. measles, whooping cough, tuberculosis; they are helpful in producing malnutrition. Apart from that loss of protein from body, infections, hemorrhage, burn or nephrosis or reduced

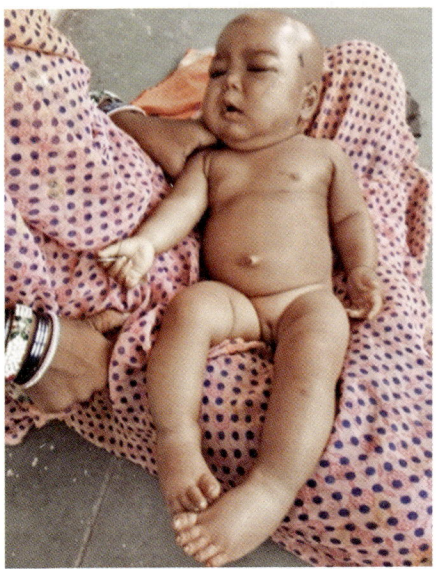

Fig. 7.2: Kwashiorkor.

protein synthesis due to liver disease are also other causes of malnutrition.

Clinical Features

Kwashiorkor occurs between 4 months to 5 years of age.

Essential Features

   i. Growth retardation
  ii. Edema
 iii. Mood changes or apathy

Complete Clinical Features

a. Early features are lethargy, apathy, irritability. He does not take interest what is happening in surrounding. Further advancements include growth retardation and loss of muscular tissue, loss of weight. At the time of edema weight may be normal.

b. Anorexia is a common feature of kwashiorkor.

c. *Edema:* It usually present from initial stage and is pitting type. It is due to low serum protein and anemia. It should be differentiated from edema of other origin (liver, heart, kidney disease). First, it is on dependent part then it involves whole body.

d. Skin changes

   i. Skin is dry and scaly and usually light colored, pyoderma occurs commonly.

  ii. Classical dermatosis is in areas of hyperpigmentation intervened by areas of raw red skin. Best characteristic of skin changes is hyperpigmentation (black patches) appear over certain localized area especially over pressure sites and flexors known as crazy pavement dermatosis. It exfoliates and peeling of plaques resemble peeling areas of paint. Hence, term 'flaky paint dermatosis'. The discoloration of skin is reddish or purple and not black.

Darkening appears in irritated areas but not those exposed to sunlight a contrast to situation in pellagra. Dyspigmentation may occur in these areas after desquamation or occur in generalized form.

iii. Other form of dermatosis dry, enelastic mosaic skin and follicular keratosis may occur but are not pathognomonic of kwashiorkor.

Hair Changes

a. Hairs become light colored, sparse, so may lead to a kind of alopecia with areas of baldness.

b. Hairs are brittle and silky and easily pluckable.

c. Hairs show bands of light and dark colors due to inadequate, adequate nutrition for long period called *'flag'* sign'. But it is occassionally seen.

d. Infections and parasitic infestations are common. Diarrhea, anorexia, worm infestation and respiratory tract infection occur frequently. Dehydration worsen the condition acutely.

e. *Muscles:* Muscles are weak, thin and atrophic.

f. *Diarrhea:* Diarrhea is common due to following reasons.

1. Reduction of digestive enzymes due to atrophy of pancreatic exocrine cells.
2. Superadded infections in the gut.
3. Atrophy of gut mucosa causing villous atrophy and malabsorption.
4. Iron deficiency associated with it causes villous damages in intestinal epithelium.

g. Liver is enlarged, soft, lower margin appear rounded. Liver initially small then enlarge afterward.

h. Sign of vitamins and mineral deficiency present. Anemia is always present. Signs of vitamins A, B, C and D complexes are also seen.

Investigations

1. **Biochemical changes**
   a. Serum protein is low especially serum albumin, gamma globulins are increased.
   b. Anemia is moderate or severe.
   c. Serum enzymes are reduced in blood (pancreatic enzymes).
   d. Serum iron and copper low.
   e. Blood cholesterol low.
   f. Water and electrolyte disturbances, decreased osmolarity of blood, low Na, potassium and magnesium, phosphate.

2. **Skiagram chest:** If childhood tuberculosis is suspected.

MARASMIC KWASHIORKOR

Mixed picture of marasmus and kwashiorkor is seen. The features of marasmus are seen more and edema is present.

Comparison between kwashiorkor and marasmus is given in Table 7.1.

Treatment of marasmus and kwashiorkor is same (*refer to* page 133)

Table 7.1: Comparison between kwashiorkor and marasmus

		Kwashiorkor	Marasmus
1.	Age	4 months–5 years	Below 3 years
2.	Growth retardation	Present	Present
3.	Muscles and loss of subcutaneous fat	Less	More
4.	Weight	Reduced	Extremely reduced
5.	Edema	Always present	Absent
6.	Hair changes	Silky, brittle, and easily pluckable	No
7.	Skin and dermatosis	Hyperpigmentation	No
8.	Appetite	Reduced	Increased
9.	Hepatomegaly	Fatty liver	No
10.	Signs of vitamins deficiency	Severe	Moderate
11.	Infections and worm	More infestation	Less
12.	Anemia	Severe	Moderate

Wasting: Wasting is divided into two:
1. Severe acute malnutrition (SAM)
2. Moderate acute malnutrition (MAM).

SEVERE ACUTE MALNUTRITION (SAM)

When child suffers from inadequate nutrition repeated infection fat of the body is utilized to meat for energy and metabolism which results reduction of fat from different parts of the body gradually and wasting of muscles.

It results following clinical picture. Wasting is assessed by skin and bone appearance of the body. Skin becomes loose due to lack of subcutaneous fat and muscle wasting which results on chest ribs are seen, loose skin on limbs, folds of skin on buttocks, *monkey face* due to loss of buccal fat, abdomen is pro-tuberant.

Edema: Edema in due to hypoproteinemia, anemia due to lack of protein and energy. It is first seen on feet then increases above and may cover whole body (anasarca).

SAM child is diagnosed by following criteria (6 months to 59 months of age) (any one)
1. Weight for length is below –3 SD
2. Mid-upper arm circumference (MUAC) is below 11.5 cm
3. Presence of edema on both feet. Exclude cardiac, renal, hepatic causes of edema.

SAM child below 6 months of age (criteria) (any one)

1. Weight for length below –3SD
2. Severe wasting
3. Edema on both feet.

Mid-upper Arm Circumference

Mid-upper arm circumference (MUAC) is reliable criteria for diagnosis of SAM and MAM. Child mid-upper arm circumference of all baby from 6 month to 5 years of age is about constant because during this period muscle develops in place of fat.

It is determined by MUAC tape. Tape has structure as shown in Fig. 7.7.

Anthropometric Measurements

Weight recording

Weight recording in an essential part of examination of malnourished child. Weight machine should be strong and durable which can record about 10 gm weight correctly. Digital (electronic) machine and which has facility of tare is useful which reduces risk of error of recording of weight.

Method (Fig. 7.3)

1. Child should be unclothed.
2. Keep a cloth on scale pan of the weight machine.
3. Keep the weight scale at zero by pressing tare button. If other machine is used having sling or pent then put at zero after putting him.
4. Keep the baby at pan slowly (or in sling or pent).
5. Weight up to when baby becomes quit.
6. Record the weight and write.

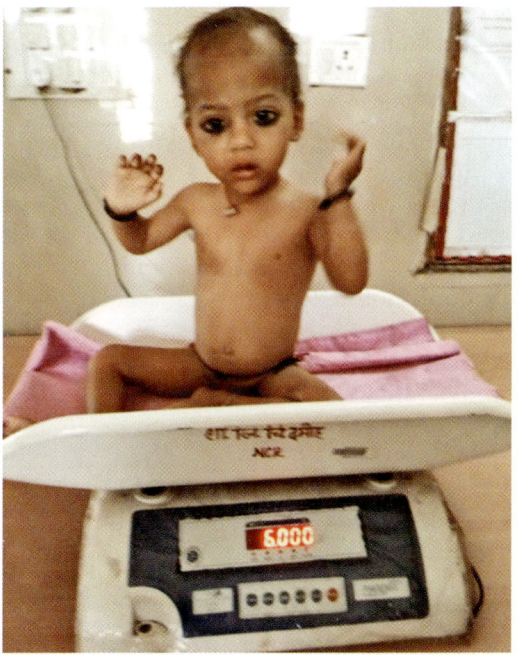

Fig. 7.3: Weight recording.

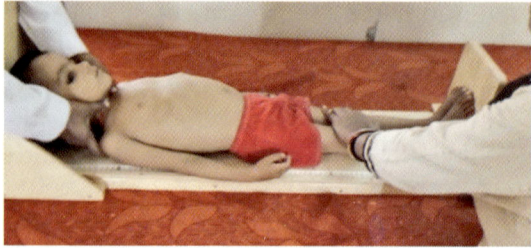

Fig. 7.4: Measurement of length.

Measurement of Length/Height

If child is less than two years age or age is not known and length is less than 87 cm then take the length in recumbent posture.

If child is more than two years of age or age in not known and length is more than 87 cm then take the height in standing position.

If child is less than two years of age and difficult to lying down then take the height in standing position and add 0.7 cm to covert it in to length.

If child is more than two years of age and cannot stand then take length in recumbent position and deduct 0.7 cm to convert in height.

Measurement of Length

Length of child is measured with the special instrument called infantometer in recumbent position or stadiometer. It consists of a head board towards head and sliding tool piece on other side. Keep the infantometer on table. keep fine cloth or paper on the board, keep shoes off and clip, etc. on hairs.

Take help of another person he/she should stand behind head board.

Keep the baby in lying down position so that his back is towards board, head is supported and keep it opposite the head board (Fig. 7.4).

Keep the head by pressing it so head is touching the head board and pressing the hairs.

Keep the head straight so that eyes of the baby face upward and vision line in at right angle to board.

Keep the baby in middle of board and do not shift him frequently.

Other person should stand along with the board he should do:
1. When baby is laid down correctly then he should support feet.
2. Press the legs strongly and gently and keep the knee straight.
   Slide the foot pad to keep the foot pad opposite to side of feet of baby strongly.
3. Record and write the length.

Measurement of Height

Stadiometer is used for measurement of height which consists of vertical back board, fixed base board and sliding head board (Figs 7.5 and 7.6).

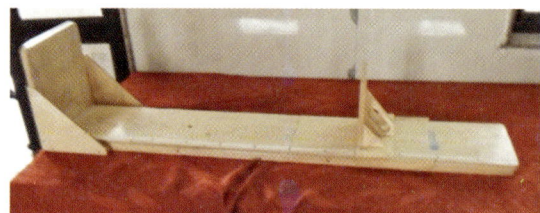

Fig. 7.5: Stadiometer.

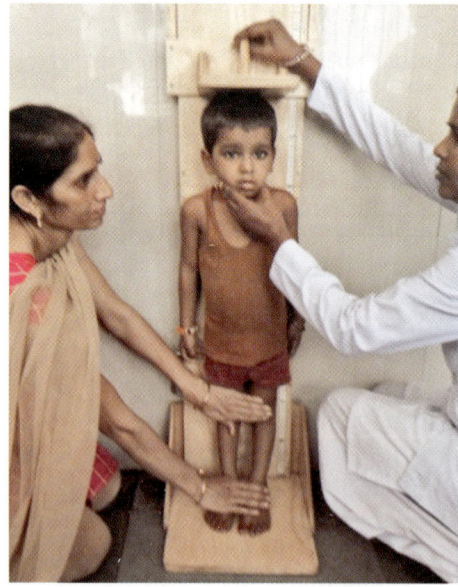

Fig. 7.6: Measurement of height.

Keep stadiometer at floor, remove socks and shoes from the baby.

Measurement of height requires help of two persons.

One person should sit near feet of baby on knee and do.

1. Help the child to stand fit to vertical board so posterior part of head, shoulder, hip, legs are adjoining to vertical board.
2. Hold to ankle and knee so lower limb should be straight and ankle flat.
3. Avoid to stand the child on finger.
4. Small child may not stand straight so push his abdomen slowly.

Second person should bent himself up to level of child's face and do

1. Keep the head of child straight so he/she see parallel, this can be done by thumb and index finger.
2. Pull the head board down so it fits and press hairs of head.
3. Measure height and write.

Measurement of MUAC (Figs 7.7 and 7.8)

1. Left upper arm is chosen for MUAC, identify acromian process, put a mark.
2. Fold the elbow at 90° angle, put a mark.
3. Put one end of the tape (MUAC tape, Fig. 7.7) at the upper part of shoulder and keep the tape (Fig. 7.8) up to folded elbow.
4. Put a mark on skin of upper arm in middle of upper part of shoulder to lower part of elbow.
5. Now keep the baby hand straight so it is straight at thigh.
6. Fold the MUAC tape around the middle of arm, keep the end of tape at slit of the tape.

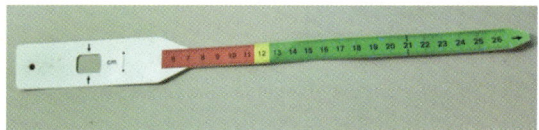

Fig. 7.7: MUAC tape.

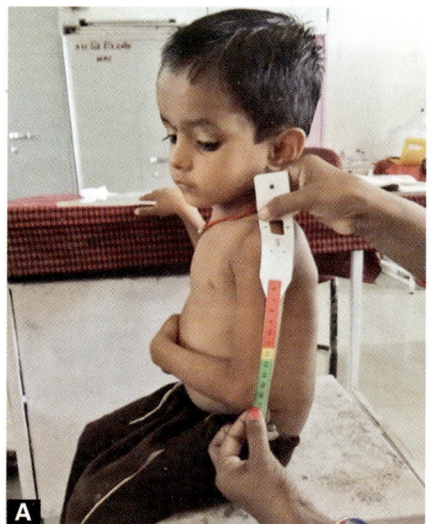

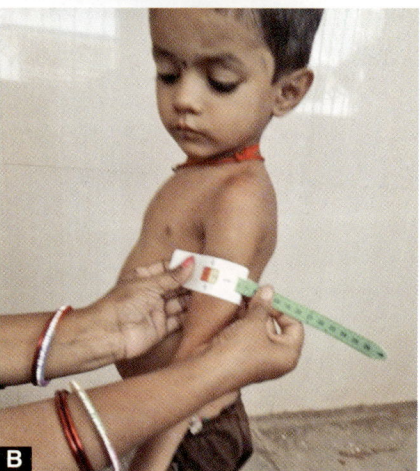

Fig. 7.8A and B: Measurement of MUAC.

7. Do not keep loose or tight around arm.
8. See the circumference from window of the tape (arrow mark).

Color

Green—12.5 cm or more good nutritional status

Yellow—11.5 to 12.4 cm moderate malnutrition

Red—below 11.5 cm severe malnutrition.

Edema: Bilateral pitting edema is diagnosed by pressing the skin by thumb, then lift thumb, pitting remains at pressure point (Figs 7.9 and 7.10).

Classification

+ edema up to feet only

++ edema at both feet, legs, knee, hands, upper limbs

+++ edema at both feet, legs, hands, upper limbs, face (anasarca).

Reactive adaptation: SAM child body adapt himself to survive in low calories by the process, called reactive adaptation since body is taking less energy. Energy is taken from fat, muscle's protein, intestinal protein.

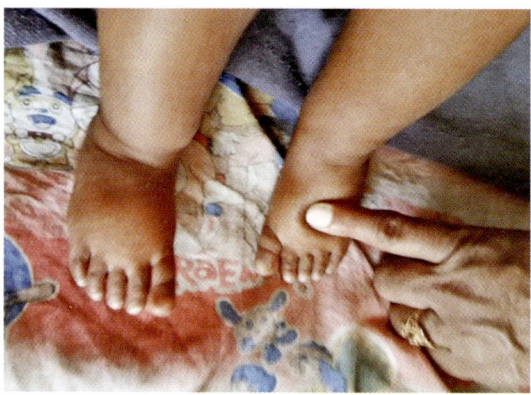

Fig. 7.9: Test for pitting.

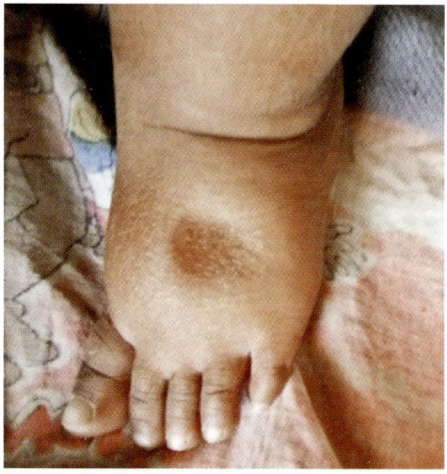

Fig. 7.10: Pitting edema.

Body change itself physically and metabolically and this process is called *reactive adaptation.*

In malnourished baby energy is spared by:
a. Decrease in physical activity and growth
b. Reduce basal metabolism by:
   • Reduce turnover of protein
   • Reduce functional reserves of oxygen
   • Slow down the sodium potassium pump at the level of cell membrane.
c. Reduce inflammatory and immune response.

Effects of Reactive Adaptation

Reactive adaptation affects every cell and organ of the body.

Liver: Glucose formation is reduced so there is always risk of hypoglycemia and hypothermia, excretion of dietary protein and toxins is reduced. It affects intake of food. SAM baby should be protected from not feeding for long duration. If he is capable to take feed, orally, give him orally or by gastric tube. Proteins are given in limited amount so it does not affect liver.

Kidney: Kidney capacity to excrete waste product and sodium is reduced so by feeding or rehydration, water comes in circulation easily.

Heart: Heart become small and weak, if there is any overload of fluid in circulation it may cause heart failure and death.

Intestine: Intestine secretes less amount of acid and enzymes. Villi become flat. Motility of intestine is reduced so bacteria stay for long time resulting injury to mucosa and reduction in bile salt conjugation.

So, at the beginning diet is given in small quantity as per intestine capacity.

To reduce excess (overload) of fluid diet should be enteral not parenteral. Intestinal mucosa repair is fast in presence of diet in the lumen of intestine. Villi regeneration is fast.

Sodium: Sodium leaks from sodium pump because their slow activity and reduced number due to lack of energy, this results excess of the sodium in cells of the body so potassium leaks from the cells and excreted through urine. It causes electrolyte imbalance, lack of appetite, fluid overload and heart failure.

So, *sodium intake should be restricted in SAM baby and potassium intake is increased.* Magnesium also should be given because it helps in potassium entry into the cells.

Muscles: Reduction of intracellular nutrients and muscle glycogen store reserve.

Red cell mass: In malnourished cell reduction in red cell mass occurs so it lefts iron. Glucose and amino acids are needed to convert harmful iron to ferritin so it can be stored.

Free iron enhance growth of pathogens and produce free radicals which harm cell membrane.

So iron is not given in initial phase of treatment of SAM child. Vitamins and minerals are given so they can help assimilating free radicals.

Reactive Adaptation and Management

Organ	Changes	Results	Management
Liver	Glucose formation less, excretion of dietary protein toxin less	Chances of hypoglycemia, hypothermia, loss of appetite	Frequent feeding, protein is given in limited amount in beginning
Kidney	Sodium, excretory product excretion less	Water comes in circulation	Restrict sodium
Heart	Small and weak	Chances of CCF more	Avoid IV fluids
Intestine	Produce less acid and enzyme, villi become flat, motility reduced	Bile acid conjugation less, absorption less, more chances of stasis of organisms, destroy much	frequent but small feed, food stimulate formation of villi
Cells	Sodium potassium pump weak	Sodium becomes in excess, potassium less (electrolyte imbalance)	Give less or no sodium, give potassium, give magnesium which help potassium entrance
Muscle	Intracellular nutrients loss	Glycogen store less	Give calories
Red cell mass	Less, leave iron, not convert into ferritin due to lack of protein, amino-acids	Free iron damage cell membrane, enhance growth of pathogens	Give no iron at beginning, give vitamins and minerals which conjugate free iron

Management of Malnutrition

Mild to moderate malnutrition.

Adequate amount of protein and calories is the basis of treatment.

1. **Calories:** Calories are provided 150 kcal/kg/day. Frequent feeding (about 6 times in a day) may be required.
2. **Proteins:** Proteins intake should be 3 g/kg/day milk or other sources of proteins

such are khichdi dal as vegetable protein mixture.

3. **Fats:** Oils are added to increase the energy.

4. **Vitamins and minerals** are given for appropriate duration.

Complications leading to death
- Hypoglycemia
- Hypothermia
- Electrolyte imbalances
- Heart failure
- Infections

Examine the clinical complications (triage)

Triage in a screening of emergency sign in sick baby.

1. Airway—any complication
2. Breathing—fast respiration, slow respiration, apnea, chest indrawing.
3. Circulation —pulse—normal or fast, signs of shock
4. Convulsion—present or not
5. Coma
6. Vomiting, diarrhea
7. Hypothermia—axillary temperature <35°C
8. Edema
9. Dehydration
10. Fever
11. Skin disorders
12. Anemia
13. Hemorrhage

Nutritional rehabilitation centre (NRC)

NRC is an institutional centre for management of SAM child. Child is admitted in these centres for feeding, treatment under supervision, daily assessment. Mother is taught how to keep cook, care of food, cleanliness and necessary precautions for it so when she returns to home she can do it herself.

Child in kept in these centres for 14 days. After discharge *follow up* is done and child is examined four times at 15 days intervals.

NRC admission criteria (any one)

1. Weight for length less than −3SD
2. MUAC less than 11.5 cm
3. Edema on both feet (pitting)

Steps in NRC

Food is given to child if baby takes at well then he passed appetite test, eagerness for feed is important not the consumed amount.

If baby resent for feed baby is failed in appetite test.

Appetite Test

- Give 35 gm of *special feed* and clean water. If baby takes all the amount he is passed in appetite test. Keep in phase 2. If he do not consume—*fail* in appetite test. Keep in phase 1.
- If child is less than 1 year of age and he has not started complementary feeding, give F-100 as per amount given in age for appetite test.

SAM child who has good appetite, without clinical complication, no edema.

These children can be managed at home or at NRC.

C-SAM: Child which has failed in appetite test and/or clinical complications are present and/or edema is present. Weight is reducing continuously for 2 weeks or weight is constant in three follow-up.

Clinical complications are diarrhea, vomiting, severe anemia, high fever, hypothermia, drowsiness, anorexia, weight loss, long-term cough.

Management

History and examination

History related to feeding, illness, breastfeeding, weaning, vomiting, diarrhea, loss of appetite, fever, cough, immunization, infections, disease, HIV infection, contact with tuberculosis.

Examination—alert, drowsy, stupor, coma, weight, length /height/MUAC, pulse, sign of shock, respiration, any clinical features of triage, hair, skin eyes (signs of vit A deficiency) pallor, sign of dehydration, general and systemic examination.

Laboratory Investigations

1. Hb%, blood glucose
2. Total and differential WBC counts
3. Urine-routine and microscope examination
4. X-ray chest
5. Mantoux test
6. Blood for malarial parasite
7. Serum electrolyte—sodium, potassium, calcium, phosphorus, serum albumin
8. HIV
9. Other investigations as per clinical condition.

MANAGEMENT OF SAM CHILD—10 STEPS

Phase 1: Stabilization Phase (0–2 Days)

Step 1. Treatment and Prevention of Hypoglycemia

Hypoglycemia in SAM is diagnosed if blood glucose level is <54 mg/dl. Clinically, it manifests as lethargy, unconsciousness, seizures, peripheral circulatory failure or hypothermia.

Management

1. Give 50 ml of 10% glucose or sucrose—orally or by nasogastric tube (50 ml water mixed with 1 tsf of sugar).
2. Give 5 ml/kg of 10% dextrose intravenously followed by 50 ml of 10% dextrose or sucrose solution by nosogastric tube.
   Assess blood glucose at every 30 min till it becomes normal.
3. Feeding: F-75 every 2 hourly given (starter diet) continued 2 hourly interval.
4. Give antibiotic because hypoglycemia, hypothermia, infection generally coexist.

Starter feed composition F-75	
Dry skimmed milk powder	2.5 gm
Sugar	7 gm
Murmura powder (without salt)	3.5 gm
Vegetable oil	3 gm
Water to make	100 ml

F-75 Second method		
Contents	*Non-cereal*	*Cereal based*
Cow milk	30 ml	28 ml
Sugar	7 gm	6.5 gm
Vegetable oil	2 gm	2 gm
Puffy rice	–	3.5 gm
Water to make		100 ml

F-75 Nutritive value per 100 ml		
Contents	*Non-cereal*	*Cereal based*
Calories	77.9 kcal	75.0 kcal
Protein	0.97 gm	1.1 gm
Lactose	1.2 gm	1.2 gm

Catch up Diets

F-100 Composition	
Dry skimmed milk powder	8 gm
Sugar	5 gm
Vegetable oil	6 gm
Water to make	100 ml

F-100 Second method		
Contents	*Non-cereal*	*Cereal based*
Cow milk	90 ml	75 ml
Sugar	7.5 gm	2.5 gm
Vegetable oil	2 gm	2 gm
Puffy rice	–	7 gm
Water to make	100 ml	100 ml

Step 2. Prevention and Treatment of Hypothermia

If axillary temperature is less than 35°C or rectal temperature is less than 35.5°C, it is called hypothermia.

Management

- Clothes the baby with warm clothes.
- Provide heat by overhead warmer or other devise heater, etc.
- Feed the child, IV glucose may be given, give antibiotic along dextrose 10%
- Give oxygen 2 hourly.

Step 3. Treatment/Prevention of Dehydration

Assess the dehydration correctly with care because sodium intake in very harmful to edematous baby.

Treatment

1. Reduced osmolarity ORS
   - 5 ml/kg every 30 minutes interval in first 2 hours
   - 5–10 ml/kg every one hour interval up to 10 hours.
2. Give feeding F-75 alternate to reduced osmolarity ORS.
   ORS–F-75: ORS–F-75 (every 30 min interval).

Prevention

Give reduced osmolarity ORS at 5–10 ml/kg after each watery stool it replaces stool losses.

Step 4. Correction of Electrolyte Imbalance

Sodium excess exists in SAM child although plasma serum may be low.

1. Restrict sodium intake during initial phase of treatment.
2. Give supplemental potassium at 3–4 mEq/g/day for at least 2 weeks orally.
3. Magnesium sulphate 50% (equivalent to 4 mEq/ml) IM 0.3 ml/kg maximum 2 ml first day IM.

   Extra magnesium 0.2–0.3 ml/kg/day for 2 weeks orally.

Step 5. Treatment of Infections

Assess the child for any infection generally fever may be absent during infection in SAM child, generally gram-negative bacterial infections are common. Hypothermia and hypoglycemia may be associated with infection.

Treatment

1. Ampicillin 50 mg/kg/dose for 2 days parenteral, followed by oral amoxicillin 15 mg/kg 8 hourly for 5 days and gentamicin 7.5 mg/kg, or amikacin 15–20 mg/kg IM or IV once daily for 7 days.

If no improvement in 48 hours give ceftriaxione or cefataxime.

If other conditions (e.g. tuberculosis) exist give appropriate antibiotic.

Treatment of helminthiasis: All children should be given

- Albendazole—age 12–23 months—200 mg (5 ml)
- Above 24 months—400 mg (10 ml)

Prevention: Good hygiene

Vaccination specially measles vaccine timely.

Blood transfusion: Packed cell if Hb <4 mg/dl.

Step 6. Correct Micronutrient Deficiencies

One day	Give vit. A orally
6–12 months	1 lakh IU
>1 year	2 lakhs IU
0–5 months	50,000 IU

If sign of xerophthalmia: Same dose, repeated next day and after 2 weeks, is given orally. Atropine is also given topically.

Folic acid	1 mg/kg (give 5 mg on day 1)
Zink	2 mg/kg/day
Copper	0.2–0.3 mg/kg/day
Iron	3 mg/kg/day after stabilization

Step 7. Initiate Refeeding

- Start feeding as soon as possible as frequent as possible as small feeds orally or by nasogastric tube in semiconscious babies.
- Continue breastfeeding.
- Start with F-75 starter feeds every 2 hourly.

Starter diet is feed which gives 75 kcal and 0.9 gm protein in 100 ml in primary phase. It gives needs for body without affecting the various systems of body. Protein and sodium is less and carbohydrate is more which in tolerated by children well as per homeostatic system of body. Weight is not increased fast.

F-100 Nutritive value per 100 ml		
Contents	Non-cereal	Cereal based
Calories (kcal)	100	100
Protein (g)	2.9	2.9
Lactose (g)	3.8	3

Duration: Give F-75, 2 hourly in low appetite and complicated child and then increased gradually 3 or 4 hourly up to 3–7 days.

If child is having edema give fluid 100 ml per kg per day.

Phase 2: Transition Phase and Rehabilitation Phase (3–7 Days) (2–4 Weeks)

Step 8. To Achieve Catch up Growth

Once appetite returns, child in taking orally, edema is lost, child in clinically improved (e.g. alertness, smile). It is generally achieved in about 7 days.

F-75 is replaced with feeds which has higher caloric density (100 k cal/100 ml) and protein 2.5–3 g/100 ml.

Catch up growth

Growth of malnourished children is lag behind well nourished children when appropriate feed is given, his growth accelerates and achieves growth of normal child it is called catch up growth.

Criteria for transition phase to rehabilitation phase:

1. No hypoglycemia
2. No hypothermia
3. Good appetite
4. No diarrhea, no vomiting
5. Edema is decreasing

When child is going from transition to stabilization phase he can take F-100 diet liberally even up to 220 ml/per/kg day. Generally all children take 150 ml/per/kg day.

Duration: Give 3 hourly feeds.

Step 9. Sensory Stimulation

Child in kept in a play full atmosphere various toys, games, are used to achieve lovely atmosphere.

Step 10. Prepare for Follow-up after Recovery

Mother promoted in NRC is:
- To prepare food
- To give feed to children
- To bath and change clothes
- To play with child
- Teach mother about.

Supplementary food to 6 months–5 years child.
1. Different feeds and nutritive value
2. Way to give food
3. Cleanliness, feeding during illness

SAM BEFORE 6 MONTHS OF AGE

Causes of severe acute malnutrition before 6 months of age
1. Mother milk—not available
2. Insufficient mother milk
3. Repeated infections
4. Neglect child

Children before 6 months of age are very delicate if method of breastfeeding is not correct their sucking power is less, child sucks less so there is less production of milk. Mother thinks it as lactation failure.

Criteria for Diagnosis

1. Weight for length in less than –3 SD
2. Edema

Mid-upper arm circumference (MUAC) is not diagnostic criteria for children below the age of 6 months.

Criteria for admission in NRC

1. Baby fulfils criteria of SAM.
2. Breastfed baby not gaining weight.
3. Problem related to breastfeeding.

Management

1. If baby is not getting sufficient breast milk, correct feeding method repeated breast feeding.
2. Encourage mother for relactation.
3. If not possible give breast milk of other lady.
4. Use SST techniques to promote milk production.
5. Give supplementary feed if necessary.

Following options for feeding (without edema)

a. Give F-75 or extracted milk to maintain basic metabolism, starter diet should be without cereals.
b. During rehabilitation phase give only breast milk, help and encourage mother. F-100 is given as supplementary feed along with breastfeeding.

Supplementary Suckling Techniques (SSTs)

These techniques help in production of breast milk in mother having insufficient milk production.

Steps

1. Make diluted F-100 mix 35 ml of water in 100 ml of F-100 to make its volume 135 ml.
2. Use no. 8 nasogastric tube to give supplementary feed.
3. Cut the tip of the tube 1 mm obliquely.
4. Keep measured amount as per weight of diluted F-100 in a cup.
5. Put another end of nasogastric tube in a cup.
6. Cut end of the tube is putted at nipple of the breast of mother.
7. Tape is used to keep the tube is place.
8. When baby sucks the nipple, milk from cup comes at baby's mouth, he takes it.
9. Keep the cup 5–10 cm below the level of nipple to prevent sudden incoming of milk which he could not swallow. If child gains weight, gradually lower the cup even up to 30 cm below the level of nipple.
10. Health worker or caretaker should help and supervise.

Mechanism of Action

When baby sucks he takes supplementary feed (F-100) and satisfies. Suckling stimulate production of oxytocin and prolactin resulting more production of milk.

Duration

- Every 3 hourly child is given breastfeed or more.
- After one hour of breastfeed give diluted F-100.
- Give diluted F-100–135 ml/kg/day (100 kcal per kg/day) in 6–8 divided feeds.

Criteria for Discharge from NRC

1. All infections and other medical complications subsided. Weight gain satisfactory—weight gain for 3 consecutive days (>5 gm/kg/day), weight gain 15% of weight at admission.
2. Edema subsided
3. Child is eating on adequate amount of nutritious food (>75%)
4. Child is provided with micronutrient and immunization is updated.

Mother/Caretaker

1. Knows how to prepare appropriate foods and to feed the child.
2. Knows how to give prescribed medications vitamins, folic acid and iron at home.
3. Knows how to prepare appropriate toys and play with child.
4. Knows how to home treatment for diarrhea, fever and acute respiratory tract infections.
5. How to recognize the signs for which medical assistance must be sought.
6. Follow-up plan is discussed and understood.

Summary of Steps of Management of SAM Child in NRC

SAM child when brought to NRC for management, following steps are taken:

a. First assess the *triage* (emergency sign)
  1. If present manage for triage then keep him in phase 2.
  2. If not present take blood sample for estimation *glucose level*.
b. If blood glucose level is less than 54 mg/dl—treat hypoglycemia, then do the appetite test.
c. If blood glucose level is more than 54 mg/dl—do the appetite test.

  Do the *appetite test* and see the medical complications, edema.

  If *pass* in appetite test and child has no medical complications edema then keep him in phase 2. Give F-100/mixed diet.

  If *fail* in appetite test and child has medical complications edema, keep him in phase 1. Give F-75. When return of appetite and reduction in edema, no medical complication then keep him in *transitional phase*. Give him F-100/SF.

  When he has good appetite and no edema then switch him to *phase 2* and give him F-100/mixed diet.

  • When child in phase 2 achieves discharge criteria—discharge him from NRC.
  • Ask to attend for *follow-up* four times at 15 days interval.

Management at Community Level

SAM with complication—phase 1 treatment in NRC.

SAM without complication—outpatient therapeutic program (OTP).

Moderate acute malnutrition—supplementary feeding program (SFP).

Prevention of Malnutrition

Political commitment, improve food production and supplies fortification of feed iodination of common salt and supplementation of feed.

At family level

• Exclusive breastfeeding.
• Complementary feeding at the age of 6 months.
• Early weaning
• Vaccination
• Birth spacing

World level with the help of WHO, FAO, UNICEF, etc. intensify food program.

Feeding of infant below 6 months of age if no possibility of breastfeeding.

If SST is failed or mother is died and thus no possibility breastfeeding then alternative feeds are given.

1. Undiluted milk of cow, goat, buffalo
2. Commercial infant formula
3. Breastfeeding of other women (who is not HIV infected).

WET NURSING

Management of HIV Infected SAM

Anti-retroviral medicine given after treatment of SAM after 2 weeks to reduce harm due to side effects.

Services Program

Integrated Child Development Services (ICDS)

This is program with integrated services of various developments for the children below 6 years, the services are provided by Aganwadi workers.

Services include supplementary health education, health check-up, referral services, nutrition and health education.

VITAMIN DEFICIENCY

Vitamins are essential nutrients that must be supplied exogenously. Incomplete or imbalance diet usually leads to deficiency of more than one vitamins. Thus, use of multivitamins preparation is increasing.

Vitamins are:

i. Fat-soluble—vitamins A and D
ii. Water-soluble—vitamins B, C and E

VITAMIN A DEFICIENCY

Vitamin A deficiency or xerophthalmia is important cause of blindness in developing countries.

Etiology

i. Deficiency of vitamin A in food as milk, greeny leafy vegetables, etc.
ii. Inadequate intestinal absorption of vitamin A. Chronic intestinal disorders, celiac disease, hepatic and pancreatic disease. Iron deficiency anemia, chronic infectious disease.
iii. *Vit A excretion increased:* Cancer, urinary tract disease, chronic infectious disease.
iv. *Low protein intake:* Due to deficient carrier protein and decrease plasma concentration of vit A.

Sources of vitamin A

Colostrum (very rich), breast milk, cow milk (satisfactory source), vegetables, fruits, eggs, butter, liver.

Clinical Features

Clinical features of vitamin A deficiency can be divided into two manifestations:
i. Xerophthalmia, or ocular manifestations
ii. Extraocular manifestations

I. Ocular Manifestations

1. **Night blindness:** Ocular manifestations develop insidiously, earliest manifestation is night blindness. Patient is unable to see in night or in dark. It is due to impairment of dark adaptation. In small child or infant, it is difficult to notice. But elder child takes quite time to see when coming from light to dim light or in dark.

2. **Conjunctival xerosis:** Bulbar conjunctiva of eye becomes dry, wrinkled and muddy devoid of shine or gloss. It is in interpalpebral conjunctiva initially. Later on whole conjunctiva is affected. Glistening and chalky brown spots are seen at conjunctiva near cornea, known as Bitot's spots. They are usually at outer aspect of eye (Fig. 7.11).

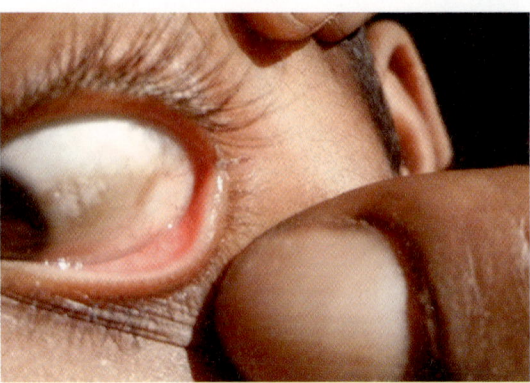

Fig. 7.11: Vitamin A deficiency (Bitot's spot).

3. **Changes in cornea:** Cornea becomes lustureless and dry (corneal xerosis). It causes photophobia. Child closes his eyes or he likes the place of dim light.

Cornea becomes dry, melting resulting necrosis and ulceration of cornea known as keratomalacia which is a irreversible change. Keratomalacia ultimately progress to perforation of cornea, panophthalmitis and destruction of not only cornea but also whole eye resulting 'phthisis bulbi' leading to complete blindness.

Keratomalacia can lead to perforation of cornea resulting in a scar and blindness.

II. Extraocular Manifestations

1. Physical and mental growth retarded, apathy, lack of interest in surrounding are other features.

2. Anemia, hepatosplenomegaly.

3. Skin is dry and scaly shows hyperkaratosis especially over the outer aspects of limbs shows follicular hyperkeratosis or phrynoderma or toad skin.

4. Increased susceptibility to the infection of urinary tract, respiratory tract and vagina. It may cause burning in micturition, hematuria, cough. It is due to squamous metaplasia of epithelium. Vit A increases resistance against infection and helping to recover damaged mucosa.

5. Increased intracranial pressure causes widening of sutures sometimes hydrocephalus and cranial nerve palsy.

Diagnosis

Depends on:
   i. Clinical features
   ii. Vitamin A level in plasma below normal.
   iii. Dark adaptation test
   iv. Vitamin A absorption test
   v. Examination of scrapping from vagina, eye.

Treatment

Specific treatment.

Oral: Treatment schedule consists of vitamin A at a dose of:

50,000 IU   for the children <6 months of age

100,000 IU for the children 6–12 months of age

200,000 IU for the children >1 year of age

   Repeat same dose after 4 weeks.

Parenteral: In case with persistent vomiting and diarrhea or severe malabsorption half of above dose up to 6–12 months of age, 75% in 6 months old child of above dose is given parenteral.

   Aqueous preparations are better than oily preparation because it causes less pain.

   Clouding of cornea is a emergency condition. Vit A should be administered immediately in a dose of 50,000 IU to 100000 IU.

   Local treatment with antibiotic eye drops and ointment and padding of eye.

   Vit A supplementation does not reduce incidence or duration of *diarrhea* but appears to reduce severity of diarrhea.

   Vit A supplementation in *measles* cases, malnourished children two doses (oral) are given on successive days (as described above). It reduces mortality in measles cases.

Prevention

• Diet—give daily requirement of vit A 1500–4500 IU.

• Foods rich in vitamin A are milk, leafy green vegetables, should be advised.

• Under National Blindness Control Program and *Bal Suraksha Program* following doses of vit A are given in 9 months of age 1 lac unit oral, 1 year of age 2 lac unit.

   Then every 6 months 2 lac unit up to the age of 5 years (total 10 doses).

Hypervitaminosis A

Toxicity of vitamin A results when more than 50,000 units of vit A is taken for several months in the form of food or vit A solution.

   It results pseudotumor cerebri (vomiting, bulging fontannel, diplopia, headache).

   In chronic cases dermatitis, alopecia, hepatosplenomegaly and hyperostosis are seen.

RICKETS

Failure of mineralization of growing bone or osteoid tissue is termed rickets.

   Failure of mature bone to mineralize called osteomalacia.

Etiology

   i. Deficiency of vitamin D in the diet.
   ii. Lack of exposure to ultraviolet rays in sunlight which convert provitamin D to vitamin D in the skin. Ultraviolet rays do not pass from ordinary window glass.
   iii. Conditions which interfere with metabolic conversion and activation of vitamin D such as hepatic and renal lesions.
   iv. Conditions which disrupt calcium and phosphorus homeostasis in any way.

Predisposing Factors

1. Rapid growing period, e.g. low birth weight infant.
2. Black children due to either pigmentation of skin or inadequate penetration of sunrays.
3. Disorders of absorption, e.g. celiac disease, etc. because of deficient absorption of vitamin D and calcium or both.

4. Anticonvulsant therapy (phenobarbitone, phenytoin) interfere in metabolism of vitamin D.
5. Corticosteroid therapy—it antagonize vitamin D in calcium transport.

Chemistry

Two forms are practically important: (i) Vitamin D_2 (calciferol), (ii) vitamin D_3 (7-dehydrocholesterol). Present in skin as provitamin D.

Both above are available synthetically.

Both D_2 and D_3 are converted into liver as 25 OH cholecalciferol and in renal cortex into 1,25 OH cholecalciferol and renal cortex into 1,25-dihydroxycholecalciferol.

Functions

Vitamin D helps in absorption of calcium and phosphorus in intestine, reabsorption of phosphorus in kidney and deposition and reabsorption in the bone. Along with parathormone and calcitonin it plays major role in calcium and phosphorus metabolism.

Clinical Features

It is common between 4 months and 2 years of age because it is common age of bone formation. Breast milk contains sufficient amount of vit D. So, it is less common in breastfed babies. Bone changes manifest after several months of vit D deficiency.

1. Earliest features are irritability, sweating over head especially at night. Occiput softened and parchment like skull bones which can be indented like a ping-pong ball. The sign should be elicited away from suture line (craniotabes). It is due to thining of outer table of skull.
2. Rachitic rosary (palpebral enlargement of costochondral junctions).
3. Thickening of wrist and ankle.

Sign of Advanced Rickets

Head

1. **Head:** Craniotabes is earliest feature.

2. Macrocephaly which remains throughout life.
3. Flattening or asymmetry of skull due to softening of skull bones.
4. Delayed closure and larger anterior fontanelle.
5. Central part of parietal and frontal bones are thickened.
6. This thickening give rise to frontal bossing or prominence giving head as box like appearance (caput quadratum).

Teeth

1. Eruption of temporary teeth delayed and defects in enamel or caries.
2. Permanent teeth show defect in calcification and enamel defects.

Thorax

1. Enlargement of costocondral junction, beading of ribs, which can be seen and palpated called rickety rosary (Fig. 7.12).
2. Sternum and adjacent cartilage seems projected (pigeon breast).

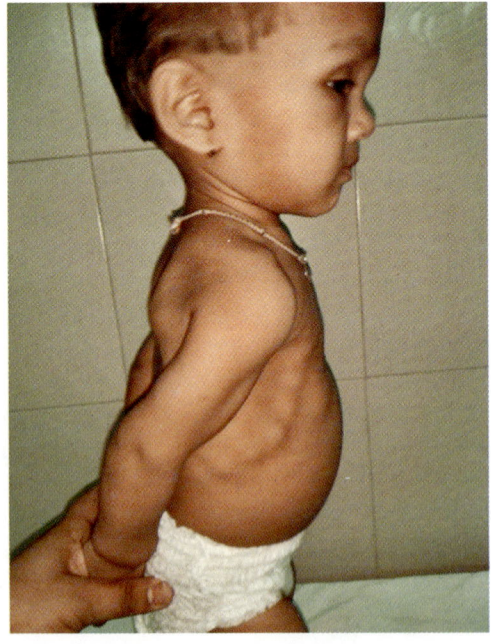

Fig. 7.12: Rickety rosary.

3. At lower part of chest of horizontal depression is seen called 'Harrison sulcus'. It corresponds to attachment of diaphragm to chest.

4. Other deformity may be seen.

Spine and Pelvis: There may be kyphosis or lordosis or scoliosis. In pelvis enterance is narrowed due to forward projection of promontory and pelvic exit is narrowed due to forward displacement of sacrum and coccyx.

Extremities

1. Changes are seen specially at wrist (Fig. 7.13) and ankle. Enlarged epiphysis is seen or palpated or seen in skiagram.

2. Bones such as femur, tibia and fibula bend due to softness resulting
   a. Either knock knee deformity (genu valgum) or bow leg deformity (genu varum) in lower limbs (Figs 7.14 and 7.15).
   b. Thigh may be bent outwards in cross-lagged sitting position on floor.
   c. Curvature is generally seen at the junction of lower and middle third of forearm.
   d. Height of the child is retarded called ricketic dwarfism.

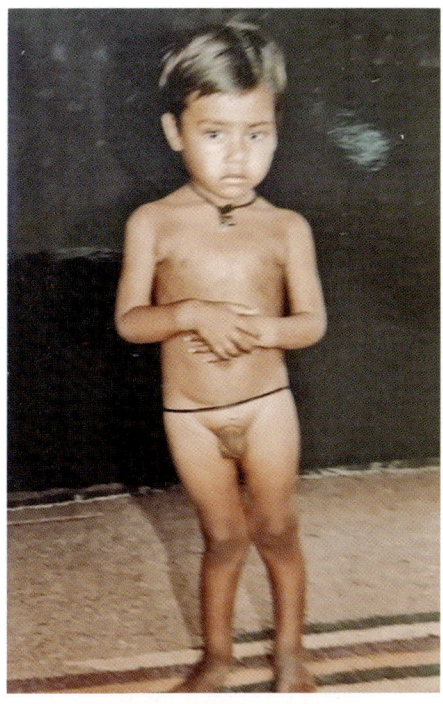

Fig. 7.14: Genu valgum.

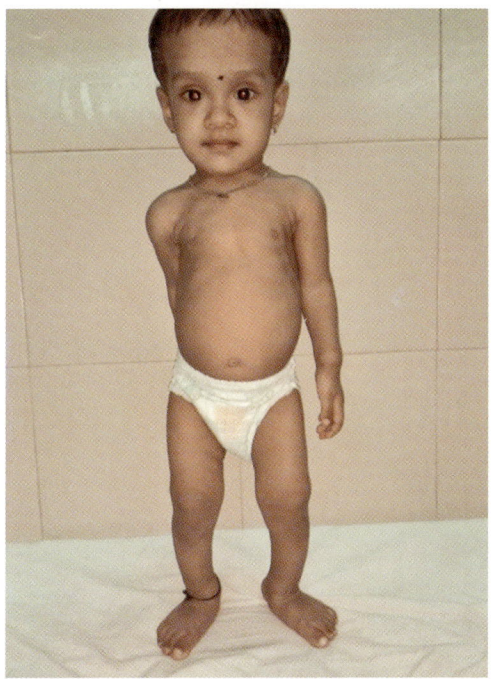

Fig. 7.15: Genu varum (bow leg).

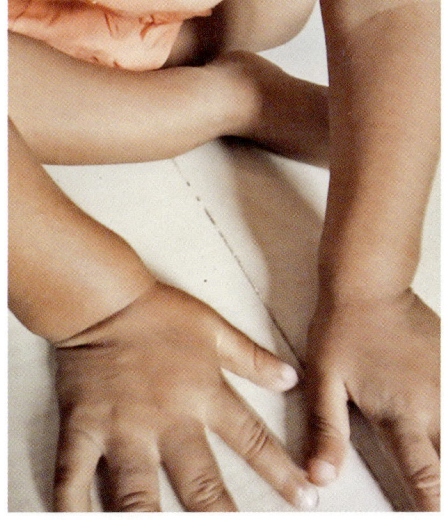

Fig. 7.13: Rickets widening of wrist.

Muscles and Ligaments

1. Due to laxity of ligaments and muscles weakness and hypotonia seen, child is late in sitting and standing (delayed mile-stones).
2. Laxity of ligaments also exaggerate knock knee, overextension of knee joints, weak ankle, kyphosis and scoliosis.
3. Flat foot and protuberant abdomen.
4. Limbs can be molded in any position due to laxity of ligaments. It is known as acorbutic rickets.

Diagnosis

Depends on:
1. Clinical features
2. Blood examination—calcium normal or phosphate less and alkaline phosphatase increased.
3. Skiagram—generally taken of wrist. Following features are seen:
   - Distal end of bone is normally convex and clearly defined but in rickets it shows concave (cupping) and flaring (Figs 7.16 to 7.18).
   - Distance between distal end of the bone and epiphysis is increased because metaphysis is broad and due to lack of calcification, it is not seen in skiagram.

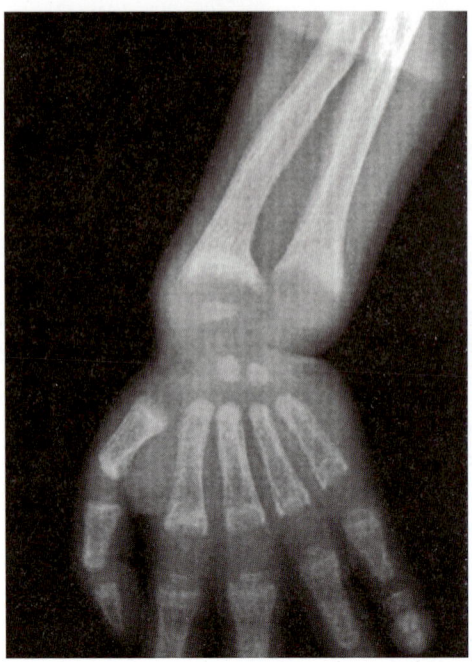

Fig. 7.17: X-ray picture of wrist showing features of rickets.

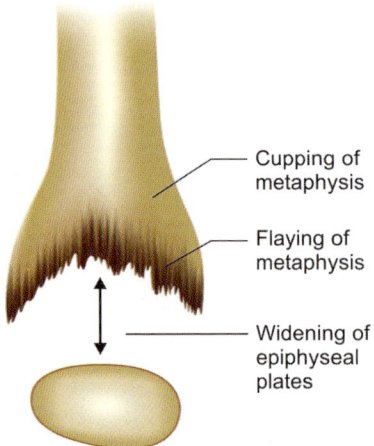

- Cupping of metaphysis
- Flaying of metaphysis
- Widening of epiphyseal plates

Fig. 7.16: Diagrammatic representation of X-ray picture of rickets.

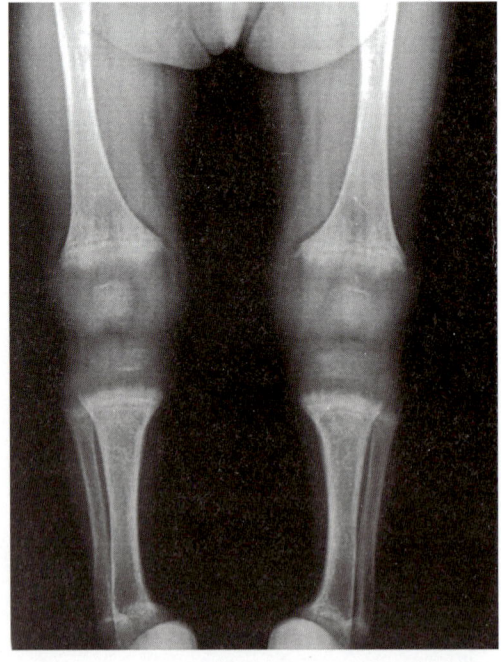

Fig. 7.18: X-ray picture of knee joint (rickets).

Laboratory Diagnosis

1. 25 (OH) D3 levels in blood. Less than 10 mg/ml. Increased level indicates deficient intake of calcium and phosphorus.
2. Alkaline phosphatase elevated.
3. Calcium and phosphatase levels—normal or low.

Management

1. Vitamin D
   Vitamin D 600,000 IU as a single oral dose or 60,000 IU daily oral dose for 10 days followed by 400–800 IU/day for 2 months.
2. Calcium supplementation: 30–75 mg/day for 2 months.
3. Mild case can be treated with daily administration of 1500–5000 IU of vitamin D.
4. Exposure to sunlight is essential. Clothes should be removed, so sunrays falls directly on skin. Ultraviolet rays cannot pass from window.

Prevention

Daily demand of 400 IU is given. Diet rich in vit D_2, e.g. milk, eggs are given and child should be exposed to sunlight properly.

Effects of therapy

If sufficient amount of vitamin D is administered healing begins within few days. Deformity corrects in variable time.

X-ray appearance—healing is indicated by line of preparatory calcification which seperates from distal end of shaft by a zone of decreased calcification (zone of osteoid tissue). Afterward osteoid tissue is calcified. The 'Shaft' grows towards the line of preparatory calcification until it becomes united with it.

Refractory rickets:

If 1–2 large doses of vitamin A fail to improve radiological changes in bones. It is evaluated for refractory rickets.

Familial hypophosphatemic rickets

It is a form of refractory rickets inherited as X-linked dominant. Clinical features of rickets are seen, the mothers of affected patient may have bowing of legs and short stature or low phosphate levels. Phosphate level in blood is less than 1.5–3 mg/dl. Serum alkaline phosphatase level increased, urinary phosphatase excretion increased.

Management includes oral phosphate in dosage of 30–50 mg/kg in divided doses and vitamin D supplementation.

Vitamin D dependent rickets:

There are autosomal recessive inherited rickets, who have receiving usual amount of vitamin D. Vitamin D and calcium supplementation required.

Other causes of rickets
1. Chronic kidney disease
2. Oncogeneous rickets
3. Metaphyseal dysplasia
4. Fluorosis

Hypervitaminosis D

Hypervitaminosis resulting from excessive dose of vitamin D for several months results features of hypervitaminosis—anorexia, nausea, vomiting, weakness, polyuria, polydipsia, azotemia, hypertension, nephrolithiasis, ectopic calcification and renal failure, hypercalcemia, hyperphosphatemia.

SCURVY

Scurvy is caused by vitamin C deficiency. Basic effects of vit C deficiency lies in collagen tissue formation, which is altered.

Etiology

i. **Deficiency in diet:** Mother's milk contains sufficient amount of vitamin C while cow milk contains less. So, baby on artificial feeding is more prone to scurvy.
ii. Demand of vitamin C is increased during fever, diarrhea and infection, iron deficiency, cold exposure, protein depletion or smoking.

Clinical Features

It may occur at any age but mostly cases are of 6–24 months of age group.

1. Early features are vague; irritability, tachypnea, loss of appetite and generalized tenderness. Due to pain child—keeps his body in specific position known as 'frog position'. In which hips and knees are semiflexed with feet rotated outwards. It shows pseudoparalysis.
2. Gums are bluish purple, spongy, mucous membrane usually seen over the upper incisors. If teeth have erupted swollen gums cover teeth. Bleeding is common from gums.
3. Rosary (beading) is seen at costochondral junction, angulation of the scorbutic beads is sharper than rachitic because it is due to subluxations of the sternal plates at the constocondral junction. But in rickets it is due to widening of the softening epiphysis.
4. Sternum appears depressed.
5. Hemorrhages are common from various sites, hematuria, malena, anemia are common, fever also present.
6. Wound healing is delayed and healed wounds may breakdown.
7. Swollen joints and follicular hyperkeratosis seen.
8. 'Sicca' syndrome (xerostomia, keratoconjunctivitis and enlargement of salivary gland).

Diagnosis

a. Clinical features.
b. Skiagram of long bones especially at distal end. Generally at knee joints show characteristic features are as follows:
   i. Trabecula of bones is not clearly seen. It is known as ground glass appearance.
   ii. Cortex of bone is reduced to 'pencil point thickness'.
   iii. Epiphyseal ends are sharply outlined as ring around epiphysis.
   iv. Thickened end of bone is irregular at the metaphysis. White line of Frankel (it is a zone of well calcified cartilage) seen at metaphysis.
   v. Periosteum is elevated due to subperiosteal hemorrhage which calcify and affected bone assume a dumbbell or club shape (Fig. 7.19).
c. Blood—ascorbic acid concentration is low in white cell platelet layer (buffy layer) of centrifuged oxalated blood. Prothrombin time increased.

Treatment

i. *Specific treatment:* Specific treatment includes administration of 100 mg of ascorbic acid orally or intramuscularly daily.

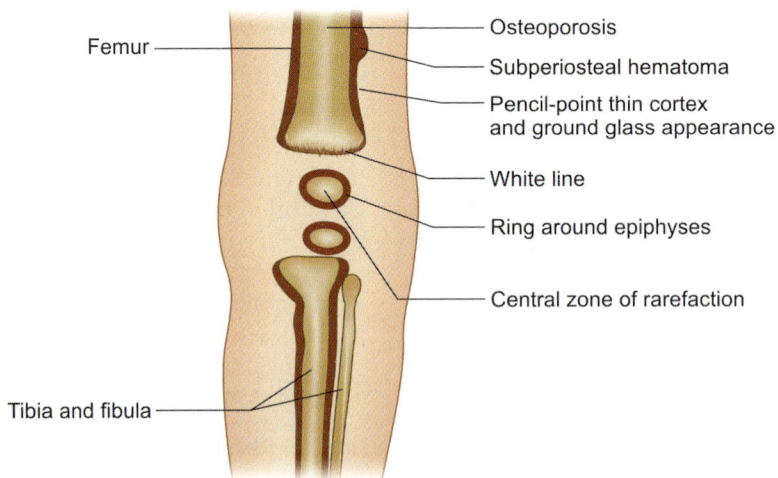

Femur

Osteoporosis

Subperiosteal hematoma

Pencil-point thin cortex and ground glass appearance

White line

Ring around epiphyses

Central zone of rarefaction

Tibia and fibula

Fig. 7.19: Diagrammatic representation of skiagram of scurvy (knee joint).

ii. Orange juice is given 3–4 ounce daily.

iii. Minimal handling is done during acute phase to avoid pain.

Prevention

Food containing ascorbic acid such as tomato, citrous fruits are given.

THIAMINE DEFICIENCY

Deficiency of thiamine causes beriberi which is of two types:

a. Dry type—characterized by apathy, peripheral neuritis and weakness of muscles.

b. Wet type—characterized by anorexia, vomiting or constipation, edema or CCF.

Deficiency of Vitamin B_2

It causes angular stomatitis. Tongue is swollen, eyes congested. Specific treatment is to give 3–5 mg of vit B_{12} daily for many weeks.

Deficiency of Niacin

It causes pellagra, skin becomes bronzed on exposed part of body. Diarrhea is common. Mental function may be affected causes dementia. Treatment consists of 50–300 mg of niacin given daily.

Deficiency of Pyridoxine

It causes vomiting, convulsions, peripheral neuritis and diarrhea. Tongue may be swollen and swelling of angles of mouth are also common. Treatment is to give 10–100 mg of vit B_6 (pyridoxine).

Deficiency of Vitamin B_{12} and Folic Acid

Causes megaloblastic anemia, treatment consists of vit B_{12} 100 mg daily and folic acid 5–20 mg daily.

Boy's and girl's weight according to length										
Boy's weight (kg)					Length (cm)	Girl's weight (kg)				
−4SD	−3SD	−2SD	−1SD	Median		Median	−1SD	−2SD	−3SD	−4SD
1.7	1.9	2.0	2.2	2.4	45	2.5	2.3	2.1	1.9	1.7
1.8	2.0	2.2	2.4	2.6	46	2.6	2.4	2.2	2.0	1.9
2.0	2.1	2.3	2.5	2.8	47	2.8	2.6	2.4	2.2	2.0
2.1	2.3	2.5	2.7	2.9	48	3.0	2.7	2.5	2.3	2.1
2.2	2.4	2.6	2.9	3.1	49	3.2	2.9	2.6	2.4	2.2
2.4	2.6	2.8	3.0	3.3	50	3.4	3.1	2.8	2.6	2.4
2.5	2.7	3.0	3.2	3.5	51	3.6	3.3	3.0	2.8	2.5
2.7	2.9	3.2	3.5	3.8	52	3.8	3.5	3.2	2.9	2.7
2.9	3.1	3.4	3.7	4.0	53	4.0	3.7	3.4	3.1	2.8
3.1	3.3	3.6	3.9	4.3	54	4.3	3.9	3.6	3.3	3.0
3.3	3.6	3.8	4.2	4.5	55	4.5	4.2	3.8	3.5	3.2
3.5	3.8	4.1	4.4	4.8	56	4.8	4.4	4.0	3.7	3.4
3.7	4.0	4.3	4.7	5.1	57	5.1	4.6	4.3	3.9	3.6
3.9	4.3	4.6	5.0	5.4	58	5.4	4.9	4.5	4.1	3.8
4.1	4.5	4.8	5.3	5.7	59	5.6	5.1	4.7	4.3	3.9

Contd...

				Boy's and girl's weight according to length *(Contd...)*						
	Boy's weight (kg)				Length (cm)		Girl's weight (kg)			
−4SD	−3SD	−2SD	−1SD	Median		Median	−1SD	−2SD	−3SD	−4SD
4.3	4.7	5.1	5.5	6.0	60	5.9	5.4	4.9	4.5	4.1
4.5	4.9	5.3	5.8	6.3	61	6.1	5.6	5.1	4.7	4.3
4.7	5.1	5.6	6.0	6.5	62	6.4	5.8	5.3	4.9	4.5
4.9	5.3	5.8	6.2	6.8	63	6.6	6.0	5.5	5.1	4.7
5.1	5.5	6.0	6.5	7.0	64	6.9	6.3	5.7	5.3	4.8
5.3	5.7	6.2	6.7	7.3	65	7.1	6.5	5.9	5.5	5.0
5.5	5.9	6.4	6.9	7.5	66	7.3	6.7	6.1	5.6	5.1
5.6	6.1	6.6	7.1	7.7	67	7.5	6.9	6.3	5.8	5.3
5.8	6.3	6.8	7.3	8.0	68	7.7	7.1	6.5	6.0	5.5
6.0	6.5	7.0	7.6	8.2	69	8.0	7.3	6.7	6.1	5.6
6.1	6.6	7.2	7.8	8.4	70	8.2	7.5	6.9	6.3	5.8
6.3	6.8	7.4	8.0	8.6	71	8.4	7.7	7.0	6.5	5.9
6.4	7.0	7.6	8.2	8.9	72	8.6	7.8	7.2	6.6	6.0
6.6	7.2	7.7	8.4	9.1	73	8.8	8.0	7.4	6.8	6.2
6.7	7.3	7.9	8.6	3.9	74	9.0	8.2	7.5	6.9	6.3
6.9	7.5	8.1	8.8	9.5	75	9.1	8.4	7.7	7.1	6.5
7.0	7.6	8.3	8.9	9.7	76	9.3	8.5	7.8	7.2	6.6
7.2	7.8	8.4	9.1	9.9	77	9.5	8.7	8.0	7.4	6.7
7.3	7.9	8.6	9.3	10.1	78	9.7	8.9	8.2	7.5	6.9
7.4	8.1	8.7	9.5	10.3	79	9.9	9.1	8.3	7.7	7.0
7.6	8.2	8.9	9.6	10.4	80	10.1	9.2	8.5	7.8	7.1
7.7	8.4	9.1	9.8	10.6	81	10.3	9.4	8.7	8.0	7.3
7.9	8.5	9.2	10.0	10.8	82	10.5	9.6	8.8	8.1	7.5
8.0	8.7	9.4	10.2	11.0	83	10.7	9.8	9.0	8.3	7.6
8.2	8.9	9.6	10.4	11.3	84	11.0	10.1	9.2	8.5	7.8
8.4	9.1	9.8	10.6	11.5	85	11.2	10.3	9.4	8.7	8.0
8.6	9.3	10.0	10.8	11.7	86	11.5	10.5	9.7	8.9	8.1
9.9	9.6	10.4	11.2	12.2	87	11.9	10.9	10.0	9.2	8.4
9.1	9.8	10.6	11.5	12.4	88	12.1	11.1	10.2	9.4	8.6
9.3	10.0	10.8	11.7	12.6	89	12.4	11.4	10.4	9.6	8.8
9.4	10.2	11.0	11.9	12.9	90	12.6	11.6	10.6	9.8	9.0
9.6	10.4	11.2	12.11	13.1	91	12.9	11.8	10.9	10.0	9.1
9.8	10.6	11.4	12.3	13.4	92	13.1	12.0	11.1	10.2	9.3
9.9	10.8	11.6	12.6	13.6	93	13.4	12.3	11.3	10.4	9.5

Contd...

Boy's and girl's weight according to length *(Contd...)*										
Boy's weight (kg)					Length (cm)	Girl's weight (kg)				
−4SD	−3SD	−2SD	−1SD	Median		Median	−1SD	−2SD	−3SD	−4SD
10.1	11.0	11.8	12.8	13.8	94	13.6	12.5	11.5	10.6	9.7
10.3	11.1	12.0	13.0	14.1	95	13.9	12.7	11.7	10.8	9.8
10.4	11.3	12.2	13.2	14.3	96	14.1	12.9	11.9	10.9	10.0
10.6	11.5	12.4	13.4	14.6	97	14.4	13.2	12.1	11.1	10.2
10.8	11.7	12.6	13.7	14.8	98	14.7	13.4	12.3	11.3	10.4
11.0	11.9	12.9	13.9	15.1	99	14.9	13.7	12.5	11.5	10.5
11.2	12.1	13.1	14.2	15.4	100	15.2	13.9	12.8	11.7	10.7
11.3	12.3	13.3	14.4	15.6	101	15.5	14.2	13.0	12.0	10.9
11.5	12.5	13.6	14.7	15.9	102	15.8	14.5	13.3	12.2	11.1
11.7	12.8	13.8	14.9	16.2	103	16.1	14.7	13.5	12.4	11.3
11.9	13.0	14.0	15.2	16.5	104	16.4	15.0	13.8	12.6	11.5
12.1	13.2	14.3	15.5	16.8	105	16.8	15.3	14.0	12.9	11.8
12.3	13.4	14.5	15.8	17.2	106	17.1	15.6	14.3	13.1	12.0
12.5	13.7	14.8	16.1	17.5	107	17.5	15.9	14.6	13.4	12.2
12.7	13.9	15.1	16.4	17.8	108	17.8	16.3	14.9	13.7	12.4
12.9	14.1	15.3	16.7	18.2	109	18.2	16.6	15.2	13.9	12.7
13.2	14.4	15.6	17.0	18.5	110	18.6	17.0	15.5	14.2	12.9
13.4	14.6	15.9	17.3	18.9	111	19.0	17.3	15.8	14.5	13.2
13.6	14.9	16.2	17.6	19.2	112	19.4	17.7	16.2	14.8	13.5
13.8	15.2	16.5	18.0	19.6	113	19.8	18.0	16.5	15.1	13.7
14.1	15.4	16.8	18.3	20.0	114	20.2	18.4	16.8	15.4	14.0
14.3	15.7	17.1	18.6	20.4	115	20.7	18.8	17.2	15.7	14.3
14.6	16.0	17.4	19.0	20.8	116	21.1	19.2	17.5	16.0	14.5
14.8	16.2	17.7	19.3	21.2	117	21.5	19.6	17.8	16.3	14.8
15.0	16.5	18.0	19.7	21.6	118	22.0	19.9	18.2	16.6	15.1
15.3	16.8	18.3	20.0	22.0	119	22.4	20.3	18.5	16.9	15.4
15.5	17.1	18.6	20.4	22.4	120	22.8	20.7	18.9	17.3	15.6

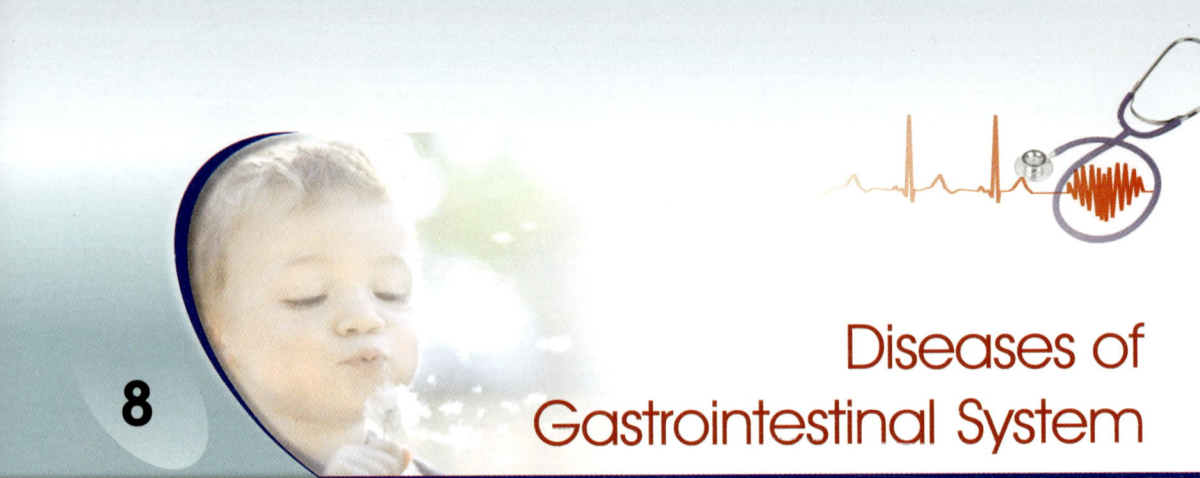

Diseases of Gastrointestinal System

8

VOMITING

Definition

Forceful expulsion of gastric contents. This should be differentiated from regurgitation, in which small amount of swallowed food is expelled out, while in vomiting, complete emptying of stomach occurs.

Causes

Neonatal Peroid

a. **Non-organic causes:** Irritation of stomach due to swallowed blood, amniotic fluid, drugs, faulty feeding techniques.

b. **Organic causes**
 - *Infections:* Septicemia, meningitis, encephalitis, intrauterine infections.
 - *Mechanical:* Hirschsprung's disease, meconium plug or meconium ileus, tracheoesophageal fistula, intestinal atresia, achalasia cardia, malabsorption of gut, volvulus, vascular rings.

c. **Neurological:** Birth injuries, hydrocephalus, birth defects, subdural effusion and bilirubin encephalopathy.

d. **Metabolic:** Idiopathic hypercalcemia, adrenal hyperplasia, hypoglycemia, galactosemia, phenylketonuria.

Infancy

1. Faulty feeding techniques.
2. Obstructive lesion (mechanical)—oesophageal atresia, achalasia, hiatus hernia, pyloric stenosis, duodenal atresia, stenosis, annular pancreas, jejunal atresia, malrotation, volvulus, diaphragmatic hernia, congenital bands, intussusception, Hirschsprung's disease, meconium ileus, ascariasis.
3. Infections—GIT, urinary tract, septicemia, meningitis.
4. Metabolic—hypocalcemia, hypercalcemia.
5. Endocrine—adrenogenital syndrome.

Management: Management of vomiting includes treatment of underlying cause, correction of dehydration. Promethazine, prochlorperazine, metochlopramide, or ondansetron are drugs used.

DIARRHEA

Definition

It is very difficult to define diarrhea. In general term 'Diarrhea' may be defined as the 'passing of liquid or watery stools'.

The stools are usually passed more than 3 times in a day. Recent change in consistency of stool is important. Frequency of passing stool is not so much important. If formed stools are passed many times such as breast-fed babies often pass loose 'pasty stools', this is not diarrhea. If stool is passed even once but it contains excessive watery portion, it is diarrhea.

Diarrhea may be acute-lasting for hours or day or chronic-lasting for weeks or months.

Types of Diarrhea

i. Acute watery diarrhea—lasting not more than 14 days, self-limiting in 7 days.
ii. Dysentery—diarrhea with visible blood in stool.
iii. Persistent diarrhea—lasting more than 14 days.

Chronic diarrhea is non-infectious in origin. In Toddler's diarrhea growth is normal and no dehydration. Traveller's diarrhea develops during travelling.

The term gastroenteritis is used when diarrhea in associated with vomiting, with or without fever.

In winter, human rotavirus is major cause of diarrhea occurring in about 25–50% of cases. Presence of bacteria in stool is not proof of being causative agent.

Incidence

No age is exempt; worldwide distribution. During the first 3 years of life a child will experience an estimate 1–3 acute severe episodes of diarrhea every year. Peak incidence occurs between 6 and 9 months of age, most frequently in rainy season, poor hygienic conditions and in malnourished children.

Incidence is less in breastfed infants as compared to artificially fed. Teething does not cause diarrhea. During this period child puts his fingers or objects into mouth to allay irritation in gums caused by erupting teeth. Thus, infections enter in gastrointestinal tract.

90% of all diarrheal episodes do not develop dehydration, while 9% of all episodes develop some dehydration; 1% develops severe dehydration.

Etiopathogenesis

Agent factor: Following organisms are responsible for enteric infections causing diarrhea.

- **Virus**
  a. Human rotavirus (20–50% of cases)
  b. Enterovirus
  c. Influenza virus
  d. Measles virus
  e. Parvovirus like agents—coxsackievirus, echovirus, adenovirus.
- **Bacteria:** *E. coli* (most common), Shigella, Salmonella, Staphylococcus.
- **Toxin:** *Vibrio cholerae, Yersinia enterocolitica, Aeromonas hydrophilia, Bacillus cereus.*
- **Parasites:** *E. histolytica, Giardia lamblia, Strongyloides stercoralis, Trichuris trichiura,* cryptosporidium
- **Fungi:** *Candida albicans.*

Reservoir of Infection

For enterotoxigenic *E. coli, Vibrio cholerae*—Man
- *E. histolytica*
- *Campylobacter jejuni*   :   Man, animal
- Virus   :   Animal

Host factor: In children 6 months to 2 years, and under 6 months if baby is fed on cow's milk, it is common.

Diarrhea is a major cause of malnutrition because

1. Body needs more nutrients than normal to cope up with infections such as diarrhea. Yet, children with diarrhea usually eat less than normal.
2. Loss of appetite, vomiting which may discourage mother from giving food.
3. Mother is feeding less or giving diluted food based on traditional beliefs or incorrect recommendation to 'rest the bowel'.
4. Absorption of nutrients may also be reduced as much as one-third during acute diarrhea. However, even though some nutrients are lost, most nutrients continue to be absorbed.

Malnutrition can make diarrhea worse because

i. Reduction of digestive enzymes occur due to atrophy of pancreatic exocrine cells.
ii. Concomitant insanitary environment conditions.
iii. Atrophy of gut mucosa and diminished resistance to infections lead to proliferation of bacteria in intestine causing diarrhea.

Bacteria cause diarrhea by two mechanisms

i. Through the action of toxins, e.g. *Vibrio cholerae*.
ii. Direct invasion of the intestinal mucosa.

Pathophysiological changes due to diarrhea

Pathology: Diarrhea leads to blunting of villi, extensive ulcerations and hyperemia of intestinal mucosa. Other changes are venous thrombosis, renal thrombosis and adrenal hemorrhage and focal changes in lung parenchyma.

Normally, water is present in extracellular and intracellular compartments. Extracellular compartment composed of blood, interstitial fluid and secretions. Diarrheal losses come from extracellular fluid.

Loss of water due to diarrhea causes reduction and shrinkage in the volume of extracellular compartment. In 70% cases, concentration of sodium in extracellular compartment remains nearly normal. Since excessive sodium in comparison to water is lost in stool, in another 20% cases. There is fall in sodium level in serum and extracellular fluid—hyponatremia. Sodium is main determinant of osmolarity of extracellular fluid; so due to hyponatremia osmolarity of extracellular fluids falls causing movement of water from extracellular to intracellular compartments (Fig. 8.1).

This causes further reduction in extracellular compartment volume.

Thus, shrinkage in extracellular water in hypo- or isonatremic dehydration impairs the elasticity of skin. Thus, on pinching, it takes few seconds for skin fold to return to normal and seems wrinkled as old man skin (Fig. 8.2).

In about 10% of diarrhea cases, especially if child is given fluid with more salt, serum sodium is elevated, so osmotic pressure of extracellular fluid is relatively higher. Therefore, water moves from inside the cells to the extracellular compartment resulting restoration of extracellular fluid. Therefore, skin turgor is not lost. Skin is soggy or leathery which is mistakenly diagnosed as mild or no dehydration, if circulatory or renal impairment is not assessed simultaneously.

Due to reduction in fluid in extracellular compartment, blood volume is reduced, resulting in low blood pressure and weak thready pulse. Extremities become cold. Due to low hydrostatic pressure in glomeruli urine filtration is reduced. So, quantity and frequency of urination is reduced.

Urine flow is an important indication of severity of illness. Renal failure may supervene.

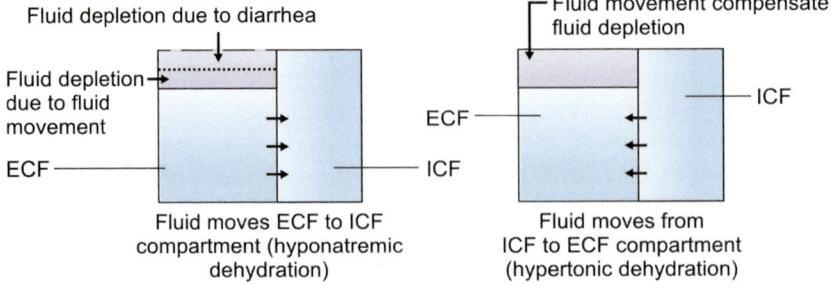

Fig. 8.1: Fluid moves from ICF to ECF compartment (hypertonic dehydration) and from ECF to ICF in hyponatremic dehydration.

Due to loss of bicarbonate in stools acidosis develops menifesting as deep and rapid breath.

Since stool contains potassium in large amount so potassium level falls in affected child.

Alkalosis—common causes are: (i) Vomiting (severe loss of HCl from stomach), (ii) therapeutic administration of potassium citrate.

Factors peculiar to infants and children: Child may loose about same amount of water and electrolyte from the body during an episode of diarrhea as an adult, because length and surface area of intestinal mucosa from where the diarrheal fluids are secreted quite large in adult. So, same loss in comparatively very small extracellular fluid compartment in children is hazardous and produce serious menifestations.

Clinical Features

Onset may be acute or insidious. On an average a child suffers 3 attacks of diarrhea in a year up to 3 years of age.

Symptoms are of gastrointestinal tract and due to dehydration. Frequency of stools may be 4–6 times to more than 100 in 24 hours.

Faeces may be loose, watery, curdy deposits may be seen; mucus may be present but blood is rare. In enteroinvasive bacterial infection, diarrhea is mixed with variable degree of pyrexia, cramps and tenesmus.

Abdominal distension is quite often due to hypokalemia. It is also feature of lactose intolerance, necrotizing enterocolitis and paralytic ileus.

Infant loses weight. In mild dehydration—less than 5%, in moderate dehydration—5–10%, in severe dehydration—more than 10%.

Dehydration: Death in acute diarrhea is mostly due to dehydration which results from excessive loss of body water and salts in stools, vomitus, urine, sweat and insensible losses. Infants, older children and adults with similar degrees of dehydration from acute diarrhea have similar fluid and electrolyte deficits per units body mass. So, rehydration solution to all age groups are similar.

Brain cells get dehydrated earlier than others, so restlessness, irritability, excessive thurst appear early if some dehydration is present. Loss of skin turgor appears afterward (Fig. 8.2). In severe dehydration child becomes drowsy, unconscious, floppy.

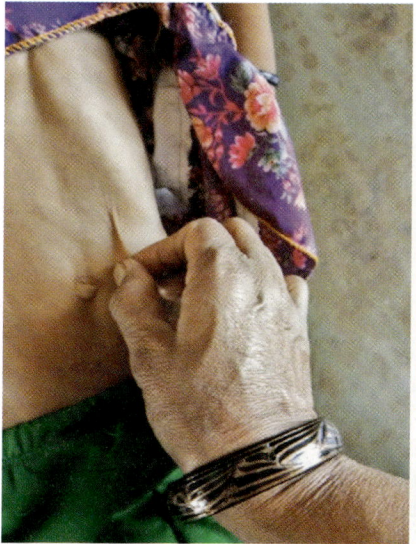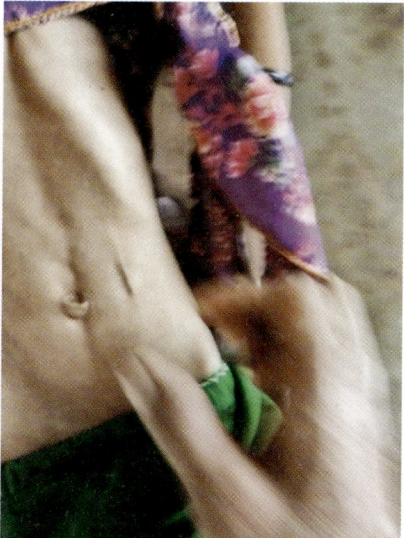

Fig. 8.2: Assessment of dehydration (loss of skin turgor).

Clinical assessement of patient history: A history is taken for following informations—

a. Duration of illness.
b. Quantity, consistency and frequency of stools.
c. Duration and frequency of vomiting if associated.
d. Time when urine was last passed. Quantity and color of urine.
e. History of fever or convulsions.
f. Food consumed during illness, type and amount of liquids taken.

Physical Examination

A complete physical examination with particular attention to signs of dehydration should be performed. Apart from it, look for:

i. *Fever:* Fever is often present in severely dehydrated babies. Take temperature by rectal thermometer as the skin may be cold despite of high fever.

ii. *Signs of dehydration:* No exact 'formula' can be given for assessing dehydration. It is done by careful assessment by history and physical examination. Best tool is experience (Table 8.1).

iii. *Fast breathing:* Rapid and deep breathing is due to acidosis. Rapid breathing may be also due to dehydration or lower respiratory tract infections.

iv. *Signs of shock:* Cold and moist extremities, rapid, feeble pulse, low or unrecordable systolic blood pressure (less than 70 mm Hg) and peripheral cyanosis.

Weighing the patient: Weighing has two purposes:

i. If weight of child is known; sudden loss of weight during the diarrheal illness gives useful indication of severity of dehydration.

ii. Weighing of patient at regular intervals during therapy is helpful in assessing the progress of rehydration.

Dehydration may be

a. Isotonic—losses of water and electrolyte are proportional. In India, mostly dehydration is isotonic.
b. Hyponatremic—a large amount of electrolyte especially sodium is lost in out of proportion to fluid losses, e.g. cholera.
c. Hypernatremic dehydration—it occurs usually homemade electrolyte solution rich in sodium is given. Loss of water is more than loss of electrolyte (Table 8.2).

Serum Sodium Values

130–150 mEq/L   Isonatremic dehydration
<130 mEq/L   Hyponatremic dehydration
Above 150 mEq/L Hypernatremic dehydration

Table 8.1: Signs of dehydration	
Grade	*Clinical presentation*
Mild (weight loss <5%)	Irritability or drowsiness; pallor, slightly sunken eyes, thirsty. Fluid deficit 40–50 ml per kg
Moderate (weight loss 5–10%)	Weak pulse, some reduction in urine volume output, pallor, depressed fontanelle, eyeball shunken, facies dry. Buccal mucosa dry, lips parched, loss of skin turgor (except in hypernatremic dehydration), thirsty. Fluid deficit 60–90 ml per kg
Severe (weight loss >10%)	Moribund, apathetic, signs of peripheral circulatory failure (cold extremities, warm body, excessive bounding, weak pulse) marked reduction in urine volume. Fontanelle markedly depressed. Eyeball shunkens markedly, facies markedly dry and parched. Buccal mucosa dry, lips parched, loss of skin turgor (except in hypernatremic dehydration). Fluid deficit 100–110 ml per kg

Table 8.2. Salient differences in various types of dehydration

Criteria	Isotonic	Hypertonic	Hypotonic
Sensorium	Drowsy	Irritable very much	Comatosed
Skin elasticity	Poor	Fair	Very poor
Feel of skin	Dry	Thickened	Clammy (moist)
Mucous membrane	Dry	Parched	Slightly moist
Pulse	Rapid, weak	Rapid, bounding	Rapid, weak
BP	Low	Moderately low	Very low

CNS disturbances such as irritability, restlessness, cloudiness of consciousness, delirium or stupor, lethargy, coma or convulsion are more common in hypernatremic dehydration.

In malnourished child—pinching of skin is not reliable criteria because loss of elasticity is present without dehydration. So, dryness of mucosa is better guide in these patients.

Clinical manifestations of various conditions associated with diarrhea are as follows:

Acidosis: Deep, rapid breathing.

Alkalosis: Shallow and slow breathing. Latent or manifest tetany, convulsions.

Hypokalemia: Abdominal distension due to paralytic ileus, ECG changes.

Hyperkalemia: Bradycardia, heart block, sudden heart stoppage, ECG changes.

Hypocalcemia: Tetany, paralytic ileus.

Hypomagnesemia: Twitching of muscles, tetany.

Hypermagnesemia: Diminished reflexes, CNS depression.

Cerebral thrombosis may result in convulsion
Anemia is common complication: Cause is unknown may be simple iron or protein deficiency or both or due to toxemia.

Laboratory Investigations

i. Examination of stool.
 • For pus cells, red cells, macrophages, cyst or vegetative form of *E. histolytica* or Giardia. pH of stool is taken—low in lactose intolerance.
 • Culture for causative bacteria.

 • Tests for presence of toxins in the organism cultured from stool.
ii. Blood examination: For pH, serum sodium and potassium estimation, Hb%, blood urea, osmolarity.
iii. Test for identification of rotavirus by electron microscope or by ELISA test.

Management

Principles of management of acute diarrhea are:

1. Rehydration and maintaining hydration.
2. Adequate feeding or maintenance of nutrition.
3. Oral supplementation of zinc.
4. Early recognition of danger signs.
5. Antibiotics and antimicrobial therapy.
6. Adjunctive anti-diarrheal therapy.

1. Rehydration and Maintaining Hydration

Correction of dehydration in acute diarrhea is achieved by using oral rehydration solutions. Dehydration is classified as:

a. No dehydration
b. Some dehydration
c. Severe dehydration.

Treatment plan A: Treatment of 'No Dehydration'. Child with no dehydration may be treated at home with the ORS. Dose is as follows:

Age	Amount of ORS after each stool
<24 months	50–100 ml
2–10 years	100–200 ml
>10 years	As child can take

Treatment plan B: Treatment of 'some dehydration' Children having sign of dehydration should be treated at health center.

Fluid requirement is calculated into following headings.

1. The daily fluid requirement

Weight up to 10 kg = 100 ml/kg
             10–20 kg = 50 mg/kg
             >20 kg = 20 ml/kg

For example child weight is 15 kg
First 10 kg   = 10 × 100 = 1000 ml
Remaining 5 kg = 5 × 50 = 250 ml

Total   = 1250 ml

2. Deficit replacement or rehydration therapy. Calculate requirement 75 ml/kg. Total fluid is given in 4 hours orally or by nasogastric tube.

   If some dehydration persists after 4 hour of ORS therapy another treatment as in rehydration therapy is given.

3. *Maintenance fluid therapy:* To replace losses. when sign of dehydration disappear, ORS should be given volume equal to diarrheal losses (maximum 10 ml/kg/stool).

Treatment plan C: Children with severe dehydration. Children suffering from severe dehydration should be treated using intravenous fluids.

- IV fluids
- Types of fluids
  - Ringer lactate with 5% dextrose, or
  - Plain normal saline, or
  - Plain Ringer solution
  - ORS should be started simultaneously, if child can take orally.

Dose

<12 months age—100 ml/kg fluid given over 6 hours.

>12 months age—100 ml/kg fluid given over 3 hours.

Assess the child clinically and take decision for further IV fluid as follows.

1. Persistence of severe dehydration—intravenous infusion is repeated.

2. Hydration is improved but dehydration is present—discontinue IV fluid, give ORS.

3. No dehydration—discontinue IV fluid, ORS is given if danger sign appear.

2. Adequate Feeding or Maintenance of Nutrition

Pathogens especially rotavirus destroy intestinal villi resulting poor absorption of water. It causes watery diarrhea, food in intestine stimulate regeneration of villi thus improves absorption of water from intestine and reduces severity of diarrhea.

Maintenance of nutrition

It is essential to replace nutritional deficit and maintain nutrition during the diarrheal illness. Nutritional deficit results from the reduced intake due to loss of appetite and with holding food and due to losses caused by vomiting and malabsorption.

There is no scientific basis for resting the bowel during diarrheal illness as thought in past. In fact fasting is harmful because it reduces further the ability of small intestine to absorb a variety of nutrients. During acute diarrhea 60% or more of the nutrients are absorbed normally even fats and oils (which provide large amount of energy).

Breastfeeding started as soon as fluid therapy for rehydration is complete in breast fed babies, while in nonbreast fed babies full strength milk formula can be started again when diarrhea is stopped.

All the children older than 4–6 months and adult as soon as their appetite return, should be given adequate diet rich in calories and easily digestible food (less fibre food), these food should be started during maintenance therapy. Do not wait up to the diarrhea stops. Food rich in potassium (e.g. fruit juices, bananas, coconut water) are also useful to consider the replacement of potassium loss due to diarrhea.

Patient who have lost their appetite in such cases frequent small meals advised. Recent studies shows that Vit A supplementation in diet reduce severity of diarrhea.

Regeneration of epithlium is better if feeding is continued. Oral rehydration therapy and continued feeding is also known as ORT-N (oral rehydration therapy-nutrition).

3. Oral Supplementation of Zinc

Zinc deficiency is common in children in developing countries. Intestinal zinc losses during diarrhea aggravate zinc deficiency. So, zinc supplementation is an essential part of management of diarrhea.

Zinc is given as sulphate, acetate or gluconate formulation at a dose of:

Age

2–6 months 10 mg per day for 14 days
>6 months 20 kg per day for 14 days

Mechanism of action of zinc

1. It regulates intestinal fluid transport, mucosal integrity.
2. It plays role in increasing immunity.

3. Zinc modify expression of gene encoding several zinc dependent enzymes such as cytokines.
4. Zinc moderate oxidative stress.

4. Early Recognition of Danger Signs

Recognize the danger signs such as septicemia, paralytic ileus, severe electrolyte disturbances, convulsions.

5. Antibiotics and Antimicrobial Therapy

Medicines

a. *Antimicrobial drugs (including antibiotics):* Mostly diarrhea is due to human rotavirus and toxigenic strains of *E. coli* which are self-limited and do not need antibiotics. Antibiotics are indicated as follows:
   i. Cholera
   ii. Severe Shigella dysentery. For amoebic dysentery, specific drug therapy may also be required when acute diarrhea is associated with another acute infection in the body (e.g. pneumonia, otitis media, etc.) (Table 8.3).

Table 8.3: Antimicrobials indicated for specific situation		
Cause	*Drug(s) of choice and dose*	*Drug(s) and dose*
Cholera	Tetracycline *Children*—50 mg/kg/day in 4 divided doses for 2–3 days	Furazolidone *Children*—5 mg/kg/day in 4 divided doses for 3 days Erythromycin *Children*—30 mg/kg/day in 3 divided doses
Note: Antibiotic therapy shortens duration of illness and excretion of organisms in severe cases.		
Shigella dysentery	Ampicillin 100 mg/kg/day in 4 divided doses for 5 days Trimethoprim (TMP) in 4 divided doses Sulfamethoxazole (SMX) for 5 days *Children*—TMP 10 mg/kg/day and SMX 50 mg/kg/day in two divided doses for 5 days	Nalidixic acid 55 mg/kg/day Tetracycline 50 mg per kg in 4 divided doses for 5 days
Note: Select antibiotic keeping in mind about resistance to antibiotic in that area. Antibiotics are especially required if infants are having persistent high fever.		
Acute intestinal amoebiasis	Metronidazole, ornidazole *Children*—30 mg per kg per day for 5 days depending on response	Tinidazole
Acute giardiasis	Metronidazole *Children*—15 mg per kg per day for 5 days	

Medicines that should not be used in diarrhea

i. Neomycin—damages the intestinal mucosa and can cause malabsorption.

ii. Clioquinol—it is associated with neurological sequelae.

b. Antidiarrheal agents though used commonly are not indicated for routine case. Absorbants (e.g. kaolin, pectin, activated charcoal, bismuth) are of no value in acute diarrhea.

Opiates and other drugs which inhibit intestinal motility (time opium, codeine, diphenoxylate, atropine, loperamide). They delay the elimination of causative organism due to slowing intestinal persistalsis. They may prove fatal if not properly used.

6. Adjunctive Anti-diarrheal Therapy

Microorganism such as *Lactobacillus casei,* strain GG or Lactobacillus GG, *L. plantarum* and strains of Bifidobacteria, *Enterococcus faecium* and yeast *Saccharomyces boulardii* has shown to some efficacy in reducing the duration of acute diarrhea if started in very early phase of illness.

Probiotics: The effectiveness of probiotics preparation is strain and dose specific, routine use is not recommended.

OTHER DRUGS

i. Stimulants such as adrenaline, nikethamide, etc. are not indicated to correct shock in diarrhea. Shock in diarrhea is hypovolemic, so must be corrected by intravenous fluids, not by drugs.

ii. *Steroids:* Steroids are not indicated, can cause serious side effects.

iii. *Purgation:* Never used. Purgation worsen diarrhea and dehydration.

iv. *Oxygen:* Expensive and unnecessary.

Associated Problems and Complications

a. **Vomiting:** If vomiting is persistent, it may better to delay feeding for a few hours and clear fluid is given in small sips, e.g. 1 teaspoonful in 2–3 minutes. Metaclopramide:

Dose: 0.1–0.2 mg per kg or phenothiazine 0.5 mg per kg may be given in cases of severe vomiting. Better avoided due to risk of phenothiazine toxicity.

b. **Protein energy malnutrition:** In such patient continues ORS solution for longer than in other patient to replace the chronic losses of sodium and potassium. In babies with kwashiorkor rehydration therapy will be closely supervised because it may increase edema already present. Nutritional rehabilitation initiated.

c. **Fever:** Treated with cold sponging or antipyretics. Underlying infection causing fever (e.g. pneumonia) must also be treated.

d. **Convulsions:** Convulsions associated with diarrhea may be due to following causes and treat the cause:

i. *Febrile convulsions.* Treated by cold sponging.

ii. *Severe dehydration.* As already described.

iii. *Hypoglycemia.* In comatose patient 20% of glucose given intravenously. 2.5 ml per kg given over 5 minutes.

iv. *Hypernatremia.* Occurs in children usually below 1 year. Cause is inadequate fluid intake and consumption of fluid with high sugar content. Due to osmotic effect solution draw water into bowel causing hypernatremia. Clinical feature is excessive thirst without typical signs of dehydration. It also occurs if ORS solution is given to patient in excessive quantity after diarrhea has stopped: Measure electrolyte if facilities are available. Treatment—give more plain water than usual.

v. *Abdominal distension.* Abdominal distension is primarily due to paralytic ileus caused by hypokalemia, necrotizing enterocolitis or septicemia.

Treatment: Patient is kept nil orally. Potassium chloride (30–40 μg per litre) is given in parenteral fluid after passing urine, intravenously. Nasogastric suction is done by nasogastric tube. Turpentine stopping.

vi. *Renal failure.* Dialysis is indicated in case of renal failure.

Prevention of Diarrhea

i. Promote breastfeeding.
ii. Care of nutrition, water supply, hygiene and preparation of food is done in hygienic way.

CHRONIC DIARRHEA

Chronic diarrhea in an insidious onset diarrhea of more than 2 weeks duration.

Clinical Features

Child passes pale bulky stool. Chronic diarrhea has insidious onset and persists more than 14 days resulting growth failure, abdominal symptoms with distension and flatulence, nutritional deficiency coexists with ill health. Symptoms related to cause of diarrhea coexist and should be investigated.

Causes

i. Malnutrition (PEM)
ii. Intestinal parasites
iii. Iron deficiency anemia
iv. Celiac disease
v. Cystic fibrosis
vi. Tropical sprue
vii. Carbohydrate intolerance
viii. Irritable colon syndrome
ix. Ulcerative colitis
x. Dietary allergies
xi. Immune deficiency

Others

• Intestinal lymphangiectasia
• Drug-induced diarrhea
• Inflammatory bowel disease
• Abdominal tuberculosis.

Management: Management of existing cause.

REHYDRATION SOLUTIONS

Oral Rehydration Therapy (ORT)

For treatment of dehydration oral rehydration solution (ORS) plays an important role. This therapy is called oral rehydration therapy.

Physiological Basis

During diarrhea due to pathogens physiological absorption of sodium becomes impaired, but glucose-dependent sodium pump remains intact. Transporting of one molecules of glucose and dragging along a molecule of sodium and one molecule of water across the mucosa resulting in repletion of sodium and water losses. So, it is called ORS coupled co-transport mechanism, this coupled to transport process of intestinal absorption continues to function normally during secretory diarrhea.

In ORS glucose and sodium are in 1:1 ratio. It is the basis of therapy.

a. It provides adequate quantities of electrolyte to correct the deficits associated within acute diarrhea. Potassium in the solution provides potassium to the body lost with acute diarrhea.
b. Glucose: The absorption of sodium and water in small intestine is more rapid in presence of glucose.
c. Citrate and bicarbonate in ORS solution which is to correct acidosis (Table 8.4).

Osmolarity of replacement fluid should not exceed that of blood (290 mmol/L), so intestinal lumen is kept in low osmolarity than blood by ORS. It results greater absorption of fluid into the blood stream across

Table 8.4: Composition of WHO ORS	
Constituents	*Gram/liter*
Sodium chloride	2.6
Glucose anhydrous	13.6
Potassium chloride	1.5
Trisodium citrate	2.9
Dissolved in one liter of water	

Table 8.5: Osmolarity of ORS

Osmole or ion	Millimole/liter
Sodium	75
Chloride	65
Glucose anhydrous	75
Potassium	20
Citrate	10
Total osmolarity	**245**

Table 8.6: Composition of intravenous infusion (Millimole/liter)

Solution	Na+	K+	Ca+	Cl−	Lactate or alactate
Ringer lactate	130	4	3	109	28
Half strength Darrow's solution	61	18	52		27
Normal saline	154			154	

concentration gradient which results electrolyte absorption by solvent drag (Table 8.5).

Since concentration of glucose increases osmolarity so it is suggested that glucose concentration should not increases 111 mmol/L (low osmolarity of ORS). Benefits of it are: (a) Reduction of stool output, (b) decrease in vomiting, (c) decrease in use of intravenous fluids without increasing risk of hyponatremia.

ORS FOR SAM CHILD

Diluted ORS is given to meet his requirement for rehydration. Ingredients are as follows:

ORS	(1 pkt) as described.
Water	2 L
Sugar	50 gm
Potklor	30 ml

SOLUTIONS FOR INTRAVENOUS FLUIDS

Following solutions are preferred:
- 'Ringer lactate solution': It is best available solution for all age group and for dehydration due to all causes.
- It provides adequate sodium and potassium.
- Lactate yields bicarbonate for correction of acidosis.

Less Suitable Solutions (Table 8.6)
- *Half-strength Darrow's solution:* It does not contain adequate sodium to correct sodium deficit.
- *Normal saline:* It will not correct acidosis and will not replace potassium losses.
- Half-normal saline in 5% dextrose. It will not correct acidosis and potassium deficit.

Unsuitable Solutions

Plain glucose or dextrose solutions. It will provide glucose and water only. They will not corrrect electrolyte losses and acidosis. So, never be used for intravenous correction of dehydration.

GASTROESOPHAGEAL REFLUX

It is a normal physiological state in which stomach contents move retrograde into esophagus.

About 60% of all infants have episodes of spitting up or vomiting not related to overfeeding or any gastrointestinal disease. It is benign. Parental education and reassurance is only required.

Gastroesophageal Reflux Disease (GERD)

It is a pathological state characterized by passage of gastric contents into oesophagus, associated with gastrointestinal (GI) or pulmonary symptoms and sequelae. About 10% of children with GER have GERD.

Pathophysiology

Normally lower oesophageal sphincter (LES) relaxes in coordinated fashion with peristalsis wave to allow esophageal content to enter the stomach. If this relaxation is inappropriate it results gastric refluxate to enter the oesophagus. Gastric emptying delay may also place role.

Clinical Features

Recurrent regurgitation of gastric contents with or without vomiting. But emesis is most common presentation.Weight loss or poor weight gain is due to lack of caloric retention.

Midepigastric pain (heart burn) that is temporarily relieved with food or antacid and exacerbated by fatty food, caffeine or supine position.

Upper and lower airway disease may be induced results hoarseness, wheezing, vocal cord nodules, subglottic stenosis.

Gastrointestinal sequelae are esophageal strictures, hematemesis, dysphagia. Sandifer syndrome is characterized by torticollis with arching of the back caused by painful oesophagitis.

Diagnosis

1. pH of esophagus is continuously monitored for at least 18 hours.
2. Combined 24 hours multiple intraluminal impedance and pH monitoring.
3. Upper GI endoscopy may show erosions or mucosal breaks is esophageal mucosa, stricture.
4. Endoscopic biopsy to evaluate the cause.
5. Nuclear scintigraphy uses a radioactive markers, e.g. (technetium 99m) mixes into age appropriate foods to measure the rate of gastric emptying. Radioactive tracer detected in lungs confirms aspiration.

Management

1. Patient should be kept in left lateral position with the head end elevated by 30° after feeding or when asleep. Dietary recommendations to patient—take frequent small meals and thickening of feed.
2. Acid inhibition by:
   a. Histamine-induced gastric secretion blockers (ranitidine)
   b. Proton pump inhibitors effective in reducing the irritation caused by refluxate.
3. Surgical therapy:
   a. Fundoplication wraps the fundus of the stomach around the distal 3.5 cm of esophagus resulting in transient lower esophageal sphincter relaxation (TLESR).

CONSTIPATION

Definition

Constipation is infrequent and or difficult evacuation of faeces. Constipation is often complained by parents but true constipation is rare in children.

It is important to interpret correctly normal bowel movement with its three variable: Frequency, consistency and volume. Stool is hard or too firm in constipation and time interval is long.

Causes

In neonates and infants
   i. Physiological: Breast fed babies may only have bowels open every 1–7 days.
   ii. Dietic
      • Underfeeding
      • Less fluid intake especially in hot weather
      • Excessive protein in food
   iii. Febrile illness
   iv. Faculty training
   v. Organic lesions
      a. Hirschsprung's disease
      b. Congenital pyloric stenosis
      c. Anal fissure
      d. Intestinal atresia
   vi. Frequent use of laxative and purgative
   vii. Cretinism
   viii. Mental deficiency
   ix. Subacute intestinal obstruction due to tuberculosis enteritis.

Features

Pain on passing stool. Abdominal distension if severe obstruction occurs with vomiting and visible peristalsis.

Treatment

   i. Treatment of cause.
   ii. Symptomatic therapy—high residue diets, proper fluid intake, milk of magnesia or liquid paraffin.
   iii. Toilet training.

HEPATOMEGALY

Causes

1. Infections
   a. *Viral:* Infective hepatitis, serum hepatitis, infectious mononucleosis.
   b. *Bacterial:* Typhoid, pneumonia, tuberculosis.
   c. *Protozoal:* Malaria, amoebiasis, kala-azar.
   d. *Parasite:* Ascariasis, hydatid.
   e. *Spirochaetae:* Weil's disease, syphilis.
2. Congestive
   a. CCF
   b. Tricuspid regurgitation
   c. Constrictive pericarditis.
3. Cirrhosis
   a. Indian childhood cirrhosis
   b. Other types of cirrhosis
4. *Hemolytic anemias:* Thalassemias and sickle cell anemia.
5. *Fatty infiltration:* PCM, severe infections, vit A excess, diabetes, cortisone therapy.
6. Neoplasm—leukemia, Hodgkin's disease.
7. *Storage disease:* Gaucher's disease, amyloidosis, Niemann-Pick disease.
8. *Tumor or cyst:* Hepatoma, secondary to embolic metastasis.
9. *Others:* Riedel's lobe, sarcoidoses, hemangioma.

ABDOMINAL PAIN

Abdominal pain is a common manifestation of multiple pathologies. It may be benign or requires urgent evaluation, diagnosis and treatment.

The abdominal pain may be acute or chronic. Stretching of visceral peritoneum due to inflammation or other cause results in pain sensation.

Causes

A. Intra-abdominal pain
   a. Inflammation: Gastritis, gastroenteritis, appendicitis, Mickel's diverticulitis, acute non-specific lymphadenitis, peritonitis, pancreatitis, hepatitis.
   b. Perforation: Typhoid ulcer, peptic ulcer.
   c. Acute intestinal obstruction.
      Mechanical
      In the lumen : Roundworm
      Intestine : Intussusception
      Toxic : Paralytic ileus
      Neurogenic : Hirschsprung's disease
   d. Colitis—renal, intestinal, appendicular, infantile colic.
   e. Psychogenic pain.
B. Extra-abdominal
   i. Thoracic condition—diaphragmatic pleurisy, pneumonia, pneumothorax.
   ii. General diseases—malaria, typhoid, leukemia, filaria, rheumatic fever, congenital hypertrophic pyloric stenosis.

Evaluation

Complete History

Complete history of child is taken trauma, infection prior to pain, surgery, worm infestation, duration and type of pain, any nocturnal episodes, blood in stool, loose motion, constipation, fever, dysuria, hematuria, weight loss, jaundice, abdominal distension, fever, history of drug intake, radiation of pain, place of pain, worsening of pain after eating.

- Pain from the stomach and proximal intestine is sensed in the epigastrium, from the midgut in the periumbilical area, from the transverse colon in the suprapubic area.
- Pain from retroperitoneal area is referred to the back of abdomen. Ureteric pain in referred to testicular area.

Physical Examination

General Examination

Restlessness may indicate colicky pain, abdominal rigidity seen in peritonitis.

Abdominal Examination

a. **Intestinal obstruction** may presents with diminished or absent bowel sounds, abdominal rigidity and rebound tenderness.

b. **Peritonitis** may presents with diminished or absent bowel sounds, abdominal wall rigidity, and rebound tenderness.

c. **Tests**

Imaging

1. Abdominal skiagram, ultrasonography, CT scan to evaluate the cause.
2. *Laboratory evaluation:* Blood—CBC, urinalysis, hepatic function test, stool examination, testing for pregnancy in adolescent, test to diagnose specific cause.

Management

Management of acute abdominal pain is according to cause diagnosed.

Chronic Abdominal Pain

Chronic abdominal pain is defined as abdominal pain that occurs each month for at least 3 consecutive months. It occurs in children or adolescents.

1. Organic—caused by disease or disorder in about one-third of cases.
2. Functional—about two-thirds of cases, more commonly in females.

Organic Causes of Chronic Abdominal Pain

1. Constipation
2. Peptic ulcer disease
3. Carbohydrate intolerance
4. Inflammation bowel disease
5. Pancreatitis
6. Parasitic infections (Giardia)
7. Worm infestation
8. Genitourinary disorders—pyelonephritis, hydronephrosis
9. Congenital structural abnormalities of gastrointestinal tract (e.g. malrotation).

ASCITES

Causes

I. *Diseases of peritoneum:* Infections: Tuberculous peritonitis and other infections.

II. *Portal hypertension*
   a. Obstruction to portal venous system.
      i. Intrahepatic: Cirrhosis, Hodgkin's disease and leukemic infiltration.
      ii. Extrahepatic: Portal or splenic vein block due to thrombosis or pressure from portal lymphadenopathy or tumors.
   b. Obstruction to hepatic vein or inferior vena cava.
      i. Intrahepatic: Veno-occlusive disease.
      ii. Extrahepatic: Hepatic vein thrombosis, constrictive pericarditis.

III. Hypoproteinemia
   a. Nephrosis
   b. Malnutrition
   c. Protein losing enteropathy

IV. Other causes. Beriberi, epidemic dropsy.

Anasarca (Common Causes)

   i. Anemia or hypoproteinemia
   ii. CCF
   iii. Nephrotic syndrome
   iv. Epidemic dropsy
   v. Beriberi.

VIRAL HEPATITIS

Hepatitis is major health problem worldwide.

Etiology

   i. Hepatitis A (HA) virus (infective hepatitis)
   ii. Hepatitis B (HB) serum hepatitis
   iii. Hepatitis; viruses other than HA, HB (non-A, non-B virus)
   iv. Virus that may cause hepatitis incidentally HIV, cytomegalovirus, herpesvirus, enterovirus, rubella virus, Epstein-Barr virus.

Modes of Infectivity

This is transmitted as follows.

Infective hepatitis
   i. Person to person contact.
   ii. Ingestion of contaminated food and water.

Serum Hepatitis Transmitted

i. By inoculation, by contaminated needles with minute amount of blood from a carrier.

ii. Transfusion of contaminated blood or blood products.

iii. Transplacental passage may effect the fetus causing neonatal hepatitis. Australia antigen has been detected in blood of patient of serum hepatitis.

INFECTIVE HEPATITIS

Onset of this type of hepatitis is from systemic complaints, e.g. fever, malaise, nausea, vomiting, anorexia and abdominal discomfort, which are mild in children and often not noticed.

Jaundice and dull pain on epigastrium and right upper quadrant develop later on. Jaundice is often presenting symptom.

Stool is clay colored or light colored, constipation is common than diarrhea, liver is enlarged and tender. Convalescence recovery is better than adult and least disability in children.

Treatment

Therapy is supportive:

i. Diet low in fat, with adequate vitamins.

ii. There is no evidence that rigid restriction of physical activity will speed recovery.

iii. Intravenous fluid to prevent dehydration in severe anorexia and vomiting.

iv. Cortiosteroids are not indicated in uncomplicated case.

v. Receive 0.5 ml of HBIG.

Complications

i. Acute fulminating hepatitis

ii. Chronic active hepatitis

iii. Aplastic aremia

iv. Nephrosis.

HEPATITIS B (SERUM HEPATITIS)

- Caused by hepatitis B virus (HBV)
- Transmission caused by:
  1. Infected mother to fetus.
  2. Parenteral route through exposure to infected blood product, following tattoing and intravenous drug use.
- Exposure to infected body (sexual contact secretions such as blood, tears, saliva, semen, vaginal secretions, urine, faeces, breast milk.

Clinical Features

Incubation period is 45–160 days; mean 90 days.

Special Features

1. Symptoms are variable asymptomatic to nonspecific hepatitis and fulminent liver failure.

2. Chronic HBV is common in young infants. It results to chronic liver disease, e.g. cirrhosis, fibrosis.

Diagnosis

1. HBV surface antigen (HBS Ag) is pathognomonic. It is also known as Australia antigen.

2. Anti-HBC

PREVENTION

i. Donated blood sample should be tested for to be free of HBV.

ii. Isolation of patient is not necessary; careful handling of blood, needle contaminated

iii. Immunoglobulins as above.
   Dose: 0.06 ml/kg

iv. Vaccines—hepatitis B, pentavalent vaccine.

HEPATITIS C

It is caused by hepatitis C virus.

Transmission

a. Perinatal vertical route from mother to fetus.

b. Parenteral route

Clinical Features

Infection is rarely symptomatic, chronic infection occurs in 80% of children suffering from hepatitis C resulting cirrhosis and hepatic fibrosis.

Diagnosis

Diagnosis of hepatitis is made by detection of anti-HCV and HCV RNA antibody.

HEPATITIS D

Hepatitis D is caused by hepatitis delta virus (HDV).

Transmission

By parenteral exposure.

Clinical Features

Hepatitis D may precipitate fulminant liver failure.

Diagnosis

Demonstration HDV antigen and antibody in serum.

HEPATITIS E

Caused by hepatitis E virus (HEV).

Transmission

By feco-oral route.

Clinical Features

Results acute hepatitis in young children and responsible for 20% mortality in infected pregnant women.

Chronic disease does not occur.

Diagnosis

Serology: Demonstration of HEL antibody.

INDIAN CHILDHOOD CIRRHOSIS

Synonym

Jamaican cirrhosis, veno-occlusive disease of liver.

Definition

This is a fatal familial disorder that occurs predominantly in rural India in middle income group hindu families.

Epidemiology

1. This occurs mostly in all parts of India, but cases also have been reported in Middle East, West Indies, Sri Lanka, Nepal, Pakistan, Burma, Israel, Indonesia, Egypt, West Africa and Central America.
2. Common ages 1–3 years.
3. Male suffers 4 times than females.
4. A definite familiar predisposition seen. Twins, siblings are frequently affected. But no recognized chromosomal or sex-linked pattern yet observed.
5. Vegetarians are more prone than non-vegetarians.

Etiopathogenesis

Cause is not known. Various hypotheses have been suggested as follows:

A. **Nutritional:** According to this theory, it is due to malnutrition but objections against it are:
   a. Patient with marasmus and kwashiorkor did not progress to ICC.
   b. Food (nutrition) does not protect it.
   c. This is common in India. In Africa, where malnutrition is prevalent, it is rare.

B. **Toxic:** Since this resemble vaso-occlusive disease caused by hepatotoxic effect of seneco alkaloid contained in bush teas in West India. It is proposed that this is also due to some toxic agents. It has been suggested that excessive dietary copper may play role in etiology owing to the use of copper and brass in cooking and for storage of water and milk.

   Copper is absorbed from the gut in excess deposited in the liver. Which is itself hepatotoxic or might make the infant more vulnerable to other hepatotoxic agents.

Many workers believe that so-called 'ghuttis' fed to infants, as ritual to keep evil spirit away in many communities, have hepatotoxic properties.

C. **Viral:** Since its features and onset resembles to hepatitis. It is supposed that this is due to virus in origin. In some cases, Australia antigen found but histological features do not resemble to chronic active hepatitis and this does not occur as complication of hepatitis in other parts of world. So, viral etiology is less likely.

D. **Genetic:** ICC family predisposition suggests that this may be genetic but definite autosomal and sex-linked correlation not yet prooved. Family predisposition may be related to environmental factor.

E. **Autoimmune:** It is supposed that ICC may be an autoimmune disease because:
   i. Antibodies against liver tissue observed in many cases of ICC.
   ii. Serum immunoglobins are high, serum complements are low, depressed and delayed abnormal cellular immune response have been observed by some workers.
   iii. Increased incidence of α-fetoprotein (AFP) also has been observed.

Pathology

Liver size is variable, color (grey and green), capsule shows patchy thickening and surface is nodular. On cut section exaggerated lobular markings with small or no parenchymal nodes seen. Portal vein, biliary passage, lymphatics remain normal.

Microscopically

Diffuse liver cell degeneration, necrosis and replacement fibrosis.
a. Formation of macronodules and micronodules clumps.
b. Poor regeneration activity indicated by regeneration nodules enriched by bands of fibrous tissue.
c. Clumps of eosinophilic hyaline are seen in the hepatocytes usually in perinuclear area and this is called Mallory's hyaline.
d. Fatty change is either absent or at its minimal.

Clinical Features

Onset may be insidious or acute. Early presentation may be symptomless or with jaundice only. Clinical manifestations are mainly due to liver dysfunction, portal hypertension or hypersplenism or in combination.

Insidious Onset

It is described in 3 stages overlapping each others.
   i **First stage:** Liver is enlarged by 3–5 cm and has a firm feel with sharp, leafy border, surface is smooth or nodular.

   Anorexia, abdominal distension, constipation, diarrhea having clay-colored stool and growth failure are vague symptoms in this stage.
   ii. **Second stage:** Manifestations of first stage exaggerated. Liver is more firm with leafy border. Jaundice is prominent feature. Sign of portal hypertension, ascites, splenomegaly, hematemesis, anemia, leukopenia, prominent superficial veins and low platelet count dominate the picture.
   iii. **Third stage:** It is terminal stage. Jaundice becomes deep, distension and ascites increases, liver is grossly enlarged or shunken. Spleen is more enlarged and hard.
   Symptoms of liver failure: Restlessness, confusion, then sign of hepatic coma seen and death occurs. Duration of illness varies from 6 months to 3 years.

Acute Onset

About one-third of cases take a fulminant course. Jaundice, fever, clay-colored stools and hepatomegaly are seen. Disease progresses to hepatic coma.

Diagnosis

Depends on:

a. Clinical picture—characteristic of hepato-splenomegaly.
b. History of siblings in family suffered from ICC.
c. Liver biopsy and other liver function tests are deranged.

Differential Diagnosis

a. Benign hepatic enlargement
b. Tuberculosis
c. Hemolytic anemia
d. Persistent hepatitis
e. Metabolic cirrhosis
f. Malaria and kala-azar
g. Veso-occlusive disease

Treatment

No specific treatment is yet known of this fatal disease.

Symptomatic treatment is given depending upon patient symptoms.

Beneficial results of steroids and gamma globulins have been suggested by some authorities. D penicillamine has been used to chelate copper from liver with some long survival.

At initial stage, adequate diet with enriched vitamins and minerals are given.

Symptomatic treatment of hepatic coma and precoma is done.

Prognosis

Prognosis is fatal inspite of all efforts.

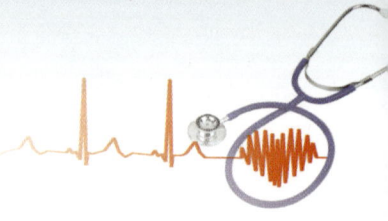

Diseases of Respiratory System

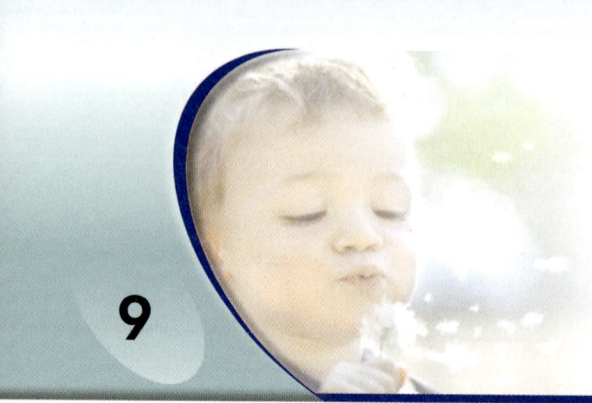

9

Applied Anatomy and Physiology

By 26–28 weeks of gestation sufficient air sac and pulmonary vasculature developed so that fetus is able to survive. Afterbirth, 90% alveolar development occurs. Alveoli increase in number until 8 years of age.

Pulmonary vascular resistance decreases afterbirth when fetal pulmonary and systemic circulations separate when the lungs ventilate first time. Infants are at higher risk for respiratory insufficiency because they have smaller air passage, less compliant lungs with more compliant chest wall and less efficient pulmonary mechanics.

Lung problems may be

- **Obstructive:** Secondary to decreased airflow through narrowed airway, e.g. asthma.
- **Restrictive:** Secondary to pulmonary process that decrease the amount of air filling the alveoli, e.g. pulmonary edema, pulmonary fibrosis.

Clinical Assessment of Pulmonary Disease

History

1. **Antenatal history:** Complication of pregnancy.
2. **Natal:** Obstructed labor, prematurity, instrumentation.

3. **Post-medical history:** Previous pulmonary disease or problem such as frequent respiratory tract infections—cough, wheeze, stridor, snoring and exercise intolerance.
4. **Present history**
   - Cough: Acute or chronic
   - Expectoration: Young children usually swallow the expectoration, older children may be able to bring out expectoration.
   - Hemoptysis
   - Respiratory noises
   - Wheeze is high-pitched voice
   - Snoring is low pitched voice
   - Inspiratory noises: Extrathoracic origin
   - Expiratory noises: Intrathoracic origin.
   - Rettling

   It is due to excessive secretion in phrarynx or tracheobronchial tree.
   - *Wheezing*: Wheezing is high-pitched whistling sounds audible without auscultation. Obstruction of bronchi or bronchiole produces wheezing.
   - *Stridor:* Indicates upper respiratory tract obstruction.
   - *Dyspnea:* Tachypnea is abnormally rapid respiration while dyspnea means labored or difficult breathing usually associated with air hunger and pain.

- *Epistaxis:* Bleeding from nose
- *Croup* is a peculiar brassy cough

Physical examination related to respiratory system

General examination

- Assess for increased work of breathing
- Tachypnea
- Nasal flaring
- Expiratory grunting
- Chest wall indrawing
- Assess ear, nose, throat, examination for sign of obstruction, infection, allergy.
- Inspiratory stridor suggest extrathoracic obstruction.
- Systemic examination of respiratory system.
- Assess for related examination of other organs.

Cardiovascular system: Murmur, tachycardia, increased second sound due to increased pulmonary pressure, clubbing at fingers, eczema, liver size.

Investigations to evaluate respiratory system.

Imaging studies

- Chest X-ray
- CT scan
- Magnetic resonance imaging (MRI)
- Nuclear studies (e.g. ventilation perfusion scan).

Arterial blood gas (ABG)

To measure oxygen (pO_2) and ventilation (pCO_2).

Pulse oximetry

It is a noninvasive technique to measure oxygen saturation.

Pulmonary function tests: To evaluate severity of lung dysfunction.

- Spirometry
- Lung volumes

Laryngoscopy and bronchoscopy

To visualize lower and upper airway, e.g. in persistent pneumonia—cough, stridor, wheezing.

Sweat chloride test

Chloride in sweat is increased in cystic fibrosis. Normal value—40 mEq/L.

ACUTE RESPIRATORY INFECTION

Definition

Acute respiratory infection (ARI) is an acute infection of any part of the respiratory tract and related structures including paranasal sinuses, middle ear and the pleural cavity. This includes all infections of <30 days duration except those of the middle ear where the duration of an acute episode is <14 days.

Incidence

A child on an average suffers from 2.5 to 6 episodes of ARI. 10–15% of these cases will progress to disease of moderate to severe intensity with case fatality rate 5 to 10%. ARI accounts 14.3% death during infancy and 15.9% of death between 1 and 5 years of age. In pediatric age group 20–24% of death are due to ARI; this is higher than due to diarrheal disease (7–12%).

Agent Factor

  i. Bacteria (60%): Streptococci, pneumo-cocci, *Haemophilus influenzae*, *Staphylococcus aureus*, *B. pertussis*, *Corynebacterium diphtheriae*.
 ii. Virus: Syncytial virus, parainfluenzae, influenzae, measles virus.
iii. Fungus: Mycoplasma

Host Factor

ARI is common in first year of life, followed by 1–4 years of age group. Male and female ratio of sufferers is 1.7 : 1.

Environmental Factor

3–4 times more common in winter than summer. Common in overcrowding, poor hygienic conditions.

Mode of Transmission

Droplet infection.

Classification of ARI

ARI is often classified in following clinical syndromes depending on the site of infection.
  i. Upper respiratory tract infections (URTIs) include common cold, pharyngitis and otitis media.
  ii. Lower respiratory tract infections (LRTIs) include epiglotitis, laryngitis, bronchitis, bronchiolitis and pneumonia.

COMMON COLD OR NASOPHARYNGITIS

It is a most common respiratory illness caused by viral infection. Rhinitis is also caused by allergy.

Virus: Adenovirus, influenza, rhinovirus, parainfluenza, respiratory syncytial virus.

Clinical Features

It manifests as fever, thin nasal discharge and irritability. Nasal discharge mucoid may become purulent. Symptoms due to airway obstruction or blocked eustachian tube are other manifestations.

Complications

Otitis media, laryngitis, sinusitis, bronchiolitis, exacerbation of asthma or bronchopneumonia.

Treatment

- Nasal decongestants: Epinephrine, xylometozoline, nasal drops of saline.
- Antihistaminic drugs are used for drying up thin secretion. Avoided in first 6 months of life.
- Non-sedating agent is used for allergic rhinitis: Loalidine, cetrizine.
- Fever is controlled by paracetamol.

Antibiotics have little value because infection is viral in origin.

LARYNGOTRACHEOBRONCHITIS (CROUP)

Croup is inflammation and edema of subglottic, larynx, trachea and bronchi.

Two Forms

Viral croup: Most common cause of stridor.

Spasmodic croup: It occurs in preschool children.

Etiology

Viral croup: Parainfluenza viruses are most common causes.

Other: Respiratory syncytial virus (RSV), rhinovirus, adenovirus, influenza A and B and *Mycoplasma pneumoniae.*

Spasmodic croup is due to hypersensitive reaction.

Clinical Features

Viral croup begins with upper respiratory tract infection for 2–3 days which are followed by inspiratory stridor, fever, barky cough worsen at night and hoarse voice. In advance cases respiratory distress, wheezing may occur.

Spasmodic croup in characterized by acute stridor usually at night. It resolves without treatment.

Management

- Systemic corticosteroid is required to children with stridor at rest.
- Respiratory distress—epinephrine aerosols.
- β_2 agonists when wheezing is present.
- Supportive care—cool, mist and fluids.

EPIGLOTTITIS

This is an acute inflammation and edema of the epiglottis, arytenoid and aryepiglottic folds.

Common in 2–7 years of age.

Causes

Bacterial Infections

- *Haemophilus influenzae* type b (Hib)

- Group AB: Hemolytic Streptococcus, *Strepto-coccus pneumoniae, Staphylococcus* species.

Clinical Features

Onset is acute. High fever muffled speech and quiet stridor, drooling and dysphagia are common clinical symptoms.

Rapidly progressive upper airway symptoms may result respiratory arrest.

Investigations

Laryngoscopy: Epiglottis appears red.

Lateral radiograph: Epiglottis appears as thumb-print.

Management

It is an emergency.
- Oxygen
- Nebulization with epinephrine (1.1000 in doses of 0.1–0.5 ml/kg with maximum 5 vials).
- Dexamethasone: Parenteral once reduce severity.
- Inhalation of budesonide useful.
- Antibiotics: Second or third generation intravenous cephalosporin.

ACUTE BRONCHIOLITIS

This is a common serious illness of lower respiratory tract infection resulting inflammatory obstruction of small airways.

This occurs most frequently below 2 years of age; maximum incidence at 6 months of age. This is a disease having more symptoms and less signs.

Etiopathogenesis

This is a viral illness
1. Respiratory syncytial virus in 50% of cases.
2. *Other viruses:* Mycoplasma, parainfluenza, adenovirus.

Bacteria cause it or not, is not confirmed. As a result of edema, accumulation of mucus and cellular debris of bronchiole, branchiolar obstruction results. This increases airflow resistance since the radius of an airway is smaller, resulting ball valve obstruction leads to early air trapping and overinflation, resulting in collapse and emphysema (Fig. 9.1).

CLINICAL FEATURES

Symptoms

Initially, infant has mild upper respiratory tract infection showing as serious nasal discharge, sneezing and mild pyrexia. Later on fever may be up to 101°–102°F, loss of appetite and gradual development of respiratory distress manifest as wheezy cough, dyspnea and irritability. Feeding is difficult due to rapid respiratory rate, sucking and swallowing is also difficult. Sometime onset is sudden with severe dyspnea which may develop within several hours.

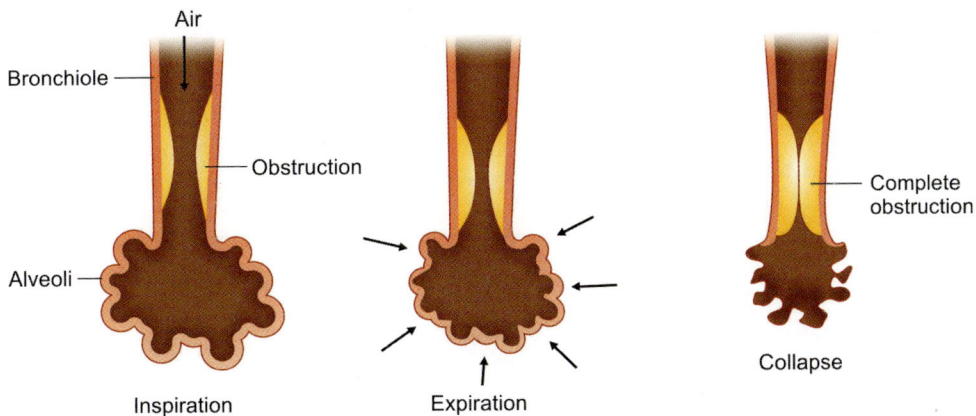

Fig. 9.1: Acute bronchiolitis—showing result of obstruction on air passage.

Signs

On examination respiratory rate is high 60–80/minute. Sign of air hunger, flaring of alae nasi, use of accessory muscles of respiration result in intercostal and subcostal retraction, which is shalow due to persistant distension of the lungs by the trapped air.

Spleen and liver is palpable due to over-inflation of lungs. Fine crepts (rales) are heard at the end of inspiration and early expiration. Expiratory phase is prolonged.

In severe cases, breath sounds are dimi-nished. Sign of CCF and cyanosis may be present.

INVESTIGATIONS

i. Skiagram chest shows hyperinflation of lungs, increased anterior posterior diameter on lateral view of chest, consoli-dation; collapse is seen in some cases.
ii. Blood count normal.
iii. Virus may be demonstrated in naso-pharyngeal secretion by immuno-fluorescence or in culture, rise in antibody titre.
iv. *Screening:* Diaphragm with limited movements, lungs overinflated, inter-costal spaces wide.

Complications

i. Anoxia, exhaustion, acidosis
ii. Dehydration
iii. CCF
iv. Secondary infections.

Treatment

Bronchiolitis is an emergency. Patient should be hospitalized. Management is mostly symptomatic.

General Measures

i. *Oxygen inhalation:* Cold and humified oxygen is given, it reduces dyspnea.
ii. Patient is kept in atmosphere saturated with water vapors.

iii. Sedation is avoided whenever possible due to risk of respiratory depression.
iv. Position in bed 30–40° angle in sitting position, chest slightly elevated and neck extended.
v. IV fluids are given for dehydration or oral fluids given. Respiratory acidosis is corrected.

Specific

i. *Antiviral agent:* Ribavirin (virazole) is effective in reducing the severity of bronchiolitis due to RSV. Injection is given in early in course of illness, administered as continuous inhalation (aerosol) for 12–20 hours/24 hours. It is given up to 2 years of age.
ii. Antibiotics are of no role except in secondary infections.
iii. *Corticosteroids:* Steroids are not beneficial and in certain conditions may be harmful.
iv. Bronchodilator drugs (e.g. epinephrine) are used but have not been tested ad-equately. Trachiostomy is not beneficial because obstruction is at bronchiole level.

PNEUMONIAS

Definition

Pneumonia is defined as inflammation of the lung parenchyma, the portion distal to the terminal bronchioles and comprising the res-piratory bronchioles, alveolar ducts, alveolar sacs and alveoli.

Pneumonia may occur alone or it may occur as secondary complication of some illness, which is more common.

Incidence

About 10% of hospital admission.

Classification

Anatomical or clinical

i. Lobar pneumonia: One or more lobe of the lung involved.

ii. Bronchopneumonia: Patchy involvement of the lungs.
iii. Pneumonitis (interstitial pneumonia): Alveoli or interstitial tissue between them affected. It is generally radiological diagnosis.

Etiology or Etiological Classification

i. Bacterial: *Pneumococcus, Staphylococcus, Streptococcus, H. influenzae,* Klebsiella, *M. tuberculosis,* Pseudomonas.
ii. Viral: Respiratory syncytial virus, adeno-virus, measles, influenza, chickenpox, smallpox, varicella, Mycoplasma.
iii. Fungal: Histoplasmosis, coccidiomycosis.
iv. Protozoal: *Pneumocystis carinii.*
v. Aspiration pneumonia.
vi. Löeffler's pneumonia.
vii. Hypostatic pneumonia.
viii. Drug/radiation pneumonia.
ix. Hypersensitivity pneumonia.

The etiology remains unknown in one-third cases of pneumonia.

PNEUMOCOCCAL PNEUMONIA

This is more common in winter, pathologically scattered area of consolidation occur which coalesces around the bronchi and become lobular or lobar.

Clinical Features

Symptoms have more rapid onset and greater severity. Fever, cough and dyspnea occurs without preceding upper respiratory symptoms.

Increased respiratory rate, decreased breath sound, grunting, chest indrawing (Fig. 9.2), difficulty in feeding and cyanosis is present.

On examination: Crepitations and decreased breath sounds, bronchial breathing, broncho-phony, whispering pectoriloque overconsoli-dation.

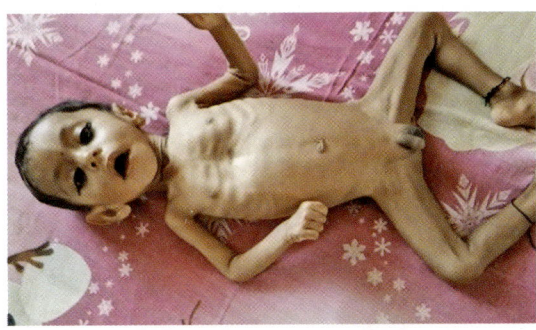

Fig. 9.2: Chest indrawing.

Diagnosis

1. Clinical features
2. X-ray chest: Lobar consolidation
3. Blood: Leukocytosis >20000 cells/mm^3 with neutrophil predominance
4. Blood culture
5. Sputum examination: Gram staining for identification of bacteria.

Treatment

Antibiotics

Penicillin

- Penicillin V 250 mg q 8–12 hr orally
- Penicillin 0.5 mg/kg/day/IV
- Procaine penicillin 0.6 MU IM daily for 7 days.

If allergic to penicillin: Cefalosporin, cefazolin 50 mg/kg/24 hr or cefuroxime 100 mg/kg/24 hr.

Amoxicillin 30–40 mg/kg/day for 7 days is alternative.

Oxygen for respiratory distress

Paracetamol for fever. If dehydration give IV fluids.

Duration of therapy: 7–10 days.

STREPTOCOCCAL PNEUMONIA

Caused by group A β-hemolytic streptococci. It is generally secondary to measles, chick-enpox influenza or whooping cough. It is also important cause of respiratory distress in newborn.

Pathology

It is an interstitial pneumonia which becomes hemorrhagic. Tracheobronchial mucosa ulcerated. Lymph nodes enlarged.

Serosanguineous pleural effusion or empyema is frequent.

Clinical Features

The onset is abrupt with fever, chills, dyspnea, rapid respiration, blood streak sputum.

X-ray chest
- Shows interstitial pneumonia
- Segmental involvement
- Diffuse peribronchial densities
- Pleural effusion
- Pneumatocele

Complications: Empyema, pleural effusion, lung abscess.

Treatment: Same as pneumococcal pneumonia

Empyema: Tube drainage

STAPHYLOCOCCAL PNEUMONIA

This is a serious and rapidly progressive infection caused by *Staphylococcus aureus*. 70% of cases are below 1 year of age. This may be primary infection of lung parenchyma or may follow septicemia.

Pathogenesis

Initially, there is pneumonic process but soon hemorrhagic necrosis results in cavitation. Destruction of lung tissue leading to formation of multiple abscesses which erode bronchial wall and discharge their contents in bronchi. During inspiration air enters in these abscesses cavity because bronchi are in dilatation. But in expiration bronchioles collapse, so air cannot moved out due to valve-like mechanism. Thus, abscess is progressively dilated resulting in pneumatocele which is characteristic of the disease seen in skiagram.

Staphylococcal pneumonia results in empyema commonly. All empyema in infant is considered almost staphylococcal until unless proved otherwise (Flowchart 9.1).

Clinical Features

Symptoms are of pneumonia. Abdomen is usually distended due to septicemia and ileus. Cyanosis may be present. Empyema is common. Pneumatocele on skiagram is characteristic. General condition may be mild despite gross radiological findings.

Blood picture shows polymorphonuclear leukocytosis.

Diagnosis

i. *Skiagram chest* (Fig. 9.3): Homogeneous consolidation, lung abscess, pneumatocele or complication picture.

ii. *Recovery of Staphylococcus from* cough swab, nose and throat swab, gastric washing, tracheal aspiration or pleural tap.

iii. *Blood*

   a. Often leukocytosis. Prognosis is poor if normal count or leukopenia.

   b. Blood culture to isolate the organism.

Flowchart 9.1

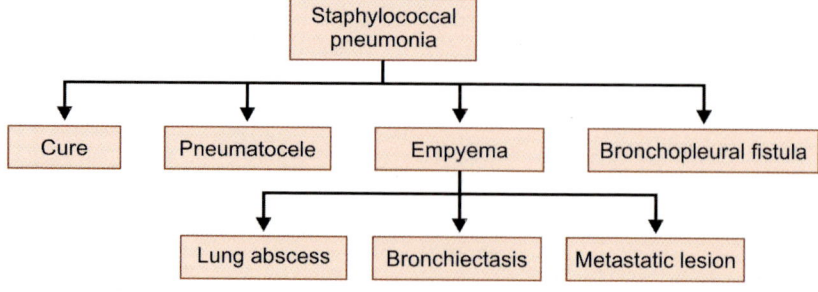

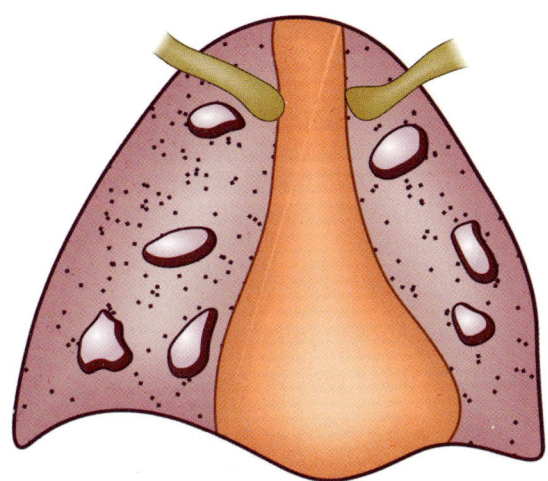

Fig. 9.3: Diagrammatic representation of skiagram of staphylococcal pneumonia showing pneumatocele.

Treatment

Must be energetic; as described earlier penicillin G 1 lakh units/kg/24 hr or semi-synthetic penicillanase resistant penicillin, e.g. methicillin 200 mg/kg/24 hr intravenously given.

If patient is sensitive to penicillin, cefazolin 30 mg/kg/24 hr is alternative.

Prognosis

Prognosis is worse.

HAEMOPHILUS INFLUENZAE PNEUMONIA

It occurs between 3 months to 3 years of age. Transplacental antibodies of the mother protects infant up to 3–4 months. Most infections are mild and confer immunity for subsequent infection.

Clinical Features

Onset is gradual as a nosopharyngeal infection. Child has fever, dyspnea, grunting respiration and retraction of lower intercostal space.

Complications: Pericarditis, empyema, meningitis, polyarthritis.

Treatment

Antibiotics

- Ampicillin 100 mg/kg/day or coamoxiclav
- Cefotaxime (100 mg/kg/day)
- Ceftriaxone (50–75 mg/kg/day)

PRIMARY ATYPICAL PNEUMONIA

It is caused by *Mycoplasma pneumoniae*. It is one of the most common causes of pneumonia in older children and adolescents.

Clinical Features

Symptoms are low grade fevers, chills, nonproductive cough, headache, pharyngitis, malaise and cough.

On examination: Widespread crepitations on lungs.

Diagnosis

1. Positive cold agglutinins are suggestive but not specific.
2. Chest X-ray: Bilateral diffuse infiltrate.
3. Elevation of serum 1 gm titre for Mycoplasma.

Treatment

Oral erythromycin, or azithromycin is drug of choice given for 7–10 days.

CHLAMYDIA PNEUMONIAE

Common in young infants. Clinically spasmodic cough is prominent feature.

Pneumonia due to gram-negative organism

Causative organism: *E. coli*, Klebsiella, Pseudomonas.

Clinical Features

Malnourished or immunodeficient children generally less than 14 years of age are affected by gram-negative organism.

Clinical features are same as other type of pneumonia but constitutional symptoms are more prominent than respiratory symptoms. X-ray chest shows consolidation or pneumatocele.

Treatment

Antibiotics

- Third generation cephalosporin (cefotaxime or ceftriaxone 75–100 mg/kg intravenous with or without glycosides.
- Ceftazidime or piperacillin tazobactam is drug to be used in Pseudomonas infection.

Viral pneumonia: Viruses are most common causes of pneumonia in all age.

Virus: Influenza, parainfluenza, and adenoviruses.

Clinical Features

Viral pneumonia often begins as upper respiratory complaints such as nasal congestion and rhinorrhea. Fever, cough, tachycardia, wheezing or crepitations are common clinical manifestations.

Diagnosis

- **X-ray chest:** Perihilar or peribronchial infiltrates.
- **Blood:** White blood cell count more than 20000 cells/mm^3 with lymphocyte predominance.
- **Management:** Supportive.

Ingestion of aliphatic hydrocarbons

Ingestion of kerosene oil may cause pneumonia because it diffuses from pharynx to lungs. Clinical features are cough, fever, dyspnea, high fever, vomiting, drowsiness, coma.

X-ray chest: Homogenous or patchy opacities.

Treatment

Gastric lavage or induced vomiting to remove the oil is avoided to prevent aspiration.

Oxygen, antibiotics or corticosteroids are not recommended for routine use.

Loeffler's Syndrome

Larva of many nematodes when enters in lungs during the lifecycle plug the bronchi with mucus and eosinophilic material due to allergic reaction.

Clinical features are fever, cough, rales.

X-ray chest shows pulmonary infiltrates.

Treatment is supportive.

BRONCHIAL ASTHMA

Definition

This is a common respiratory allergic disorder characterized by recurrent attacks of dyspnea, and wheezing due to bronchial spasm. This is regarded as diffuse obstructive lung disease with:

1. Hyperactivity of airways to a variety of stimuli.
2. A high degree of reversibility of the obstructive process which may occur either spontaneously or in response to treatment.

Etiopathogenesis

Age

80–90% of asthmatic children have first symptom before 4–5 years of age. One-third cases of asthma commences before the age of 10 years. Incidence falls slowly as age advances.

Sex

Male children tend to suffer more since they have smaller airway which is also inherited. At least twice in males than females up to puberty. Afterward incidence is same.

Obstruction of the airflow is caused by:
i. Spasm of smooth muscles of bronchi.
ii. Edema and inflammation of mucous membrane lining the airways.
iii. Intraluminal exudation of mucus, inflammatory cells and cellular debris. As a result of this, obstruction of bronchi

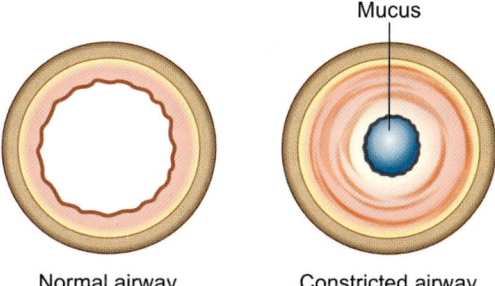

Mucus

Normal airway   Constricted airway

Fig. 9.4: Bronchial asthma constricted airway.

increases. As muscles of inspiration are more powerful than those of expiration, lungs tend to fill and airway closes prematurely during expiration. As a result, lungs are hyperinflated leading to temporary emphysema (Fig. 9.4).

Sometimes complete obstruction to a small bronchus occurs owing to tenacious mucus resulting in segmental collapse. Acidosis develops due to rise in arterial pCO_2.

As attack subsides, muscular spasm relaxes. Mucus is coughed out and breathing returns to normal.

Predisposing Factors

1. Hereditary: Family history of asthma or other allergic disorders often present.
2. Respiratory tract infections like measles and whooping cough.
3. Emotional: A asthmatic child is usually labile, overconscious.
4. Endocrine factor: Asthma attacks are more in relation to menses particularly premenstrually or at menopause and in thyrotoxicosis patient.

Exciting Factors

Allergy to certain foreign substances known as allergens. They may be:
  i. Inhalants: Pollens, house dust, feathers, moulds, dandruff (human or animal).
  ii. Foods: Protein food (egg, meat, chocolate).

iii. Drugs: β-adrenergic blocking agent, aspiration.
iv. Viral and bacterial infections.
  v. Psychological (emotional): Stress, worry.
vi. Exhaustion.

Immunofactors (IgE, Cytokines, Allergens)

Triggering factors:
• Viral infection
• Exercise
• Whether changes: Cold air
• Emotional factor
• Food allergy
• Endocrine factor: In puberty endocrine changes increase symptoms of asthma.

Clinical Features

1. Onset is often sudden and in night. Sometime insidious. Obstruction develops within minutes when child is exposed to irritant (e.g. cold air, etc.).
   If attack is precipitated by viral infections, it is slower and severity increases.
2. During early course of disease features are cough which sounds light and non-productive, wheezing and tachypnea and predominantly expiratory dyspnea but dyspnea is inspiratory also. Signs of use of accessory muscles of respiration present.
   Cyanosis and hyperinflation of chest, tachycardia develops as disease advances; widespread rhonchi heard during auscultation; wheezing is cardinal sign.
3. As severity advances respiratory distress increases. Shortness of breath, difficulty in walking and talking occurs. Child assumes position of sitting.

   Wheezing may be absent, which is ominous sign shows worsening of disease, wheezing may appear after treatment or improvement. Child sweats profusely, has a low grade fever and is exhausted.

   Pigeon chest deformity or clubbing is rarely present in long-standing cases.

After the attack, child becomes symptomless and shows no sign of lung disease.

Status Asthmaticus

Status asthmaticus is clinical diagnosis, defined by increasingly severe asthma not responsive to drugs that are usually effective. Attack generally lasts one hour or two hours normally, but in this condition attack lasts for many hours.

Investigations

   i. Eosinophilia of blood and sputum
  ii. Immunoglobulin concentration: IgE increased.
 iii. Skiagram chest: Evidence of emphysema.
  iv. Allergy skin testing for articles to which body is allergic, tested if positive.
   v. Exercise testing is characteristic.
  vi. Pulmonary function test: Evaluated.
 vii. Therapeutic trials: Trials of epinephrine or other bronchodilators are given and seen the response. If favorable response, it suggests asthma. But validity of test is not established.

Lung function tests: Not very significant, FEV1 spirometry is commonly used parameter for diagnosis of severity.

FEV25–75: Sensitive to airway obstruction
1. FEFR: Abnormal.
2. Eosinophil count: Often normal
3. X-ray chest may show hyperinflation, patchy thickening, patchy at alectasis.

Diagnosis

The disease is diagnosed on the basis of clinical picture. Search to the allergan should be made. "All that wheeze is not asthma." Diagnosis of asthma is mainly depends on clinical features, therapeutic response to bronchodilator drugs.

Differential Diagnosis

Cardiac asthma, bronchiolitis, foreign body inhalation, tropical eosinophilia, hypersensitivity pneumonitis and other conditions give rise to wheezing.

Acute wheezing: Causes:
1. Asthma
2. Hyersensitive reaction including anaphylaxis.
3. Bronchiolitis
4. Pneumonia
5. Foreign body aspiration
6. Acute aspiration of stomach contents
7. Environmental irritants

Management

Treatment of asthma depends on severity of symptoms and trigger factor. Self management with normal lifestyle is the primary goal.

Management of acute asthma is done by following ways:
1. Control of trigger factor
2. Pharmacotherapy
3. Education of parents and patient. About nature of disease and steps for prevention.
4. Assessment and monitoring of asthma.

Bronchial asthma	Asthmatic bronchitis
1. Onset—5–10 years of age mostly.	1. Infant mostly.
2. Allergy is cause in most cases.	2. Non-allergic in origin.
3. Dyspnea is expiratory predominantly.	3. Dyspnea is inspiratory and expiratory.
4. Family history present.	4. No family history.
5. Infections may or may not be present.	5. Infections always present.
6. Emphysematous changes in skiagram.	6. Non-specific changes.

Control of Trigger Factor

Avoidance of casual allergens, dust mites, molds, animal dander, cockroach, pollen, smoke, tobacco smoke, pollution, irritants (wet paints, disinfectants).

Pharmacotherapy

Medication of bronchial asthma acts by following ways:

a. Relax smooth muscle and dilate the airway.
b. Decrease inflammation so prevent exacerbation.

Drugs

a. Bronchodilator
b. Steroids
c. Mast cell stabilizers
d. Leukotriene modifier
e. Theophylline

Bronchodilators

1. Salbutamol oral, parenteral, inhalation.
   Dose
   - MDI (100 µg/per puff) 1–2 puff q 4–6 hr
   - Respirator solution 0.15–0.2 mg/kg/dose (5 mg/ml)
   - Respules nebulization (2.5 mg/3 ml)
   - Dry powder 1 cap q 4–6 hr (capsule 200 mg)
2. Terbutaline
   MDI (250 µg per puff) 1–2 puff 12–24 hr
   Oral, parenteral, inhalation.
3. Salmetrol
   MDI (25 µg per puff) dry powder (50 mg) 1 cap q 12–24 hr long acting.
4. Formoterol
   MDI (25 µg per puff) 1–2 puff 12–24 hr long acting
5. Theophylline (oral tab) 2.5–7.5 mg/kg/ q 12 hr
6. Cromolyn MDI 1–2 puff q 6–8 hr mild to moderate asthma, exercise-induced asthma (5 mg/puff)
7. Nedocromil inhalation
8. Ketotifen 1 mg q 12 hr oral route

These drugs are safe, duration of improvement may be evident after 14 weeks of therapy.

Salbutamol is drug of choice for acute attack and to prevent exercise-induced bronchospasm.

Long acting bronchodilators are used for long-term prevention of symptoms.

Formoterol used with inflammatory therapy. Formoterol and salmeterol are safe after 4 years of age, they may be used for chronic control of asthma.

Side effects of drugs

- Adrenaline is α and β stimulants which have higher cardiac side effects then terbutaline and salbutamol, which are β-agonist hence has less cardiac side effects (tachycardia, tremors, headache, hypokalemia, hyperglycemia.
- Inhalation routes have quick action and less side effects.
- Side effects of corticosteroids are growth retardation.
- Adrenaline is given subcutaneously.

Mast Cell Stabilizers

Mechanism of action reduces bronchial reactivity and symptoms induced by irritant, antigens, and exercise. Anti-inflammatory prophylaxis is induced by inhibition of activation of inflammatory mediator.

There is no effect on acute symptoms but may prevent exacerbation.

Leukotriene Modifiers

Indication: Mild to moderate persistent asthma and exercise-induced asthma.

Drugs
Montelukast (tab 4, 5, 10 mg)

Dose

2–5 years	4 mg q 24 hr
5–12 years	5 mg q 24 hr
>12 years	10 mg q 24 hr

Used in children above 1 year of age.

Zafirlukast—used in children at 12 years of age.

- Theophylline: Mechanism of action
  1. Bronchodilator
  2. Anti-inflammatory
  3. Immunomodulatory

Indication: Used as second line therapy along with glucocorticoids in moderate, persistent asthma in children 5 years age or elder children as adjunctive therapy mainly for control of nocturnal symptoms.

Dose: 2.5–7.5 mg/kg q 12 hr (oral 100, 150, 300 mg)

Corticosteroids

Corticosteroids used in inhaled form are better because they have less systemic side effects. Steroids used in asthma are:

- Beclomethasone
- Budesonide
- Fluticasone

Drugs	Dose
Beclomethasone MDI (50, 100, 200 µg per puff)	50–800 µg/day in 2–3 divided doses
Fluticasone MDI (25, 25, 125, µg per puff) *Respules* (0.5, 1 mg/ml) Rotacap (100, 200, 400 µg)	25–250 µg q 12 hr
Ciclesonide MDI (80,160 µg)	1 puff q 24 hr

Immunotherapy: It is occasionally used under special supervision. If allergen in known administer gradually increasing allergen extract to ameliorate the symptoms.

Inhalation Devices

Medicines of bronchial asthma can be given by inhalation devices or oral route. Drugs used with inhalation devices have rapid action and less side effects. So, these are preferred than other way.

Metered dose inhaler

It deliver fixed amount of drug in aerosol form in a manner—press and breath.

Use: Exacerbation and maintenance therapy.

Method to use of MDI (Figs 9.5 and 9.6)
1. Remove the cap of inhaler.
2. Shake the inhaler in vertical position 3–5 times.

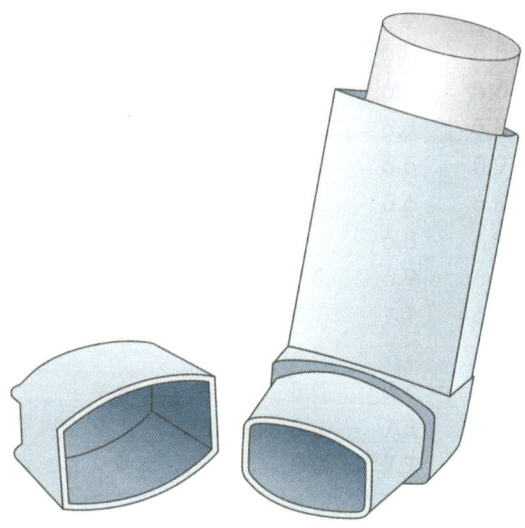

Fig. 9.5: MDI with spacer.

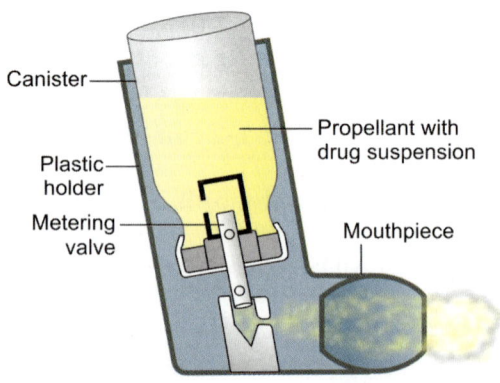

Fig. 9.6: MDI—internal view.

3. Breathe out gently.
4. Put mouthpiece in mouth.
5. Press the top of MDI and continue to inhale deeply.
6. Hold the breathe for 10 seconds or as long as possible.
7. Breathe out slowly.
8. Wait for few seconds before repeating the inhalation.

Metered Dose Inhaler with Spacer (Fig. 9.7)

MDI use may not be possible in correct way in young children. Large proportion of drug is deposited at oropharynx.

So, MDI with spacers is better in young children.

Metered dose inhaler with spacer with facemask

Facemask attached with MDI space is choice of device in very young infant.

Dry powder inhalers

They are breath activated devices, a capsule is inserted into square hold. Make sure that top of the capsule in level with top of hole. Hold inhaler horizontally. Twist barrel clockwise and anticlockwise, this twisting action break the capsule into two.

Breathe out gently, put mouth end of rotahaler in mouth and take deep inspiration. Remove rotahaler from mouth and hold breathe for 10 seconds.

Method to use of rotahaler (Fig. 9.8)

- Rotahaler is a dry powder inhaler which is very easy to use.
- It contains rotahaler and rotacap. Rotacap contains dry powder of medicine, upper part of rotacap in colored and lower part in transparent.
- Rotacap is inserted upside down at square, transparent part is lower at square so that the upper part comes at the level.
- Turn the lower part of rotahaler. Lower part of rotacap separate from upper part.
- Breathe out.
- Inhale powder from mouth closed properly cracking sound is produced means proper working of inhaler.
- Hold breathe for 10 seconds or as long as you can.
- Breathe out slowly
- If powder in left in inhaler, again inhale.

Nebulizer

Medication can be given with the help of nebulizer.

Indication for use—severe asthma in young children.

Method to use of nebulizer (Figs 9.9 and 9.10)

1. Connect compressor to mains.
2. Connect compressor to nebulizer chamber by the tubing provided with nebulizer.

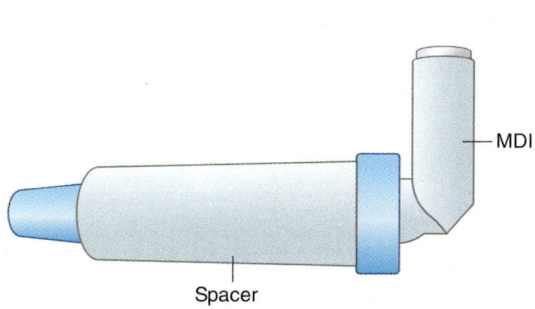

Fig. 9.7: MDI with spacer.

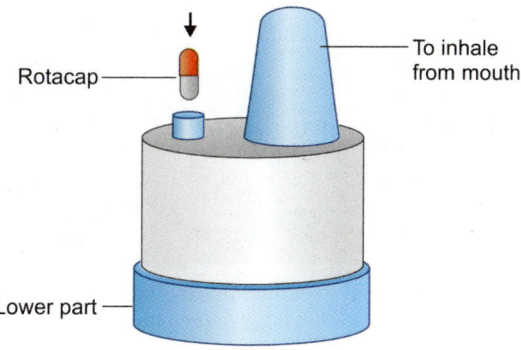

Fig. 9.8: Rotahaler.

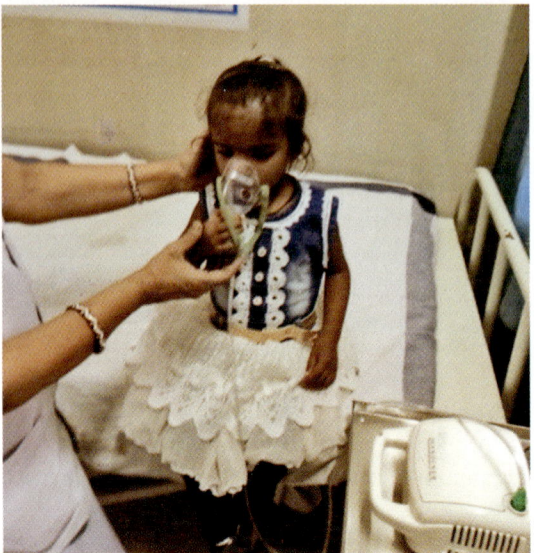

Fig. 9.9: Nebulization.

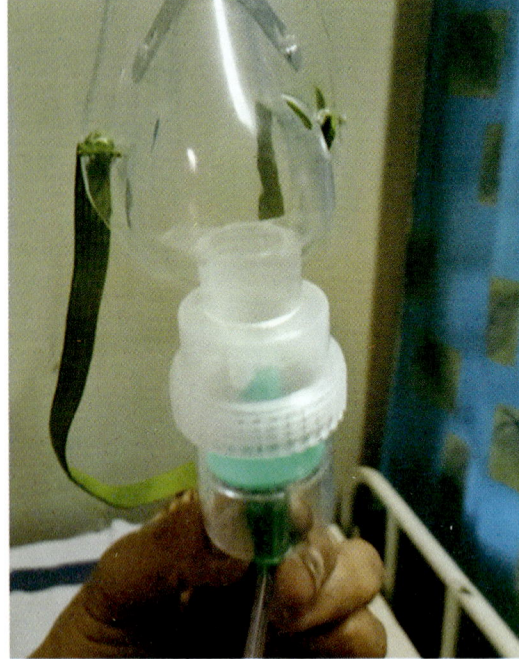

Fig. 9.10: Medicine chamber with mask.

3. Put measured amount of drug prescribed in the nebulizer chamber and add normal saline to a total of 2.5–3 ml.

4. Connect tubing with mask at its distal end (use appropriate size of mask to cover nose and mouth).
5. Switch on the compressor and look on aerosol coming out from the other end.
6. Encourage the baby to take gentle breathe with open mouth.

Guidelines

- Children below 4 years old—MDI with spacer with face mask.
- 4–12 years old—MDI with spacer
- Above 12 years old—MDI

Pharmacological Management Guidelines

Before beginning of pharmacological management assess:
1. Severity of disease
2. Selection of medication
3. Selection of inhalation device
4. Monitoring of effects

1. Severity of Disease

As per severity patient of asthma can be classified in 4 groups:
1. Intermittent
2. Mild persistent
3. Moderate persistent
4. Severe persistent

Step 1: Intermittent

Daytime symptoms, attack less than one time in a week.
- Asymptomatic
- Normal FER between attacks
- Nighttime symptoms—about 2 time in a month
- Peak expiratory flow rate >80%

Step 2: Mild persistent

- Daytime symptoms—more than one time in a week but less than one time a day.
- More than 2 times in a month.
- Peak expiratory flow rate >80%
- Nighttime symptoms >2/min.

Step 3: Moderate persistent

- Daily attacks affect activity. Daily use of β-agonist needed.
- Nighttime symptoms more than one time in a week.
- Peak expiratory flow rate >60% and 80% predicted.

Step 4: Severe persistent

- Continuous, limited physical activity.
  Night symptoms frequent.
  Peak expiratory flow rate <60% predicted.
  Stage: Drugs used are per stage of asthma.
  Intermittent—inhaled short acting β-agonist for symptomatic relief.
  Mild persistent—inhaled short acting β-agonist + inhaled budesonide, fluticasone or inhaled beclomethasone 100–200 µg 12 hr or cromolyn sodium or sustained release theophylline or leukotriene modifier.
  Moderate persistent inhaled short acting β-agonist + inahaled beclomethasone 100–200 µg 12 hr, if needed salmeterol, 50 µg q 12–24 hr and sustained release theophylline.
  Severe persistent inhaled short acting β-agonist + inhaled budesonide, fluticasone or beclomethasone 200–400 µg 12–24 hr + salmeterol or formoterol and/or sustained release theophylline + oral dose of prednisolone on alternate day, if symptoms persist with above treatment.

Supportive Treatment

1. Rehydration
2. Treatment of infection
3. Avoid provoking factors

Mild Acute Asthma

Such children should be given β$_2$-agonist by nebulizer or MDI or with spacer at the rate one puff every minute up to 10 puffs, if improves.

Oral β-agonists may be given 6–8 hr.

If no improvement treat as acute moderate asthma.

Acute moderate and severe asthma

- β-agonist inhalation repeated every 20 min, if improves every 30 min.
- Oxygen
- Oral prednisolone for 5–7 days

No improvement

- Salbutamol inhalation add
- Ipratropium 250 µg every 20 min
- Hydrocortisone 10 mg /kg/IV

No improvement

Magnesium sulfate infusion in 5% dextrose.

No improvement

Mechanical ventilation.

Improvement administer a single dose of prednisolone (1–2 mg/kg) and transfer to hospital.

Life-threatening Asthma

Peak expiratory flow is less than 33%, O$_2$ saturation less than 92%, poor expiratory effort, silent chest, exhaustion, cyanosis, altered consciousness are clinical features suggestive of life-threatening asthma. Screen for pneumothorax, acidosis, infection.

Management

a. Oxygen: High flow.
b. Terbutaline or adrenaline injection given subcutaneously.
c. Salbutamol or terbutaline via oxygen driven nebulizer.
d. Hydrocortisone 5 mg/kg intravenous.

If improvement

- Salbutmol or terbutaline inhalation
- Continued (20–30 min interval)
- Hydrocortisone (3–5 mg/kg) continued every 6–8 hr till child can take orally.

If no improvement

1. IV infusion of magnesium sulfate (50 mg/kg) is given over 30 min
2. Theophylline is infused.
3. If no improvement mechanical ventilation.

Exercise-induced bronchoconstriction

Many children suffer from bronchoconstriction after exercise short acting β-agonists should be taken before exercise and long acting β-agonists leukotriene modifiers should be taken at morning which continue to prevent it throughout daytime.

Seasonal Asthma

In a particular season child gets symptoms of asthma medications depends on severity. Maintenance treatment started two weeks in advance.

Education of Parents

Parents should be educated about:
a. Minimize over, avoid triggering factor.
b. Maintain record about symptoms, sleep disturbances and medications required.
c. Use of spacer and side effects of drugs.
d. Peak flow monitoring.

Home treatment of acute exacerbation

Acute exacerbation is defined by increase in cough, wheeze and breathlessness. PEF is measured which may be decreased.

Such patient requires administration of short acting β_2-agonist by MDI with or without spacer with or without face mask. One puff is given at a time and repeated every 30–60 seconds (max 10 puffs.)

If improvement continue salbutamol or terbutaline every 4–6 hr.

CHRONIC WHEEZING

Causes

1. Asthma
2. Aspiration
3. Congenital anomalies of respiratory tract
   - Tracheomalacia or tracheal stenosis
   - Bronchomalacia
   - Subglottic hemangioma
   - Lobar emphysema
4. Compression of airway
   a. Vascular
      - Vascular ring or sling
      - Anomalous vessel
   b. Tumor or lymph node
5. Congestive cardiac failure
   Pulmonary edema
6. Hypersensitivity pneumonitis
7. Cystic fibrosis
8. Immunodeficiency diseases
9. α_1-antitrypsin deficiency.

TUBERCULOSIS

This is a common chronic infection of children, and important cause of mortality and morbidity in children, caused by *Mycobacterium tuberculosis.*

Epidemiology

A. Tuberculosis is common among urban, low socioeconomic group but it may be seen in any socioeconomic group.

B. High risk group includes immigrants, residence of homeless individuals, institutions, correctional facilities and immunodeficiency conditions (e.g. HIV), chronic disease, immunosuppressive medication.

In HIV patient tuberculosis is 10 times higher than others.

C. Children younger than 12 years are generally not contagious because their cough in minimal and their pulmonary lesion is small.

Incidence

1 in 50, according to ICMR survey. 5–8% of pediatric OPD patients are of tuberculosis.

Etiopathogenesis

Bacteria: Tuberculosis is caused by most common tubercle baccilli *Mycobacterium tuberculosis. Myobacterium bovis* and *M. africanum* are rare cause of tuberculosis. This is a straight, aerobic, non-motile, non-sporing rod. Bacilli contain fatty material which make staining difficult particularly decolorizing actions of alcohol or acid, bacilli therefore called acid-fast bacilli (AFB). They are stained by Ziehl-Neelsen stain. Bacilli appear as red rods against blue backgrounds.

Route of infection: A child is infected by inhalation of airborne infected droplet, derived from sputum of open case of tuberculosis usually an adult. Common site is lungs being for primary infection. Other sites may be lymph nodes, skin, tonsils, intestines, etc.

Pathogenesis: As soon as infection enters, polymorph accumulates at the site. It is followed by epithelioid cell formation. At the end, tubercle formation takes place. It has feature of surrounding layer of mononuclear cells and occassional giant cells with central area of necrosed and caseous or cheesy material. It is described as Ghon's focus. It is about a centimeter in diameter.

Primary complex: From the primary focus, bacilli traverse to regional lymph nodes via lymphatics. Primary focus, inflammation of lymph nodes and inflammation of lymphatics are together is known as primary complex.

Inflammatory reactions in lymph nodes are marked in comparison to primary infection. Midzone of lungs is common site of primary infection because it is an area of maximum ventilation and sub-pleural because current in peripheral part of lungs is more sluggish and bacilli stay here longer time. Right lung is more affected, because right bronchus is more vertical and has more pulmonary volume.

Fate of Primary Complex

a. Lesion may heal completely and disappear, if resistance is good and conditions are favorable.
b. May enlarge or caseate; later calcification may occur; living bacilli lurk in apparently healed focus; fibrosis occurs around.
c. Inflammation progress in continuous area of lung parenchyma, pleura, lymph nodes, if host resistance is poor. It is called progressive primary complex.
d. Inflammed lymph nodes compress bronchi resulting collapse of lung or obstructive emphysema.
e. Lesion erodes bronchi and spread to other parts of lungs—segmental tuberculosis.
f. Hematogenous spread occurs due to caseous gland proximity of the lesion rupture into large vein. Thus, large number of bacilli enter into blood stream. Spread due to blood dissemination results lesion in other part of body, e.g. lung, liver, brain, spleen, etc. (Fig. 9.11).

PRIMARY FOCUS

Secondary or post-primary tuberculosis (adult) results from either overwhelming new infections or reactivation of existing dormant lesion. Even calcified lesion may contain living bacilli.

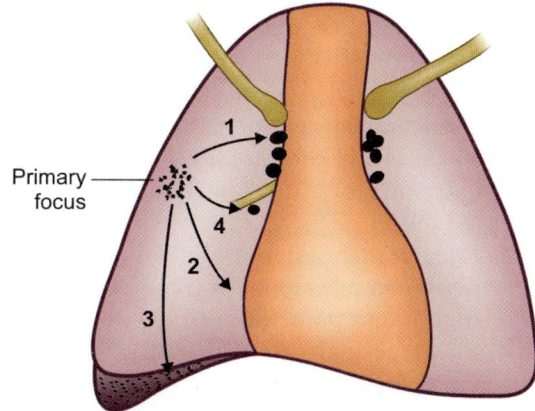

Primary focus

Fig. 9.11: Spread of primary focus to: 1. Hilar lymph node. 2. Lung parenchyma. 3. Pleura. 4. Hematogenous.

Clinical Features

Clinical types are as follows:

i. Intrathoracic
   a. Primary pulmonary tuberculosis.
   b. Progressive primary pulmonary tuberculosis.
   c. Reactivation tuberculosis.
   d. Pleural effusion.
ii. Extrathoracic
   a. Tuberculosis of upper respiratory tract.
   b. Tuberculosis of lymph nodes.
   c. Miliary tuberculosis.
   d. Tuberculous meningitis.
   e. Tuberculosis of heart and pericardium.
   f. Abdominal tuberculosis.
   g. Tuberculoma of skin.
   h. Skeletal tuberculosis
   i. Urogenital tuberculosis.
   j. Tuberculosis of eye.

A. PRIMARY PULMONARY TUBERCULOSIS

Incubation period is 4–8 weeks. Clinical features are as follows:

a. Usually, there is no symptom or symptoms are not specific, e.g. mild fever, reduced appetite and weight loss. Diagnosed by positive skin test or radiograph of chest.
b. Symptoms due to massive enlargement of lymph nodes causing compression, obstruction of chest structures.
   1. Oesophageal compression: Dysphagia, recurrent aspiration.
   2. Blood vessel compression: Edema of an extremity or superior vena caval syndrome.
   3. Recurrent laryngeal nerve or phrenic nerve compression: Vocal cord paralysis, diaphragm paralysis.
   4. Paratracheal, parabronchial nodes enlargement: Recurrent cough, stridor, wheezing, segmental collapse, emphysema.
   5. Bronchial erosion and discharge of material: Symptoms of acute pneumonia.

Older children and adolescents present as infiltration and cavitation of upper lobes, while in young infant and children up to three years sign and symptoms are of miliary tuberculosis.

Segmental lesion (epituberculosis): Sometimes collapse due to bronchial compression by lymph nodes occurs, more common in children due to soft cartage. Patients have high temperature, sometimes wheezing and in long-standing cases of bronchiectasis.

Investigations

i. Tuberculin test positive.
ii. **Radiologically**: Skiagram of chest is often normal. Abnormalities are:
   a. Enlarged hilar shadow: Massive, unilateral, hilar lymphadenopathy with or without parenchymal lesion is usually seen in middle and lower lobe. Calcification on healing. Hilar lymph nodes opposite the side of Ghon's focus are rarely seen.
   b. Ghon's focus is sometimes seen as blurred opacity.
   c. Widening of mediastinum (superior) due to paratracheal adenitis.
   d. **Skiagram in segmental collapse**: The collapsed portion of lung results in an opacity. In children, in addition, there is crowding of bronchi and vessels in that region with a shift of the hilum, trachea, oesophagus towards the collapsed portion of lung.
iii. **Sputum examination:** Acid-fast bacilli may be seen or on culture on special media. It is difficult to get sputum for examination in young children because it is often swallowed. It is obtained by following way: Gastric contents are gently aspirated out in the morning, in a fasting child through nasogastric tube and placed in a sterile container. Gastric lavage is done with 30 ml of water and again aspirated material is added to previous one. Material is examined,

culture and guinea pig inoculation is done. It is done for two occasions on separate days. Sensitivity of the test varies from 12 to 32% only.

iv. **Blood**: ESR is raised during active phase of disease, it is not diagnostic. ESR may remain high even after recovery.

B. PROGRESSIVE PRIMARY COMPLEX

The child is very sick and toxemic having high temperature, malaise, anorexia, weight loss

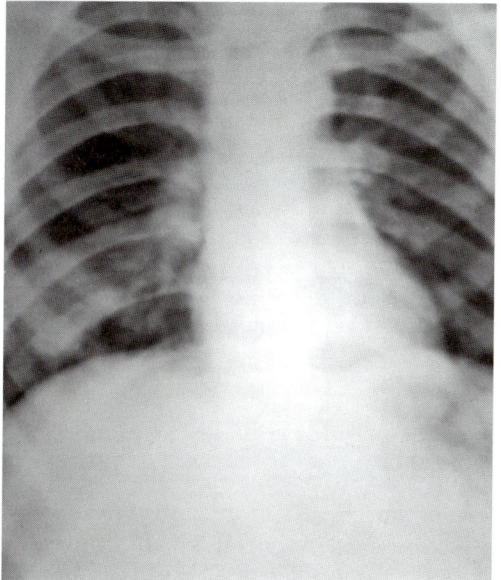

Fig. 9.12: Progressive primary complex: Skiagram chest showing hilar lymphadenitis and radiopaque shadow on right lung (consolidation).

and productive cough, physical signs and radiography shows sign of pneumonia, (commonly on middle and lower lobe) consolidation or cavity formation and hilar lymphadenopathy. Diagnosis by bacterial examination is confirmatory (Fig. 9.12).

C. REACTIVATION TUBERCULOSIS (REINFECTION)

Characteristic symptoms are low grade fever and night sweats. General symptoms are malaise, fatigue and weight loss, cough is productive often associated with mild hemoptysis.

Signs are fine rales or post-tussive rales at the apex. Skiagram of chest suggests homogenous shadow, consolidation or cavity (Table 9.1).

D. PLEURISY AND PLEURAL EFFUSION

Dry pleurisy is common in tuberculosis rarely give rise to clinical symptoms.

Pleural rub is characteristic sign.

Pleural Effusion

This is caused by discharge of tubercle bacilli into pleural spaces from subpleural focus or from hematogenous spread.

Effusion is due to enterance of bacteria in pleural space and exaggerated (allergic) response resulting in production of large quantity of fluid.

Symptoms

Symptoms are pyrexia, weight loss, chest pain and discomfort on the affected side. Pain

	Primary complex (childhood tuberculosis)	Adult tuberculosis (reactivation, reinfection)
Etiology	From inhalation, or rarely ingestion or innoculation of *T. bacilli*	By reinfection or reactivation of old focus
Pathology	Regional lymphadenopathy collapse, consolidations are common pathology	Cavitation is common pathology
Site	Commonly at lower part of lung	Commonly at apex of the lung
Skin test	Positive 4–8 weeks after primary complex	Positive even previous to reactivation
Symptoms	Cough with expectoration less common	Cough with expectoration more common
Spread	Hematogenous spread common	Hematogenous spread rare
Intectivity	Not infective except rarely	Infective in most cases because sputum positive

Table 9.1: Differences between primary complex and adult type of tuberculosis

becomes worse on coughing. Decreased chest movements, mediastinal shift opposite side, dullness on percussion, pleural rub, diminished breath sounds and vocal fremitus are diagnostic signs clinically.

Investigations

i. **Aspiration of fluid:** Confirms the diagnosis. It is exudate.

ii. **Skigram of chest:** Homogenous well defined opacity with concave upper border. The lateral edge is higher than the medial edge. Mediastinum may be shifted to opposite side. Early sign is obliteration of costophrenic angle. The fluid collects in the most dependent portion of thorax. Hence, a decubitus view may be used for confirmation of free fluid (Fig. 9.13).

iii. **Sonography:** Occassionaly, pleural effusion may be loculated and can be confirmed by sonography.

iv. **Culture and identification of organism:** Generally not identified by staining. Culture is positive in 50% cases.

v. **Pleural biopsy:** Granuloma in majority.

EXTRATHORACIC TUBERCULOSIS

A. TUBERCULOSIS OF UPPER RESPIRATORY TRACT

Rarely, larynx, epiglottis and middle ear involved. Symptoms may be croupy cough,

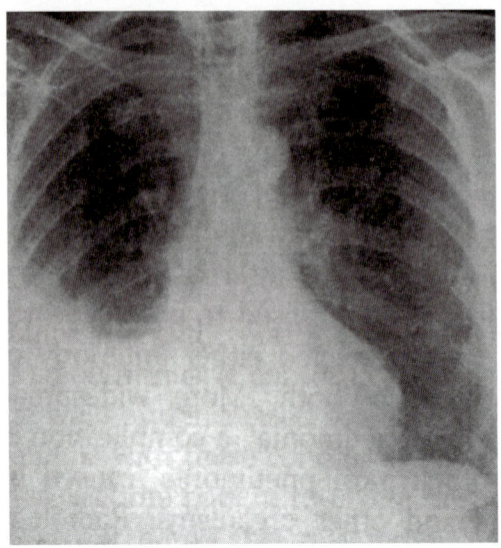

Fig. 9.13: Pleurisy with effusion (right side).

sore throat, horseness and pain. Swelling due to involvement of larynx present. Ear infection presents as profound hearing loss, absence of pain with pre- or postauricular adenopathy. Membrane is thickened with one or more perforations.

B. TUBERCULOSIS OF LYMPH NODES

Source of infection

- *Infected lymph nodes due to local spread:* Hilar nodes, paratracheal, supraclavicular, deep cervical, abdominal nodes (Fig. 9.14).

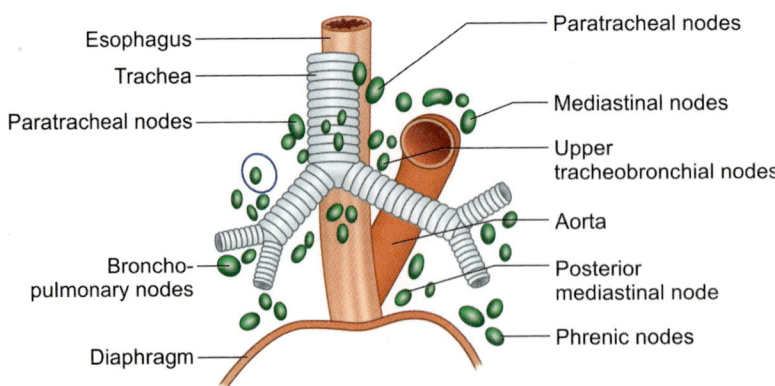

Fig. 9.14: Lymph nodes of the respiratory tract.

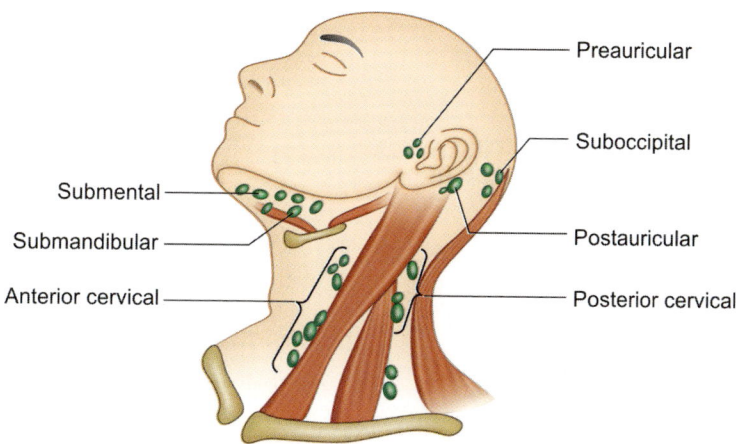

Fig. 9.15: Lymphatic glands of neck.

- Secondary to primary focus: Inguinal or axillary.
- Following hematogenous spread or lymphatic spread.

Tuberculosis of Cervical Lymph Nodes

Not common under 3 years of age, upper deep cervical most frequently involved. Anterior and posterior cervical, supraclavicular, sub-mandibular and occassionaly preauricular and submental nodes are in order of decreasing frequency (Fig. 9.15).

Pathology

May be bilateral but one side always worse than other. When caseation occurs pus tracks outwards through fascia via small opening and forms 'cold abscess' under the skin and caseating lymph nodes collectively called 'collar stud abscess'.

Clinical Features

Insidious onset: Symptoms are enlarged lymph nodes in neck which gradually increase in size, constitutional symptoms, e.g. fever, malaise, weight loss and anorexia. Lymph nodes become matted, immobile, only slightly tender (Fig. 9.16). They are multiple and may remain enlarged for months and eventually calcify. Cold abscesses are seen. The glands may caseate and discharge its necrotic material

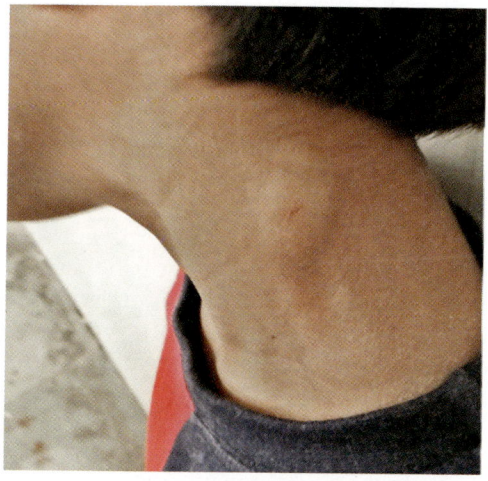

Fig. 9.16: Cervical lymphadenopathy.

into the skin resulting in an crusted and exudative lesion scrofuloderma.

Investigations

i. Total excisional biopsy of lymph nodes for histological examination and bacterio-logic culture of AFB.
ii. Fine needle aspiration cytology (FANC).

C. MILIARY TUBERCULOSIS

Definition

Miliary tuberculosis results from hemato-genous spread of *M. tuberculosis* from a established focus, producing infections that progress to necroses and caseation in multiple organs including CNS.

Nomenclature

Called 'Miliary' because lesion resembles appearance of millet seeds.

Etiology

1. Most commonly occurs at the age of 1–3 years less common after 6 years of age. Occurs 1–3 months of primary lesion.
2. *Organs involved*—lungs, spleen, liver, kidney, pleura, peritoneum, mesentery, bone marrow, rarely retina, brain and skin.
3. Also occurs in acquired immunodeficiency syndrome (AIDS).

Clinical Manifestations

Onset is acute with high temperature 102–104°F, weakness, malaise, anorexia, weight loss. Signs are lymphadenopathy, hepatomegaly and splenomegaly as a non-specific finding.

Later on cough, tachypnea is common. Diffuse rales over both sides of chest is common feature. Toxemia and wasting is marked. Choroidal tubercle is seen in eye. Nuchal rigidity is seen due to meningeal irritation.

Diagnosis

i. Blood (WBC)—normal, elevated or depressed. ESR raised, anemia.

ii. Mantoux test (skin test): Positive in initial stage, later on becomes negetive.
iii. Radiograph of chest: Multiple miliary lesions in both lungs characteristic multiple minute dots, when they blend give snow storm appearance (Fig. 9.17).
iv. Culture of urine, gastric aspirate, CSF for identification of organism.
v. Lung biopsy.

D. CNS TUBERCULOSIS

It is most dangerous form (*see* page 221).

E. TUBERCULOSIS OF HEART AND PERICARDIUM

This results from rupture of mediastinal lymph nodes into pericardial sac or hematogenous spread. Patient often presents with pyrexia, chest pain, tachycardia, dyspnea. Signs are friction rub, cardiomegaly, distant heart sounds. Enlarged liver and edema are common features.

Electrocardiogram and echocardiogram are abnormal. Pericardiocentesis: Clear fluid with

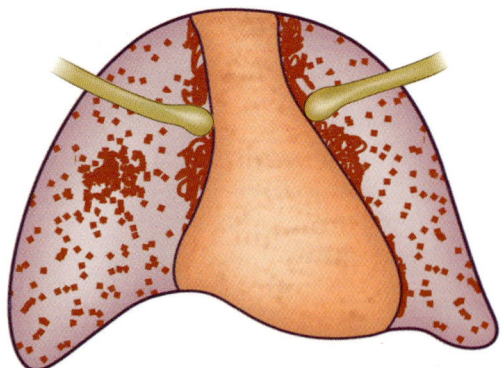

Fig. 9.17: Diagrammatic representation of skiagram of chest in miliary tuberculosis.

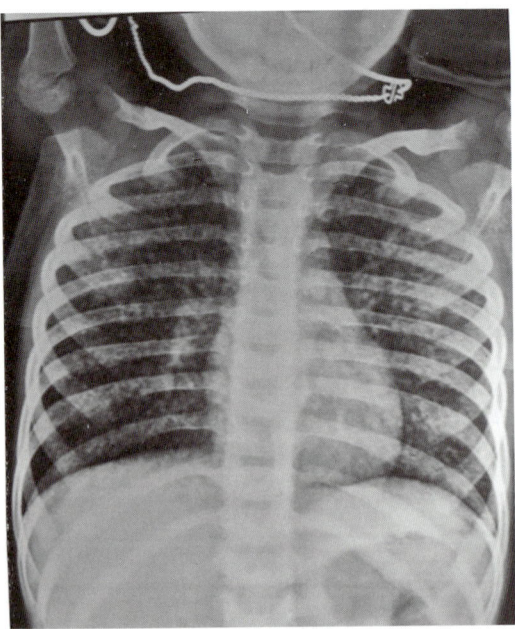

Fig. 9.18: X-ray picture—miliary tuberculosis.

characteristic exudate. Organisms are usually negative but culture is positive; biopsy and histological examination shows characteristic signs.

F. ABDOMINAL TUBERCULOSIS

Sources

a. Secondary due to swallowing of infected secretions, e.g. cough of lungs.
b. Spread from peritoneal, mediastinal lymph nodes.
c. Hematogenous spread.
d. Primary after swallowing of infected milk (bovine type) rare.

Clinical Features

Involvement of esophagus and stomach: Dysphagia, abdominal pain obstruction.

Small intestine: Obstruction, perforation and hemorrhage, fistula formation, malabsorption.

Caecum: Painful, tender mass at right lower quadrant, hemorrhage, obstruction or diarrhea.

Anal: Obstruction, perforation or hemorrhage.

Anal: Fistula or abscess formation

Liver: Hepatitis

Peritonitis

Fever, anorexia, abdominal pain, weight loss and abdominal distension common.

Plastic type: Abdomen distended with characteristic doughy feel of abdomen. Rolled up omentum or mesenteric lymph nodes may be felt as mass. Signs of obstruction may be found.

Ascitic type: Abdominal distension, ascites present, fluid gradually absorb releaving plastic form.

Investigations

a. Skin test positive.
b. Peritoneal fluid after paracentesis examined for bacilli, culture.
c. Biopsy: Histological and microbiological examination.

d. Barium meal examination:
  • Lack of barium retension in diseased segment of ilium, caecum.
  • Narrow stream of barium in small bowel
  • Areas of obstruction seen as delay into dilatation and emptying.

G. TUBERCULOSIS OF SKIN

Lesion is small papule, which later becomes ulcerated. Ulcer takes months to heal. Scrofuloderma and erythema nodosum are another features. BCG vaccination can be classified as primary tuberculosis of skin.

H. SKELETAL TUBERCULOSIS

Always due to hematogenous spread. Spine, hip joints, knee joints, fingers and toes are common sites.

I. UROGENITAL TUBERCULOSIS

Dysuria, frequency and urgency of micturition are common presenting features, urine examination shows painless hematuria; culture and identify organism.

Allergic Manifestations of Tuberculosis

Most commonly follow 6–8 weeks after primary infection due to sensitivity of *M. tuberculosis*.

  i. *Erythema nodosum:* Characteristic skin manifestations are painful, raised, red nodules occurring in crops mostly front of shin of leg. It is nonspecific reaction occurs due to other organisms and drugs.
  ii. *Phlyctenular conjunctivitis and keratitis:* Photophobia and phlyctenules in eye. Small greyish nodules surrounded by area of conjunctivitis. Ulcerate and cause scarring of cornea.

Diagnosis of Tuberculosis (Flowchart 9.2)

Based on

  i. Clinical features
  ii. History of contact with infected case of tuberculosis in family and neighbors.
  iii. Hypersensitivity to tuberculin (skin tests)

Flowchart 9.2: Diagnostic algorithm for pediatric pulmonary TB

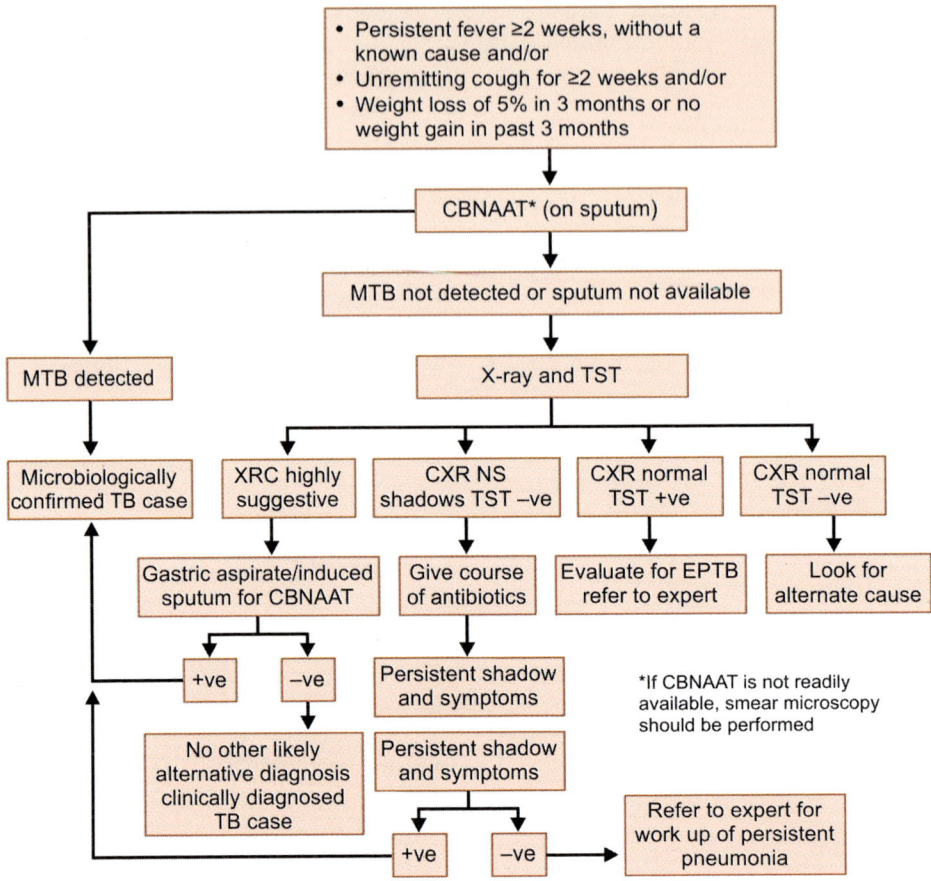

iv. Radiological features:
1. Ghon's focus is sometime seen as blurred opacity associated with increased hilar shadow due to enlarged lymph nodes. Opacity may show calcification afterward.
2. Infiltration in lung parenchyma.
3. Marked widening of mediastinum in X-ray film produced by paratracheal lymphadenitis.
4. Radiopaque shadow of consolidation or collapse.
5. Uniform opacity with curved fluid line or horizontal line when coexisting air present. Costophrenic and cardiophrenic angle obliterated and media-stinal shift to opposite side due to pleurisy.
6. Hilar nodes, opposite side of Ghon's focus, are rarely involved. Mediastinal nodes are involved bilaterally.
7. Multiple minute dots which may blend called 'snow storm appearance' in miliary tuberculosis.
8. Calcification due to healed lymph nodes.
9. Differential diagnosis of widening of superior mediastinum.
   a. Superior vena cava seen in young children and if film is not straight or taken in expiration.
   b. Normal thymus: Borders of thymus are straight while borders of

mediastinal lymph nodes are convex.

c. Abnormal vessels: Anomalous subclavian artery, right-sided aorta.

d. Enlarged lymph nodes due to other diseases, e.g. Hodgkin's disease, lymphosarcoma.

e. Encysted effusion, tumor.

10. *Collapse:* Tubercular collapse is lobar rather than segmental, upper lobe rather than lower lobe. While non-tubercular collapse is segmental and lower lobe mainly.

11. Rarely translucency due to emphysema.

12. Reactivation after measles or whooping cough or adult type may show cavity and calcification.

v. Laboratory investigations: Raised ESR.

vi. Lumbar puncture: CSF examination in meningitis.

vii. Demonstration of bacilli in sputum, gastric aspirate, bronchial, laryngeal lymph node discharge, or aspirate, pleural fluid, pericardial fluid, culture and guinea pig inoculation.

• Early morning gastric aspirate is obtained by using a nasogastric tube before child arises.

• Young children are not able to produce sputum. Following overnight fast patient receives salbutamol by nebulizer afterward 3% or 5% hypertonic saline by nebulization is given. At the end of the process children may produce expectoration.

• Nasopharyngeal aspirate is collected, stain and culture.

Polymerase chain reaction (PCR)

PCR is used to diagnose tuberculosis by identifying DNA from the *M. tuberculosis.* It is a rapid test with specificity 80–100%.

Identification of acid-fast bacilli by cartridge based nucleic acid technique (CBNAAT).

It gives results within 2 hours and provides sensitivity to rifampicin.

Culture on lower stein—Jensen egg medium or newer dobesilic acid—agar medium takes 6–12 weeks for isolation, recently less time taking techniques like slide chamber (8–10 days), radio-respiratory techniques (3–4 days) are employed for evidence of growth of bacilli.

viii. *Biopsy:* Histological examination of lymph nodes, pleural and pericardial tissue.

ix. Examination of eye for choroid tubercle.

x. Immunodiagnosis: Specially very useful in children, where there is high suspicion of tuberculosis but all other routine investigations are negative.

a. ELISA test: Antigen or antibody can be detected up to nanogram level, but what is lacking is a nonspecific antibody or antigen. With the use of PPD, and TBc ID test, sensitivity up to 80–85% and specificity up to 90–100% has been observed.

b. Polymerase chain reaction (PCR): PCR is being considered as a major advancement in the diagnosis of tuberculosis. It is highly specific and sensitive test but due to contamination, false positive results have been recorded.

It is not necessary to do all investigations in every case they are done according to need.

Mantoux Test

BTU of PPDs or 2 TU of tuberculin PPD RT 23 is used. 0.1 ml of glycerinated purified protein derivative (PPD) which is injected intradermally over the anterior aspect of forearm. A wheel should be raised at the time of injection (Fig. 9.19).

Interpretation

Extent of palpable area of induration, not erythema, is read after 48 to 72 hours, note the diameter.

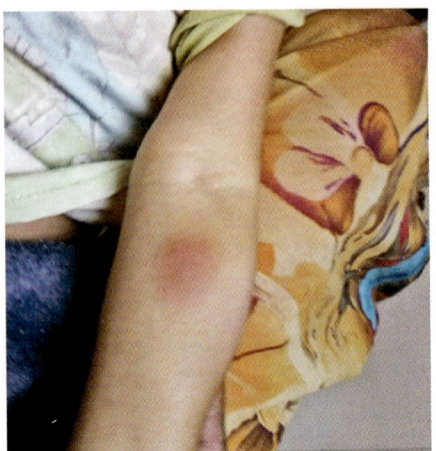

Fig. 9.19: Mantoux test—positive.

- Under 5 mm diameter—negative reaction
- 5–10 mm—'suspicious'
- >10 mm (10–20 mm)—positive reaction
- 20–30 mm—moderate reaction
- 30–40 mm—severe reaction.

Positive reaction indicates
   i. Infection of tuberculosis present
      a. Under 2 years of age.
      b. Under 6 years of age if child is exposed to known case of tuberculosis
      c. Conversion of negative to positive recently.
   ii. BCG already given to child.

False Negative Reaction

In spite of presence of infection test is negative when sensitivity is depressed, causes are:
   i. Gross PCM and debilitating states
   ii. Advanced tuberculosis—miliary tuberculosis, tuberculosis meningitis
   iii. Steroid therapy
   iv. Convalescent stage of whooping cough, measles
   v. Neoplastic disease—Hodgkin's disease
   vi. Incubation period
   vii. Extreme age (less than 6 months)
   viii. Poor techniques.

False Positive Reaction

   i. Repeated testing with PPD or XT
   ii. Previous immunization (BCG)

Positive reaction due to BCG test shows induration which rarely exceeds 10 mm and strongest first few years after immunization. Any reaction that exceeds 10 mm in diameter and occurs more than 10 years following immunization should be considered due to tuberculosis infection.

Management (See Table 9.2)

	Name	Dose	Frequency of administration	Side effects
Table 9.2: Antitubercular drugs				
1.	Isoniazid	10–15 mg/kg maximum up to 300 mg	Once daily oral	Peripheral neuritis, hepatitis, hyper-sensitivity
2.	Rifampicin	10–20 mg/kg maximum 600 mg	Once daily oral	Hepatitis, febrile reaction, purpura
3.	Ethambutol	15–25 mg/kg	Once daily oral	Optic neuritis, blurred vision, skin rash
4.	Pyrizinamide	15–20 mg/kg	Once daily oral	Hyperuricemia Hepatotoxicity
5.	Streptomycin	20–25 mg/kg	Single IM	Auditory or vestibular dysfunction
6.	Ethionamide, Cycloserine	15–20 mg/kg	Oral	

DAILY TREATMENT GUIDELINE (RNTPC)

Drugs are given daily as per Table 9.3

Category I (suggested for children)
- Pulmonary primary complex
- Progressive primary disease
- Tubercular lymphadenitis
- Pleural effusion
- Abdominal TB

Category II
- Relapse
- Treatment failure
- Interrupted treatment

Total duration of chemotherapy—drugs are given in two phases:
A. *Intensive phase*—INH, rifampicin, pyrazinamide and ethambutol
   Duration: 2 months (8 weeks)
B. *Continuous phase*—INH, rifampicin and ethambutol
   Duration: 4 months (16 weeks)

Corticosteroids

Prednisolone 1–2 mg/kg/day for 4–6 weeks.

Special situation

Management of infant born to mother with tuberculosis.

Cause: Congenital rare.

If mother is suffering from tuberculosis child acquires the disease by hematogenous spread through umbilical vessels, ingestion of infected amniotic fluid.

Examine: Clinical symptoms, X-ray chest, tuberculin test.

Prophylaxis dose: Isoniazid 10 mg/kg/day.

Management of a child in contact with adult with tuberculosis.

Children who are in contact with sputum positive should receive INH prophylaxis dose—10 mg/kg/day for 6 months.

Monitoring

Monitoring of response of treatment is done after 2–4 weeks then 4–8 weeks on following basis:
1. **Improvement in general symptoms:** Fever, cough, chest finding improvement. Weight gain and improvement in appetite and activity.
2. **Radiological criteria:** X-ray chest should be done after 4 weeks of therapy (after intensive phase) and observe clearance of finding mild to complete. If no improvement assess for treatment failure or drug resistance.

Do not wait for complete clearance it may continue even after complete course of therapy.

Table 9.3: Drugs regimen for different categories of tuberculosis

Category I: Daily regimen	WHO		
• Pulmonary primary complex	• New sputum positive	Intensive phase	Continuation phase
	• Pulmonary TB	2HRZE + 4HRE	
	• Serious extrapulmonary		
• Progressive primary disease	• Osteoarticular TB		
• Tubercular lymphadenitis	• Genitourinary		
• Pleural effusion	• Central nervous system		
• Abdominal TB	• Pericardial		
Category II			
• Relapse	2SHRZE + 1HRZE + 5HRE		
• Treatment failure			
• Interrupted treatment	Return after defaults		

H: Isoniazid E: Ethambulol R: Rifampicin S: Streptomycin Z: Pyrazinamide
2 means 2 months, 4 means 4 months, 5 means 5 months.

3. **Microbiological criteria:** Assess every time for persistence of AFB during therapy.
   - General measures
   - Surgical treatment
   - Drug resistance
   - Prevention

Recommended daily dosages of essential first line anti-TB drugs (daily)

Drugs	Range	mg/kg
Isoniazid	7–15	10
Rifampicin	10–20	15
Streptomycin	12–18	15
Ethambutol	15–25	20
Pyrazinamide	30–40	35

Isoniazid Prophylaxis

<6 years of age, contact of smear positive TB, after ruling out active TB disease, irrespective of BCG status (Table 9.4).

Isoniazid 10 mg/kg/daily for 6 months.

Table 9.4: Pediatric dosing chart		
Weight range (kg)	Number of 100 mg tab	Dose (mg)
<5	Half tab	50
5.1–9.9	One	100
10–13.9	One and half	150
14–19.9	Two	200
20–24.9	Two and half	250
>25	Three or one Adult tab	300

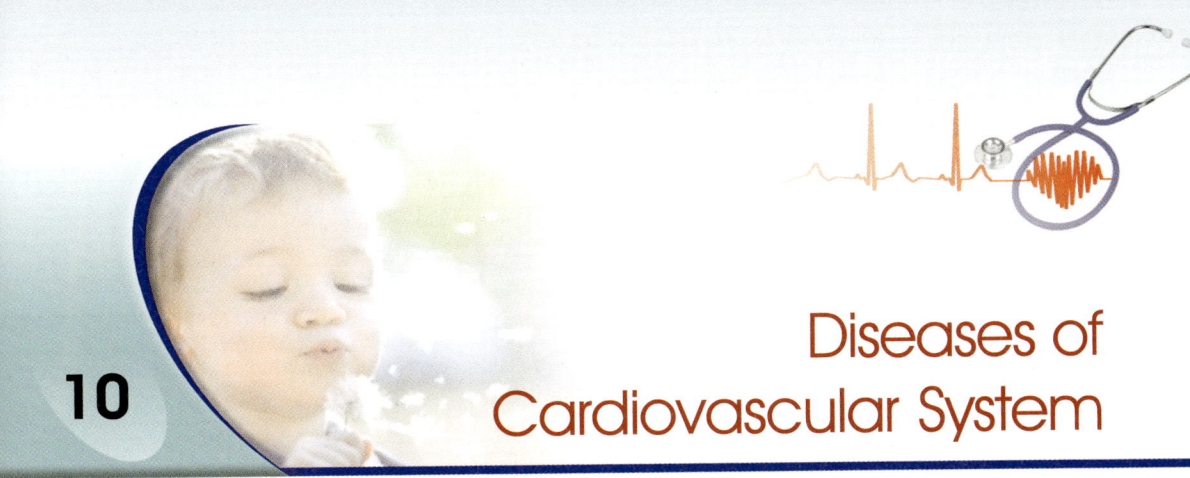

Diseases of Cardiovascular System

10

CONGENITAL HEART DISEASE

Incidence

8/1000 live births. Sex—ASD, PDA more common in females; transposition of great vessels more common in males.

Etiology

The cause of congenital heart disease is rarely known in individual case. In most instances, there is combination of genetic and environmental influences, maternal rubella, high altitudes, drugs as thalidomide.

Classification

i. Acyanotic (left to right shunt) without cyanosis
ii. Cyanotic (right to left shunt).

VENTRICULAR SEPTAL DEFECT

This is most common congenital heart disease. In this, there is communication between two ventricles. In most of the cases defects are in membranous part of the ventricular septum, while in others, it is in muscular part.

Acyanotic	*Cyanotic*
1. Ventricular septal defect	1. Fallot's tetralogy
2. Atrial septal defect	2. Transposition of great vessels
3. Patent ductus arteriosus	3. Eisenmenger syndrome
4. Coarctation of aorta	4. Truncus arteriosus
5. Vascular rings	5. Hypoplastic left heart syndrome
6. Valvular pulmonary stenosis	6. Tricuspid atresia
7. Anomalous origin of coronary artery	
8. Congenital mitral incompetence	
9. Dextrocardia	
10. Congenital aortic stenosis	
11. Congenital mitral stenosis	

Hemodynamics

Blood flows from left ventricle to right ventricle during systole. Left ventricle is dominant. Evidence of pulmonary hypertension found in most cases. But it is not related to amount of left to right shunt (Fig. 10.1).

Clinical Features

i. If defect is small, patient may be asymptomatic. It is detected in clinical examination.

ii. Large defect causes recurrent chest infections, dyspnea, failure to thrive and attacks of congestive cardiac failure. Feeding difficulties are also seen. On examination:

1. Pulse pressure wide.
2. Systotic thrill on left sternal area.
3. Pansystolic murmur loud, maximum intensity at the left sternal border in 3rd, 4th or 5th intercostal space (Fig. 10.2).
4. 2nd sound loud, widely split.
5. Heart size is moderately enlarged.

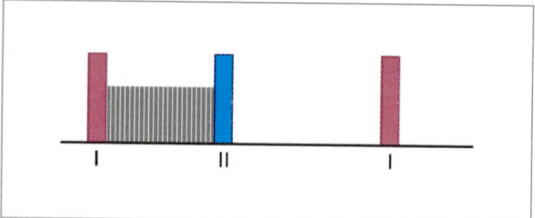

Fig. 10.2: Auscultatory events in ventricular septal defect.

Investigations

A. X-ray chest
   i. Both ventricle and left atrium enlargement
   ii. Pulmonary artery enlargement and overvascularity of lung fields
   iii. Pulsation in pulmonary vessels increased (hilar dance). It may or may not be present. In mild case—normal

B. ECG: In mild case, normal but shows biventricular hypertrophy in other.

C. Two-dimensional echocardiography— position and size of shunt seen.

D. Left ventriculography by contrast media shows site and number of defects.

Complications

Infective endocarditis, CCF, pulmonary hypertension.

Treatment

i. About 30–50% of small defects close spontaneously, mostly during first year of life; so parents should be assured about benign nature of the condition.

ii. Antibiotics prophylaxis for surgery and dental extraction to prevent infective endocarditis.

iii. Medical management of large VSD is aimed to control cardiac failure, repeated chest infections, prevention and treatment of anemia and prevention of infective endocarditis.

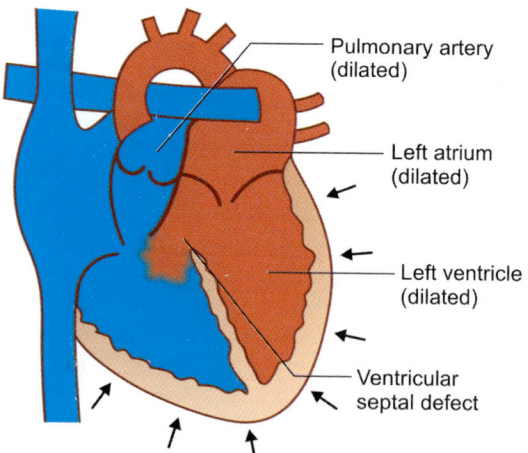

Pulmonary artery (dilated)

Left atrium (dilated)

Left ventricle (dilated)

Ventricular septal defect

Fig. 10.1: Ventricular septal defect.

iv. Surgical closure is indicated in large defect, above 2 years age and in person with signs of pulmonary hypertension and if there is pulmonary stenosis along with VSD.

ATRIAL SEPTAL DEFECT

Opening in interatrial septum due to deficiency in septal tissue.

Classification

a. *Ostium secundum:* Defect in middle portion of the atrial septum—most common type.
b. *Ostium primum:* Defect in lower portion of atrial septum.
c. *Sinus venosus:* Defect is high in the septum near the junction of right atrium and superior vena cava.

Pathophysiology: Blood flows across the septal defect from left atrium to the right atrium (e.g. left to right shunt). Blood therefore, flows from areas of higher resistance to areas to lower resistance. This leads to increase in size of the right atrium and right ventricle and to increased pulmonary blood flow (Fig. 10.3).

Clinical Features

Symptoms are minimal. But baby with ostium primum defect who develop mitral regurgitation results CHF have symptoms.

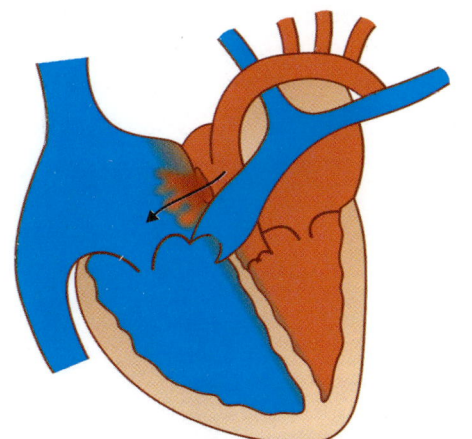

Fig. 10.3: Atrial septal defect. Direction of flow of blood from left atrium to right atrium.

Physical Examination

1. Increased right ventricular impulse, visible and palpable right ventricle.
2. Ist sound often accentuated and split with loud.
3. Fixed-split second heart sound.
4. Systolic ejection murmur best heard at the mid and left sternal borders.

A mid-diastolic filling rumble representing excessive blood flow through tricuspid valve may also be heard.

Investigations

1. *Chest radiograph*
   - Dilatation of trunk of pulmonary artery and its larger branches.
   - Absence of LA enlargement
   - Hilar dance in fluoroscopy
2. *ECG:* Incomplete RBBB
3. *Echo:* Drop out in area of interatrial septum. Doppler color flow imaging defines atrial septal defect along with other intracardiac shunts.
4. *Catheterization:* High saturation in RA, RV and pulmonary artery because of blood flow from left to right.

Associated Lesions

1. Lutembacher's syndrome: Associated MS
2. Pulmonary stenosis
3. Anomalous pulmonary venous drainage
4. Holt-Oram syndrome: Skeletal deformity of forearm.

Complications

1. Pulmonary hypertension
2. Reversal of shunt (Eisenmenger's syndrome)
3. Infective endocarditis rare.

Management

- Closure by open heart surgery to prevent right-sided failure and complications.
- Some centers close ASD using interventional catheterization procedures.

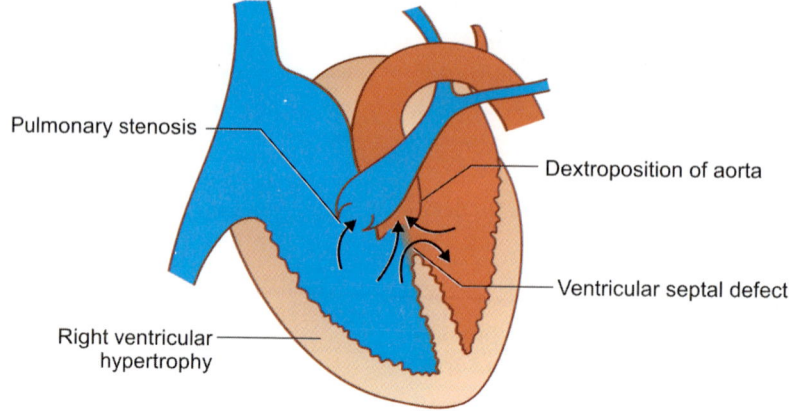

Fig. 10.4: Anatomical lesion in Fallot's tetralogy. Direction of blood flow is shown by arrows.

FALLOT'S TETRALOGY

This is the most common cyanotic congenital heart disease. Incidence is 75% of all cyanotic heart disease.

Tetralogy of Fallot (TOF) classically consists of combination of:

  i. Obstruction to right ventricular outflow: Pulmonary stenosis
  ii. Ventricular septal defect
  iii. Dextroposition of aorta
  iv. Right ventricular hypertrophy.

Hemodynamics

During ventricular contraction, due to resistance at the pulmonary stenosis, right-sided blood is shunted through the ventricular septal defect into left ventricle and then into aorta. It results in mixing of deoxygenated blood into oxygenated blood, resulting cyanosis. Blood flow is reduced in pulmonary artery, resulting poor pulmonary vascularity (Fig. 10.4).

Very rarely right to left shunt is not present, so no mixing of blood and no cyanosis. This is called acyanotic or pink Fallot's tetralogy.

Clinical Features

Cyanosis: Cyanosis may not be present at birth in mild cases. In severe cases, cyanosis in neonatal period is evident. Cyanosis is seen in mucous membranes of the lips and mouth, fingernails and toenails. Older children have dusky skin in case of extreme cyanosis.

Clubbing develops about the age of 2 years (Figs 10.5 and 10.6).

Dyspnea: Dyspnea occurs on exertion. During playing or during physical effort, infant and todders sit or lie down. Characteristically he assumes squatting position for the relief of dyspnea and assume normal activity within two minutes.

Hypoxic or blue spells (paroxysmal hyper-cyanotic spells): They occur particularly during first two years of life, most frequently in morning and after exercise. Child becomes dyspneic and restless, rate of respiration increases, gasping respiration and cyanosis increases. It is followed by with or without syncope. They are rarely fatal.

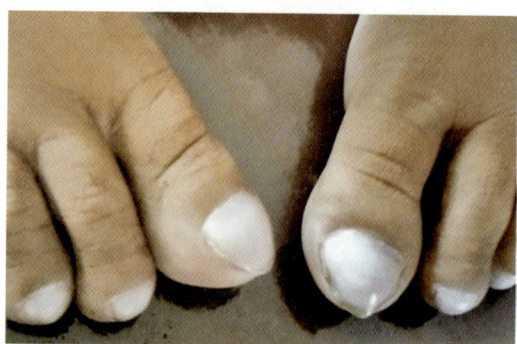

Fig. 10.5: Clubbing of the toes.

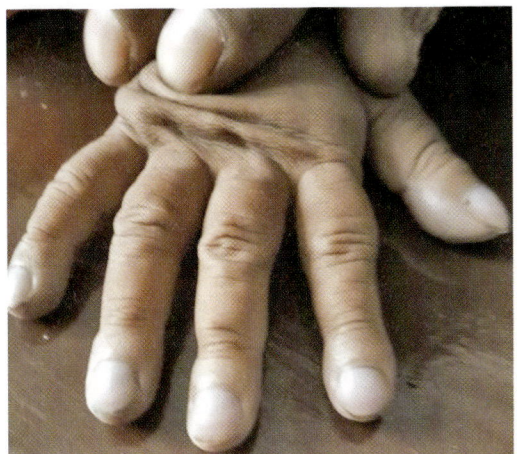

Fig. 10.6: Fallot's tetralogy: Clubbing of fingers.

One attack last from few minutes to few hours and followed by generalized weakness and sleep. Occasionally, convulsions and hemiplegia occur. It is due to increased concentration of CO_2 in blood, resulting hypoxia.

Growth and development are delayed. Pulse normal. Hemithorax bulging, parasternal heave present. Systolic thrill at left sternal border in the 3rd and 4th parasternal space. Murmur is systolic loud and harsh intense at the left sternal border, may be preceded by click, widely transmitted.

Second heart (A_2) sound is single due to closure of aortic valve. P_2 is soft and delayed, inaudible.

Investigations

a. Blood: Polycythemia
b. X-ray chest
   i. Rounded apical shadow situated high above the diaphragm due to hypertrophy of right ventricle called wooden shoe (boot-shaped appearance) (Fig. 10.7).
   ii. Concavity in left-border of heart in the region of main pulmonary artery (hypoplastic pulmonary artery).
   iii. Hilar areas and lung field are relatively clear due to diminished pulmonary vascularity.
   iv. Aorta is large.
c. ECG: Right ventricular hypertrophy with beaked 'P' wave.
d. Two-dimensional echocardiography is helpful in diagnosis.
e. Cardiac catheterization and angiography decide anatomical and structural abnormalities.
f. Selective ventriculography demonstrates the anatomy of Fallot's tetralogy.

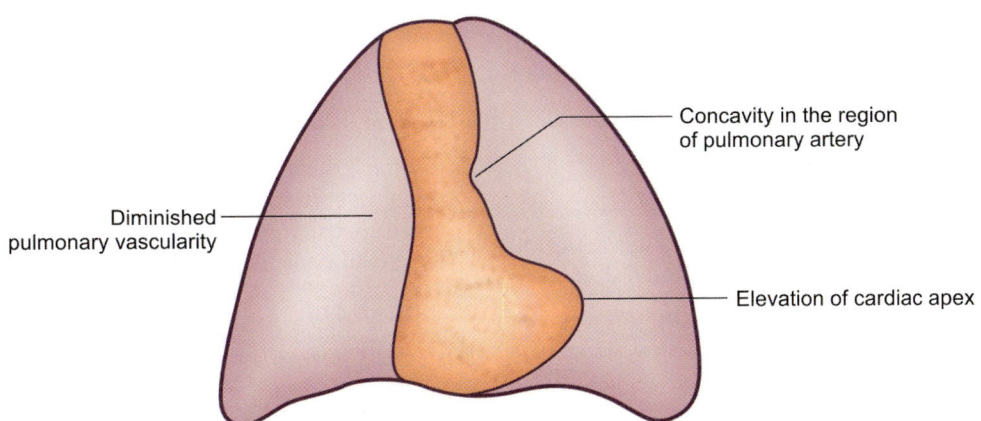

Fig. 10.7: Diagrammatic representation of X-ray chest of Fallot's tetralogy showing classical features.

Complications: Cerebral thrombosis, cerebral ischemia, brain abscess, bacterial endocarditis.

Treatment

Medical management consists of correction of iron deficiency anemia, correction of dehydration to avoid hemoconcentration and thrombotic episode and antibiotics for bacterial infections.

Anoxic spells are managed as: Place the child on abdomen in knee chest position. Clothes are loosened, oxygen inhalation, morphine injection (not excess than 0.1 mg/kg), correction of metabolic acidosis by intravenous sodium bicarbonate. In severe cases, some patients require IV propranolol 0.1 to 0.2 mg/kg. Oral propranolol is given 0.5–1.0 mg/kg 4–6 hourly to decrease frequency and severity. Methoxamine (vasopressor) also indicated for severe case, given IM or IV in drip.

Surgery

a. Palliative surgery is possible, if pulmonary artery is of adequate size. Anastomosis of pulmonary artery with systemic artery (with subclavian artery (Blalock-Taussig operation); descending aorta (Pott's operation) with Waterston shunt.

b. Definitive operation—closing the septal defect and resecting the infundibular obstruction.

Prognosis

After successful total correction, patient lives symptomless, unrestricted life.

COARCTATION OF AORTA

Narrowing of the aortic arch just below the origin of the left subclavian artery in the region where the ductus arteriosus joins the aorta.

Pathophysiology: The narrowed segment of aorta obstructs or diminishes flow from the proximal to distal part of aorta.

Clinical features: Depends upon severity of obstruction.

1. Neonates or infants: Symptoms are minimal but symptoms of CHF develop.
2. Older children or adolescents: No symptom or headache or weakness and cramps in legs.
   - Blood pressure in upper extremities may be elevated and low in lower extremities before the onset of CHF.
   - If CHF develops pulses are poor, hypotension may develop.

Femoral pulses are weak and delayed in comparison with the radial pulse.
- Systolic murmur is heard posteriorly at coarctation at left upper back near the scapula.
- Ejection click and systolic murmur in aortic area.
- Due to aortic narrowing, collateral form many in periscapular, intercostals arteries, internal mammary artery. These may result in localized bruits.

Investigations

1. *Chest X-ray:* In early childhood normal but later age shows changes in the contour of the aorta (indentation of the descending aorta, '3' sign) and notching of the under surface of ribs from collaterals.
   MRI: Ideal for detection.
2. *IV DSA:* It shows a narrowed aorta and extensive collaterals, large mammary artery.
3. *Echo:* Interruption of aortic arch distal to left carotid, left subclavian or left innominate and poststenotic dilatation of aorta.
4. *ECG:* Left ventricular hypertrophy.
5. *Cardiac catheterization:* Significant systolic pressure differences across the aorta angiography will demonstrate site and length of coarctation.

Management

Surgical Correction

- Surgical correction is advised in all but the mildest cases done in early in childhood to avoid persistent hypertension.

- Balloon angioplasty may be successful that have not undergone surgical correction and is the therapy of choice for recurrent coarctation.

Prognosis: Excellent.

Complications

1. Aortic rupture
2. Infective endocarditis
3. Heart failure

TRICUSPID ATRESIA

Tricuspid atresia is a plate of tissue located in the floor of the right atrium in the location of tricuspid valve. An ASD or PFO is always present.

Clinical Features

a. Patient with VSD have VSD murmur.
b. ECG: RAH, left axis deviation (LAD) and left ventricular hypertrophy (LVH).

Management

In the fontan procedure: Flow from inferior vena cava is directed into the pulmonary arteries usually by means of extracardiac conduct or intra-atrial baffle or tunnel.

It is done at 3–6 years of age.

TRUNCUS ARTERIOSUS

When aorta and pulmonary artery originate from a common artery, the truncus. VSD is always present.

Clinical Features

a. Sign and symptoms of CHF are common
b. Physical examination
   i. Systolic ejection murmur at the base
   ii. Diastolic murmur at the apex
   iii. High pitched systolic murmur at the base.

Management

Medication for CHF
  Surgical—during early infancy to close VSD, and place a homograft between right ventricle and pulmonary artery.

PATENT DUCTUS ARTERIOSUS

In the fetus, the ductus arteriosus connects pulmonary artery to the aorta. After birth, the ductus normally fibroses. If it remains open, it is termed patent (persistent) ductus arteriosus (Fig. 10.8).

It is common in preterm infants.

Pathophysiology: In a patent ductus arteriosus (PDA), blood flows from the aorta to pulmonary artery through the ductus leading to increased pulmonary blood flow.

Clinical features: Depends upon severity of PDA.

a. Small PDA usually produce no symptom and pulmonary pressure is normal. Survival without symptom is possible.
b. Moderate or large PDA generally results sign and symptoms of congestive cardiac failure due to increased pulmonary blood flow.

Signs: The continuous murmur at the upper left sternal border (machinary-like) murmur (Fig. 10.9).

In large PDA, there may also be diastolic rumble of blood flow across the mitral valve at the apex.

- Widened pulse pressure.
- Brisk pulses

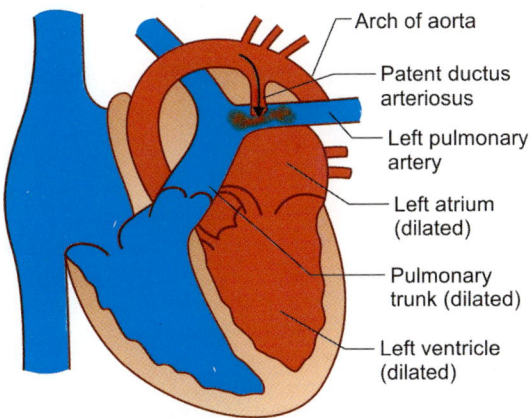

Fig. 10.8: Patent ductus arteriosus.

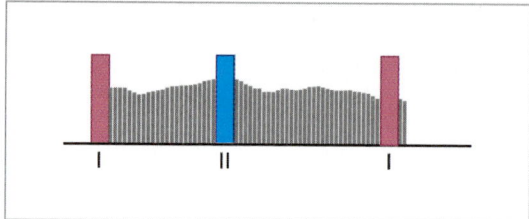

Fig. 10.9: Auscultatory events in patent ductus arteriosus.

- Continuous thrill at pulmonary area
- Pulsation at suprasternal notch.

Persistent ductus with reversed shunting. If pulmonary vascular resistance increases and become equal or increase to pulmonary artery pressure. The shunt may then reverse causing central cyanosis (Eisenmenger's syndrome). which is more apparent on toes and feet than upper arm of body.

Investigations

1. *X-ray chest:* Pulmonary plethora proportional to degree of left to right shunt enlarged aortic knuckle.
2. *ECG:* Normal but in reversed shunting right ventricular hypertrophy.
3. *Echocardiography*
   - Ductus can be imaged from pulmonary artery to aorta
   - Doppler color flow mapping shows diastolic flow from ductus to pulmonary artery.
4. *Cardiac catheterization:* Pressure in pulmonary artery elevated.

Complications

1. Subacute bacterial endocarditis
2. Pulmonary hypertension and reversal shunt
3. Congestive cardiac failure

Management

- Indomethacin is used in premature infants to close a PDA medically.

- Surgical closure: Close a patent ductus with a implantable occlusive device.
- Ligation of ductus in thoracotomy.

TRANSPOSITION OF GREAT ARTERIES

When aorta arises from the right ventricle and main pulmonary artery from the left ventricle (Fig. 10.10).

Clinical Features

Cyanosis, left ventricular hypertrophy, loud S2 with systolic ejection click, short systolic ejection murmur of pulmonary stenosis or systolic regurgitant murmur due to ventricular septal defect or no murmur heard.

Management

a. Neonates may require initial management with PGA to improve oxygen saturation but keeping ductus patent, or by emergency balloon atrial septostomy (Rashkind procedure), or PFO.
b. Definitive repair in the switch operation in which the great arteries are incised above the respective valve and implanted in the opposite root. The coronary arteries are attached to original aorta.

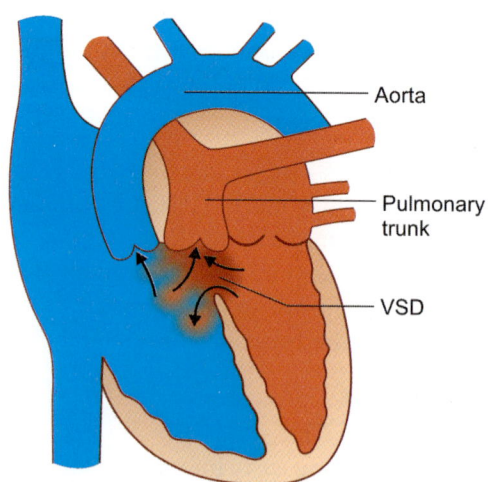

Fig. 10.10: Transposition of great vessels.

TOTAL ANOMALOUS PULMONARY VENOUS CONNECTION

Total anomalous pulmonary venous connection (TAPVC) occurs when the pulmonary veins drain into systemic venous side rather than into the left atrium.

Clinical Features

a. Cyanosis is present and severe, may indicate obstruction of pulmonary venous return.
b. Pulmonary flow murmur at midsternal border.

Management

Surgical repair: Pulmonary veins are anastomosed to the back of left atrium and the PFO, ASD is closed.

ACQUIRED HEART DISEASES

1. Acute rheumatic fever
2. Infective endocarditis
3. Pericarditis
4. Myocarditis
5. Cardiomyopathy
6. Kawasaki disease.

RHEUMATIC FEVER

Rheumatic fever is a systemic disease involving more frequently joints and the heart and less frequently central nervous system, skin and subcutaneous tissue.

This is most common immunologic, collagen disease initiated by group A beta-hemolytic streptococcus. This has tendency to recur, lesions are not suppurating.

Etiology

Preceding history of sore throat presents in 50% of cases.

Predisposing Factors

a. **Age and sex:** All ages except infancy. Peak is at age of 5–15 years; equal in both sexes.
b. **Season:** Winter and early spring.

c. **Genetic factor:** May be involved because it runs in families and high incidence is in monozygotic twins than dizygotic twins.
d. **Socioeconomic status:** Dampness, overcrowding and poor undernutrition is associated with greatly increase in incidence.
e. **Worldwide distribution:** In developing countries, 30–40% of heart diseases are due to rheumatic fever.

The etiology is unknown; strong evidence support that this is a hypersensitivity (altered immunological reaction) to beta-hemolytic streptococcus because:

i. History of upper respiratory infection preceding rheumatic fever is present in 50% of cases.
ii. Incidence of rheumatic fever high after epidemic of untreated severe exudative pharyngitis.
iii. In majority (more than 85%) of acute rheumatic fever cases, raised antistreptolysin titre seen.
iv. Penicillin prophylaxis prevents recurrence of rheumatic fever.
v. This is more common in situation where chances of infection are more, e.g. dampness crowded population, winter spring season, etc. As it is widely accepted, rheumatic fever is an autoimmune disease, streptococcal antigen, which are similar to human tissue antigen may elicit antibodies known as 'antiheart' antibodies. These have been found in case of rheumatic fever but also in non-rheumatic fever. It is yet to be proved.

Pathology

There is widespread exudative and proliferative inflammatory reactions in the connective tissue of heart, joints, skin, around muscles or tendons.

Clinical Features

Frequently, history of sore throat or respiratory tract infection is present 10–14 days prior to acute attack.

Onset is acute with polyarthritis, while insidious when carditis and chorea are presenting features. Acute abdominal pain, epistaxis, pain in limbs so-called 'growing pains' are also presenting features.

I. Joints Symptoms

It is most common presenting symptom. When pain in joints is present without objective findings, it is known as arthralgia.

Arthritis involving the larger joints like knee, ankles, elbow and wrists are commonly affected while smaller joints may also be involved. Involvement of joints is successive, (one after another) rather than together, is termed characteristic migratory polyarthritis or polyarthralgia. No suppuration occurs. Swelling, redness and heat are prominent features which subside spontaneously in few days and all joints symptoms disappear in 3–4 weeks without any deformity.

II. Carditis

Rheumatic carditis is pancarditis involving pericardium, myocardium and endocardium. Incidence is 50–60% of all cases of rheumatic fever. It may be associated with arthritis or other symptoms or may be sole manifestation. Develops as early or within 2 weeks or more of onset of rheumatic fever.

At the onset of carditis child appears more ill, pyrexia higher, tachycardia is disproportionately higher to fever especially sleeping pulse rate. Pallor increased, patient may be dyspneic or have precordial pain.

Signs

i. Murmurs
   a. Systolic murmurs of mitral regurgitation usually present with active carditis at apex.
   b. Mid-diastolic murmur (Carey Coombs murmur due to active mitral valvulitis).
   c. Rarely diastolic murmur of aortic regurgitation. Important point is change in character of any murmur is sign of active disease.

ii. Cardiac enlargement
iii. CCF in absence of other causes
iv. Pericarditis occurs in severe form, arrhythmias present.
v. ECG prolongation of PR interval
vi. X-ray chest: Cardiac dilatation.

III. Chorea

It is a late manifestation occurs about 3 months after the onset of rheumatic fever. Occurs in 10–15% of patients as only sign or in others with other manifestations. Preliminary symptoms may be deterioration in hand writing, poor coordination, emotional liabilities, which are followed by involuntary, quasipurpose or purposeless movements, random, non-rhythmic movements, affecting any group of muscles but mostly face and upper extremities. This is a self-limiting disease; affected muscles are weak for 2 weeks to 3 months.

IV. Subcutaneous Nodules

These are round, hard, freely movable, transparent, painless nodules, usually appear at bony prominences. Size is pinhead to 2 cm in diameter, appear in crops especially in extensor surface of elbow, dorsum of hand or foot, skull, scapula or other bony prominences, occurs often when severe carditis is present. They are better seen than felt.

It is a late manifestation occurs after 6 weeks of onset of attack lasts for few days to weeks but has been unknown to last for about a year.

V. Erythema Marginatum

Most characteristic lesion occurs in skin, lesion is slightly red, raised, nonpruritic macules which extend to make wavy lines or rings with sharp margins. Sites are over trunk, flexor surface of joints, inner surface of arms and legs. This is recurrent and appear from time to time along with other manifestations of acute rheumatism. Sometimes appears as an isolated physical finding.

Fever

Fever always present at the onset of acute attack, fever may rise up to 101–103°F with daily variation of 1–3°F. Low grade fever in insidious onset and absent in rheumatic chorea.

Abdominal Pain

May precede attack but may be quite severe.

Epistaxis

Presenting frequently previously, now rare.

Laboratory Investigations

A. *Evidence of preceding streptococcal infections*
  1. Tests for streptococcal antibodies:
     i. Antistreptolysin titre (ASO) titre— rising or elevated titre >300 units (normal 200–300 units). It is suggestive of recent streptococcal infection, and not the rheumatic fever. Positive in 80% cases of acute onset.

        It begins to decline in 2 months, so in cases of gradual onset of carditis and chorea it have returned to normal.
     ii. Other streptococcal antibodies, e.g. anti-DNase B.

        If these tests are not available, then multiple antibody test (streptozyme) positive in dilution 1:200.

B. *Tests for measurement of presence and degree of inflammatory process*
  i. ESR
  ii. C reactive proteins more reliable than ESR.

C. *Miscellaneous*
  i. *Blood:* Anemia—normocytic normochromic.
  ii. *ECG:* Prolonged PR interval due to pericarditis.

D. *Therapeutic test:* Appropriate doses of salicylates (aspirin) bring dramatic change and relieve joints pain within 48 hours and bring down temperature.

E. *X-ray chest:* Cardiac enlargement and pericardial effusion.

F. *Throat swab culture:* Often negative. If taken just after attack it may be positive for group A β-hemolytic streptococci.

Echocardiography shows evidence of carditis such as decreased ventricular function, valvular insufficiency or pericardial effusion.

Diagnosis

No single clinical feature or laboratory investigation is characteristic. For the need to bring uniformity in diagnosis; TD Jones formulated criteria for diagnosis are given in Table 10.1.

Major manifestations: Clinical signs most useful in diagnosis.

Minor manifestations: Clinical signs less characteristic, but helpful in diagnosis.

Table 10.1: Jones criteria (revised) for guidance in the diagnosis of rheumatic fever

Major manifestations	Minor manifestations
1. Carditis	*Clinical*
2. Polyarthritis	1. Fever
3. Chorea	2. Arthralgia
4. Erythema marginatum	3. Previous rheumatic fever or rheumatic heart disease
5. Subcutaneous nodules	*Laboratory*
	1. Acute phase reaction increased ESR
	2. C reactive protein
	3. Prolonged PR interval

They are as in Table 10.1 plus supporting evidence of:

i. Preceding streptococcal infection
ii. Increased ASO or other streptococcal antibodies
iii. Positive throat culture for group A streptococcus
iv. Recent scarlet fever.

Interpretation

One major two minor or two major one minor plus supporting laboratory evidences of streptococcal infection are important for a presumptive diagnosis of rheumatic fever.

Differential Diagnosis

a. Juvenile rheumatoid arthritis
b. Acute osteomyelitis
c. Henoch-Schönlein purpura
d. Acute poliomyelitis
e. Acute leukemia
f. Streptococcal tonsilitis
g. Collagen disease
h. Sensitivity reaction to drugs

Complications

a. Chronic rheumatic heart disease
b. Subacute bacterial endocarditis

Treatment

i. Bedrest

It is essential in the management of a child with rheumatic fever. It is required till the rheumatic activity disappear (about 1–3 months).

Periodical assessment of ESR is a simple and practical criteria of activity of acute rheumatic fever. But persistence of ESR more than 6 months should not be considered sign of rheumatic activity, if no clinical signs are present.

Signs of activity

a. Joints symptoms.
b. New organic murmur.
c. Enlarging heart size.
d. Sleeping pulse rate more than 100.
e. Subcutaneous nodules.
f. Congestive cardiac failure in absence of chronic valvular lesion.

ii. Anti-inflammatory Drugs

a. **Salicylates:** Cause dramatic improvement by lowering fever, pain and swelling of joints.
   Dose: 100–200 mg/kg/24 hours in 4–6 divided doses for first and second weeks. It is better to give with antacid, avoid giving in empty stomach.

b. **Other drugs:** Phenylbutazone or Indomethacin is substituted in place of salicylate intolerance.

c. **Steroids:** Recommended for carditis with cardiomegaly or CCF.
   Dose: Prednisolone 2 mg/kg/24 hours for 2 weeks and taper over 2 weeks. Chorea is treated with haloperidol, barbiturate and chlorpromazine. Steroids are not recommended unless signs of rheumatic inflammatory process present.

d. **Penicillin:** Penicillin is indicated for eradication of streptococcal infection.
   i. Procaine penicillin 4 lac units IM daily for 10–14 days,
   ii. Oral penicillin 4 lac units every 4–6 hours for 10–14 days
   iii. If patient is sensitive to penicillin; Erythromycin or tetracycline is given for same period.

e. Treatment of complications, e.g. CCF and good nursing care is essential.

Supportive Therapy

a. Congestive cardiac failure is treated with diuretics, dietary salt restriction, digoxin and bedrest.

b. Rheumatic chorea: If severe may be treated with haloperidol.
   1. Bedrest, salicylates, 10 days course of penicillin.

2. Sedatives: Phenobarbitone 5 mg/kg/day. Alternatively chlorpromazine 2–3 mg/kg/day or haloperidol 0.2 mg/kg/day.

c. Severe valvular dysfunction requires valve replacement or valvuloplasty.

Prognosis

1. Cardiac inflammation often leads to valvular dysfunction or stenosis (usually more than 3 years after rheumatic fever)
2. There is no chronic sequalae of the joint, skin and CNS manifestations.

Prevention

Once diagnosed, antimicrobial prophylaxis should be started to prevent streptococcal infection and recurrence of rheumatic fever.

  i. Benzathine penicillin 1.2 million units every 4 weeks IM is drug of choice or oral penicillin 2 lac units twice daily.

  ii. Sulfadiazine: In case patient is allergic to or cannot tolerate penicillin.
Dose
  a. 0.5 gm daily in children less than 30 kg
  b. 1.0 gm daily in others.

  iii. Initial attack of pharyngitis treated with penicillin to prevent rheumatic fever.

Duration of preventive treatment

Continued throughout childhood and adolescence for a minimum of 5 years or until the age of 21 years.

MITRAL INCOMPETENCE (INSUFFICIENCY)

This is a most common valvular affection following rheumatic fever. Insufficiency of the mitral value is the result of structural changes that include some loss of valvular substance, and shortening and thickening of the chordae tendineae.

During ventricular systole blood regurgitates from the left ventricle to the left atrium. In view of increased volume of blood that left atrium and left ventricle are forced to handle both the chambers enlarge (Fig. 10.11).

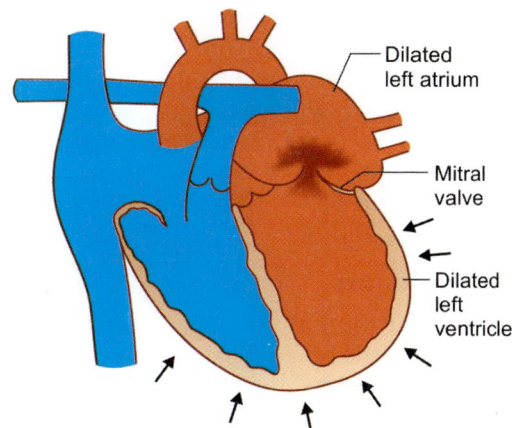

Fig. 10.11: Mitral regurgitation.

Clinical Features

Most of the patients present with exertional dyspnea, fatigue and signs of left ventricular failure. Pathognomonic signs are heaving apical impulse, systolic thrill and blowing apical pansystolic murmur which are transmitted to the axilla and even to the scapula (Fig. 10.12).

Radiology: Normal if lesion is small, in severe lesion left ventricular enlargement. Roentgenogram chest shows left artium and left ventricular enlargement.

ECG: May show bifid 'p' wave and signs of left ventricular hypertrophy (sometimes right ventricular hypertrophy also.)

Treatment

Consist of management of heart failure and prophylaxis against rheumatic fever. Surgical

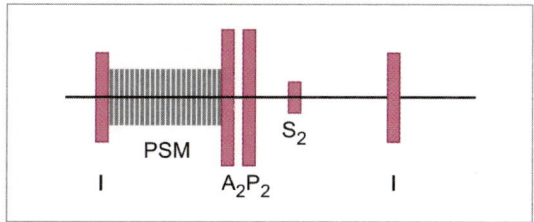

Fig. 10.12: Auscultatory events in mitral regurgitation.

treatment is indicated in severe cases (annuloplasty or valve replacement).

MITRAL STENOSIS

This is not infrequent in children, develops relatively late in children with rheumatic carditis (Fig. 10.13).

Hemodynamics

Sclerosis of the base of mitral ring causes obstruction to the flow of blood from left atrium to the left ventricle during diastole. There is incomplete emptying of left atrium resulting hypertrophy of this chamber. After-ward due to back pressure pulmonary and congestive cardiac failure may occur (Fig. 10.13).

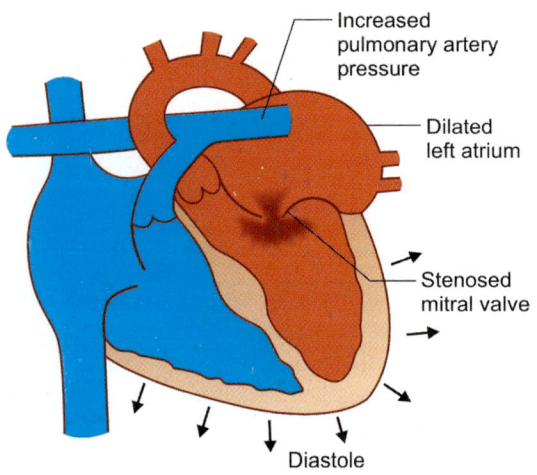

Fig. 10.13: Mitral stenosis.

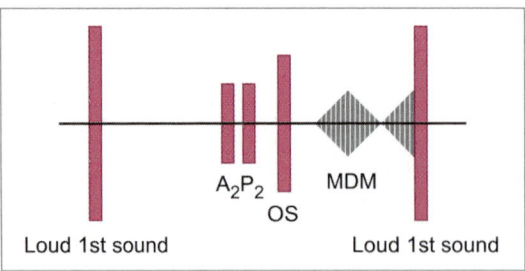

Fig. 10.14: Auscultatory events in mitral stenosis.

Clinical Features

Most of the patients are in the 4 to 10 years of age group. Exertional dyspnea, hemoptysis, congestive cardiac failure are common clinical manifestations. Important physical findings are presystolic thrill, loud first sound, with or without opening snap. Characteristic murmur is mid-diastolic murmur intensity is maximum at apex, low pitched and rumbling. P_2 is loud and in cases where right ventricular hypetrophy is present it is best heard in left lateral position and by using bell of stethoscope (Fig. 10.14).

Radiology: Heart may be normal or enlarged in size. The main pulmonary artery is enlarged and in some cases left atrium as well, which is confirmed by barium swallow.

ECG: Characteristic broad and notched P wave (P mitrale), right axis deviation and right ventricular hypertrophy.

Cardiac catheterization: Reveal significant elevation of pulmonary artery and right ventricular pressures.

Treatment

Medical management includes treatment of congestive cardiac failure, control of respiratory tract infection and prophylaxis against rheumatic fever (uptil puberty).

Surgical treatment is indicated in isolated mitral stenosis, left atrial and right ventricular enlargement, and in patient who has been free from rheumatic fever for at least 6 months.

Aortic Stenosis

Aortic stenosis is narrowing of the aortic valve. Aortic stenosis appears a commissural fusion of the three normal leaflets leading to bicuspid or unicuspid valve.

Pathophysiology: Aortic stenosis results in reduced left ventricular output due to obstruction. This may lead to myocardial ischemia.

Clinical Features

a. Neonates with severe stenosis: Neonates at birth appears normal but at 12–24 hours develop clinical features of CHF.
b. Older children have no symptoms until stenosis becomes severe. Symptoms due to exercise intolerance, chest pain syncope, and even sudden death.

Signs (Fig. 10.15)

1. Sustained or heaving cardiac impulse
2. Systolic thrill in second right intercostal space and sometimes along the right cervical vessels.
3. Ejection systolic murmur of aortic area at midsystolic and tapering off before second sound.
4. Quit 1st heart sound, 2nd heart sound delayed with reverse splitting
5. BP low with narrowed pulse pressure.

Investigations

- ECG: LV hypertrophy
- X-ray chest
    a. Prominent rounded left ventricle
    b. Post-stenotic dilatation
    c. Aortic valve calcification
- Echocardiography shows stenosed valve.

Management

1. Prophylaxis against infective endocarditis
2. Balloon valvoplasty in elder patient gives transient relief.
3. Aortic valve valvotomy is confined to congenital AS. Required 5–10 years after palliative valvoplasty.

The aortic valve is replaced with a prosthetic valve (Ross procedure).

AORTIC INSUFFICIENCY

The aortic valve is the second most frequently valve involved in rheumatic fever. Pathologically sclerosis of aortic valves leads to distortion and retraction of the cusps.

Aortic incompetence causes generally no symptoms and children may present with pallor, forceful optical impulse. A soft decrescendo blowing diastolic murmur often heard in the aortic area, the apex, as well as in 3rd left intercostal space. Evidence of wide pulse pressure such as Corrigan pulsations may be seen in carotid arteries (Fig. 10.16).

Radiology may show cardiomegaly with left ventricular hypertrophy, prominence of aortic knob.

ECG shows features of left ventricular hypertrophy.

Management consists of treatment for heart failure, and prosthetic replacement of the valve.

Tricuspid Regurgitation

1. Functional
2. Organic—rare

Symptoms: Tiredness on effort—hepatic pain on exertion peripheral edema. Pansystolic murmur in tricuspid area that increases with respiration or exercise.

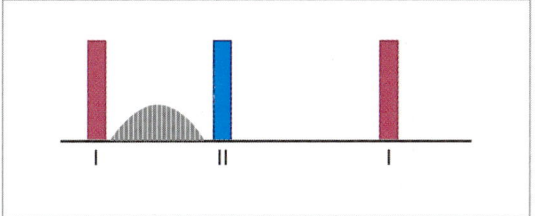

Fig. 10.15: Auscultatory events in aortic stenosis.

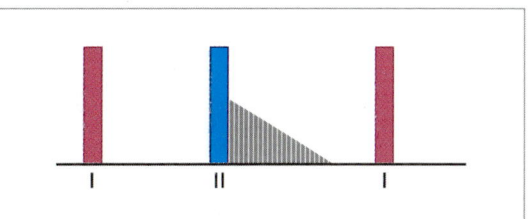

Fig. 10.16: Auscultatory events in aortic incompetence.

Investigations: Echo-systolic prolapsed, ruptured chordae, or vegetation. Doppler echo can give estimate of regurgitation and systolic pressure.

Treatment

Functional TR: Bedrest, digitalis, diuretics vasodilators.

Organic TR: Replacement of value.

Tricuspid Stenosis

Causes

1. Rheumatic
2. Congenital
3. Carcinoid tumor
4. Functional

Symptoms: Hepatic pain on exertion, peripheral edema, dyspnea on exertion.

Signs: IVP raised, first sound loud, diastolic murmur at left sternal edge.

ECG: Enlarged liver RA hypertrophy but no RVH.

Treatment: Replacement of value.

Pulmonary Regurgitation

1. Congenital
2. Acquired: With idiopathic pulmonary hyperplasia, MS, IE, rheumatic fever, syphilis, carcinoid syndrome, aneurysm of pulmonary artery and pulmonary hypertension.

Signs: Early diastolic murmur conducted to left sternal border.

ECG shows RVH

X-ray chest: Enlargement of pulmonary artery.

Pulmonary Stenosis

It is narrowing of the pulmonary valve. Pathologically fusion of valve commissures are seen.

Pathophysiology: Pulmonary stenosis results in increased right ventricular pressure due to obstruction in flow and right ventricular output.

Clinical Features

1. Ejection click
2. Systolic ejection murmur at pulmonary area.

Severe pulmonary stenosis in the neonates may be manifested by cyanosis. But in most of the children symptoms are absent.

ECG: RVH

X-ray chest: Prominent main pulmonary artery.

Echocardiography: Narrowed valve detected.

Management

1. Balloon valvuloplasty for symptomatic patient and critical pulmonary stenosis.

BACTERIAL ENDOCARDITIS

Subacute bacterial endocarditis occurs at all age groups of infancy and childhood, including neonatal period.

In most of the instances the infection is superimposed upon endocardial lesion: Congenital or acquired and some cases in relation to some disruptive immunologic factors. It is especially associated with rheumatic valvular disease. The causative agents are *Streptococcus viridans* (most frequent), Staphylococcus, *Staphylococcus epidermidis* and certain fungi.

Clinical manifestations include fluctuating fever (101–103°F), anemia, weight loss and splenomegaly, new and changing heart murmur are common. Increased ESR, ester's nodes and clubbing of figures are other features. Emboli in other parts of the body (spleen, lungs and brain) may be the only presenting features.

Other features such as hepatomegaly, leukocytosis, microscopic hematuria, joint pains, etc. may also be observed.

Treatment consists of rest in bed, attention to diet, intake of fluids and administration of antibiotic (penicillin). Penicillin in massive doses is continued for 6 weeks after the clinical symptoms have subsided. Surgery is indicated for surgically correctable lesion, e.g. PDA.

Prevention is done by prescribing antibiotics during minor surgical procedures like tooth extraction, adenotonsillectomy, etc. in children.

CARDIOMYOPATHY

Cardiomyopathy is defined as an abnormality of cardiac muscle manifested by systolic or diastolic dysfunction.

Types

1. Dilated cardiomyopathy
2. Restrictive cardiomyopathy
3. Hypertrophic cardiomyopathy

Dilated Cardiomyopathy

This is a primary myocardial disease characterized by ventricular dilatation and reduced cardiac function.

Etiology

1. Idiopathic—frequently
2. Viral myocarditis
3. Mitochondrial abnormalities
4. Creatinine deficiency
5. Nutritional deficiency such as selenium and thiamine deficiency
6. Hypocalcemia
7. Chronic tachydysrhythmias
8. Anomalous origin of left coronary artery from the pulmonary artery
9. Medications—doxorubicin

Clinical Features

Same as sign and symptoms of congestive cardiac failure.

Diagnosis

1. Viral serology
2. Serum creatinine
3. ECG: Tachycardia, low cardiac voltage and ST segment and T wave changes.
4. Echocardiography: It shows dilated left ventricle with poor ventricular function.

Management

1. Medical management of congestive cardiac failure.
2. Treatment of underlying metabolic or nutritional disorders.

3. Surgical repair of ALCAPA (implantation of left coronary artery into aortic sinus)
4. Cardiac transplantation if CHF is unresponsive to medical management.
5. Antiarrhythmic medications for arrhythmias
6. Dual chamber pacing to reduce septal hypertrophy.

Restrictive Cardiomyopathy

It is defined as excessively rigid ventricular walls that impair normal diastolic filling.

Etiology

1. Amyloidosis
2. Inherited infiltrative disorders

Clinical Features

1. *Symptoms:* Exercise intolerance, weakness and dyspnea.
2. *Physical examination:* Edema, hepatomegaly and ascites and elevated central venous pressure.

Management

Treatment is related to reduce CVP with diuretic and improve diastolic compliance with β-blockers and calcium chain blockers.

Hypertrophic Cardiomyopathy

Left ventricular hypertrophy in absence of systemic and cardiac diseases.

Etiology

It is autosomal dominant inheritance in about 60% cases.

Clinical Features

1. *Symptoms:* Chest pain and exercise intolerance, syncope or sudden death.
2. *Physical examination:* Harsh, ejection systolic murmur at apex which is accentuated antiphysiologic work (standing, Valsalva).

Investigations

- *ECG:* LVH, ST segment and T wave changes, deep and wide wave.
- *Echocardiogram:* It shows hypertrophy.

Treatment

Patient having symptoms:

1. Beta-adrenergic blockers or calcium channel blockers decrease myocardial contractility thus reduce LVOT obstruction and improve diastolic compliance.
2. Surgical myomectomy is suggested for severe cases not responding to medical management.

PERICARDITIS

Inflammation of pericardial space known as pericarditis.

Etiology

1. Infections
   a. Viral infections: (Most common cause) coxsackievirus, echovirus, adenovirus, influenza, parainfluenza and Epstein-Barr virus (EBV).
   b. Purulent pericarditis: *Staphylococcus aureus, Streptococcus pneumoniae.*
      It may be either primary or secondary from pneumonia or meningitis. In this type of pericarditis constrictive pericarditis develops frequently.
   c. Post-pericardiotomy syndrome: After open heart surgery
   d. Collagen vascular disease.
   e. Uremia

Pathophysiology: Inflammation of parietal and visceral layers of pericardium leads to exudation or transudation of fluid. Which impair venous return and cardiac filling, cardiac temponade or critically impaired left ventricular output may occur.

Clinical Features

Symptoms: Fever, malaise, dyspnea and chest pain intense while supine and relived when sitting position.

Signs

- Pericardial friction rub, distant heart sound.

- Pulsus paradoxus (reduction of pulse pressure more than 10 mmHg on deep inspiration)
- Hepatomegaly

Investigations

- Pericardiocentesis: Needle is inserted into pericardial sac and fluid is withdrawn for diagnosis and culture sensitivity.
- ESR: Elevated
- X-ray chest: Enlarged heart shadow with large effusion
- ECG: ST segment changes
  QRS: Low voltage
- Echocardiography: It shows the extent and quality of pericardial effusion.

Management

a. Antibiotic: As per sensitivity report.
b. Anti-inflammatory agents: As per or steroids for viral origin.
c. Drainage of the pericardial effusion by placement of pericardial catheter or surgical window.

MYOCARDITIS

Inflammation of myocardium. It is most common cause of sudden death in children.

Etiology

1. Virus: Enterovirus, coxasckievirus
2. Bacteria
   - *Corynebacterium diphtheriae*
   - *Streptococcus pyogenes*
   - *Staphylococcus aureus*
   - *Mycobacerium tuberculosis*
3. Fingi: Candida, Cryptococcus
4. Protozoa: *Trypanosoma cruzi*
5. Autoimmune diseases: SLE, rheumatic fever, sarcoidosis
6. Kawasaki disease

Clinical Features

1. Dyspnea and malaise.
2. Tachycardia, muffled heart sounds, gallop heart rhythm, hepatomegaly, tachypnea and pulmonary rales.

Investigations

- ESR: Elevated
- Creatine kinase (CK) raised
- C-reactive protein (CRP) raised
- Endomyocardial biopsy
- ECG: T wave and ST segment changes
- Echo: Global ventricular dysfunction.

Management

Medical: Supportives which include use of inotropic agents, diuretics, afterload reducing agents.

Cardiac transplantation: In cases refractory to medical management.

CONGESTIVE CARDIAC FAILURE (CCF)
(CONGESTIVE HEART FAILURE)

Definition

Congestive cardiac failure is defined as the state of which the heart cannot produce the cardiac output required to sustain the metabolic needs of the body without evoking certain compensatory mechanism.

Pathophysiology: Signs and symptoms are result of compensatory responses of the body due to heart failure.

1. Hypoperfusion of end organs stimulates the heart to maximize contractility and heart rate in an attempt to increase cardiac output.

Hypoperfusion also stimulates the kidneys to retain salt and water through the renin-angiotensin system in an attempt to increase blood volume.

2. Catecholamines released by sympathetic nervous system also increase heart rate and myocardial contractility.

Classification (Causes)

i. Low output failure means heart failure due to primary heart failure:
   - Congenital heart disease
   - Rheumatic heart disease
   - Myocarditis
   - Systemic hypertension (essential)
   - Cardiac arrhythmias
   - Cardiac temponade (pericardial effusion)
   - Large intracardiac shunts.

ii. High output failure means heart failure due to primarily noncardiac disturbances; non-cardiac causes:
   - Anemia
   - Acute nephritis
   - Sepsis, septicemia
   - Deficiency disease, e.g. beriberi
   - Metabolic disorders: Hypoglycemia, hyperthyroidism, glycogen storage disease.
   - Respiratory disease: Acute bronchiolitis, bronchopneumonia, pneumothorax, etc.

Common Causes

Infants	Children
1. Congenital heart disease	1. Rheumatic heart disease
2. Myocarditis and primary myocardial disease	2. Complication of congenital heart disease
3. Paroxysmal tachycardia	3. Hypertension
4. Anemia	4. Myocarditis and primary myocardial disease
5. Others: Infections, neonatal asphyxia, hypoglycemia, hypocalcemia, upper respiratory obstruction	5. Upper respiratory obstruction

Etiology

Causes

Infants

1. Congenital heart disease (CHD)
   a. Increased pulmonary blood flow
      - Large ventricular septal defect (VSD)
      - Large patent ductus arteriosus (PDA)
      - Coarctation of aorta
      - Interrupted aortic arch
      - Hypoplastic left heart syndrome
   b. Obstructive lesions
      - Severe aortic, pulmonary, mitral valve stenosis
      - Coarctation of aorta
      - Interrupted aortic arch
      - Hypoplastic left heart syndrome
   c. Other causes
      - Arteriovenous malformations
      - Mitral and tricuspid regurgitation
2. Acquired heart diseases
   - Viral myocarditis common cause
   - Others cardiac infections endocarditis, pericarditis
   - Metabolic diseases (e.g. hyperthyroidism)
   - Medications (e.g. doxorubicin)
   - Cardiomyopathies
   - Ischemic diseases
   - Dysrhythmias including tachycardia, bradycardia
   - Myocardial diseases
   - Glycogen storage disease
   - Endocrinal fibroblastosis
   - Medial necrosis of coronary arteries
   - Anomalous left coronary artery from pulmonary artery
3. Miscellaneous causes
   a. Infections
   b. Severe anemia
   c. Rapid infusion of intravenous fluids
   d. Obstructive airway disease
      - Enlarged tonsils, adenoids
      - Laryngomalacia
   - Cystic fibrosis
   - Infections of respiratory tract

Hypoglycemia, neonatal asphyxia and hypocalcemia may result CCF in neonates, pulmonary hypertension.

Children

- Rheumatic heart disease
- Congenital heart disease with anemia, infection, endocarditis
- Systemic hypertension
- Myocarditis
- Pulmonary hypertension.

Clinical Features in Children

1. *General symptoms:* Fatigue, effort intolerance, anorexia, abdominal pain and cough.
2. Dyspnea and orthopnea.
3. Raised jugular pressure.
4. Liver enlargement.
5. Edema on dependent part or anasarca.
6. Cardiomegaly.
7. *On auscultation:* Basal crepitations, finding of basic lesion.
8. Peripheral cyanosis.

In Infants

1. General symptoms are feeding difficulties, excessive perspiration, irritability, weak cry, poor weight gain. Sign of dyspnea and tachypnea.
2. JVP raised but difficult to ascertain at short neck of infant and difficulty of relaxed state in infant.
3. Edema not clinically detectable generally because it is generalized.
4. Liver enlargement present. Heart may be normal or enlarged.
5. Sign of pulmonary congestion seen.

Pneumonitis common. Collapse may be or may not be present.

Diagnosis

It is a clinical state due to underlying primary disease.

Investigations

i. **Blood:** ESR is low. Polycythemia may be present.

ii. **Urine:** Albumin and casts seen. Specific gravity raised.

iii. **Roentgenogram of the chest:** Cardiac enlargement; pulmonary vascularity variable, depending upon primary lesion other features seen.

iv. **ECG:** Helpful in diagnosis of underlying disease.

v. **Echocardiography:** For assessment of ventricular function.

Management

Goals

1. To reduce cardiac output
2. To augment myocardial contractility
3. To improve cardiac performance
4. To correct underlying cause

Underlying cause of congestive cardiac failure is removed or corrected if possible. Medical management is required for disease before surgery in surgically correctable disease and in case of cardiomyopathies unless cardiac transplantation is indicated.

i. Bedrest

The best position is 'semi-upright' at an angle of 45° for the relief of breathlessness.

ii. Oxygen

It is best given in a tent; if not available, may be given by nasal catheter.

iii. Digitalization

Digoxin is given intravenously, intramuscularly or orally (Table 10.2).

Above dose is for oral administration of the drug, parenteral dose should be about 75% of oral dose.

Rapid digitalization: It is carried out parenterally, one-half of the total calculated dose should be given stat. Divide the remaining half in two doses. Each half is given at 8 hours interval.

Table 10.2: Total digitalization and maintenance dose of digoxin

Age group	24-hour dose/kg
Neonates	0.05 mg (0.03–0.04 mg)
Premature	0.04 mg (0.02–0.025 mg)
Infants (1–12 months age)	0.08 mg (0.04–0.06 mg)
Adolescent or adult (after 1 year age)	0.06 mg (1.0–1.5 mg) in divided doses

Maintenance dose will be one-fourth or one-third of total digitalizing dose. This is given as a single dose or in two divided doses daily. In *slow digitalization* initiation of maintenance doses without overloading doses will achieve digitalization in 7–10 days. Digitalis is useful in low output type cardiac failure, whether rhythm is regular or irregular.

iv. Diuretics

Diuretics should be started after complete digitalization. Frusemide is most commonly used diuretic in patients with cardiac failure.

Dose: 1–2 mg per kg orally, 0.5–1.5 mg per kg parenterally IM or IV.

It gives prompt improvement, particularly if pulmonary congestion is present.

Chlorothiazide used for less severe cases dose 20–50 mg per kg per 24 hours or alternate day in divided dosage.

v. Potassium

Every patient of CCF who is digitalized should be given potassium supplements because diuretics causes potassium depletion.

- *Vasodilators*
  Mechanism: Vasodilators relax veins and aterioles so they counteract the compensatory mechanism at work to improve the inadequate cardiac output such as arteriolar and venous vasoconstriction mediated through catecholamines which maintain blood pressure by increasing systemic vascular resistance which increases work of heart.

Sodium nitroprusside IV

- 0.5–8 mEq/kg/min infusion
- Captopril, enalapril (ACE inhibitors)
- Beta blockers (metaprolol, carvedilol)
- Carvedilol is preferred.

Dose: 0.08–0.4 mg/kg/day increased gradually depending upon tolerability maximum 1 mg/kg/day.

Phosphodiesterase inhibitors—*milrinone.*

Specific indications

a. Acute mitral or aortic regurgitation
b. Ventricular dysfunction due to myocarditis
c. Anomalous coronary artery from pulmonary artery
d. Postoperative

- *Inotropic medications:* In severe CHF Dopamine is given if blood pressure is low as an intravenous infusion dose 5 µg/kg/min.

  It causes peripheral vasodilatation, increases myocardial contractility and renal flow resulting natriuresis.

  Dobutamine

  Dose: 2.5–40 µg/kg/min

  It should be increased gradually till the deserved blood pressure is achieved.

- *Interventional catheterization:* These procedures may be required for underlying cause of cardiac heart failure, e.g. balloon valvuloplasty or critical aortic and pulmonary valve stenosis.

- *Surgical repair:* It is often a definitive treatment of CHF secondary to congenital heart disease.

- *Heart transplantation:* Indicated in ischemic or dilated cardiomyopathies.

- *Prostaglandin:* Newborn has critical coarctation, aortic stenosis, interrupted aortic arch, administration of prostaglandin to open the closing duct has better prognosis.

vi. General

i. Caloric intake should be increased due to increased demand.

ii. Salt restricted diet is not practical in children due to unavoidability of such baby food, he cannot be forced or reduced food intake affects adversely. In extreme situation, low sodium diet is advocated when digitalization and diuretics fail.

iii. Sedation: Restlessness and anxiety should be controlled with morphia, pethidine, diazepam.

iv. Antibiotics: Antibiotics are given to control infection causing congestive cardiac failure.

v. Drugs which reduce ventricular load, e.g. nitroprusside, hydralazine are used to reduce ventricular load and they enhance myocardial contractability.

HYPERTENSION

Systemic hypertension is not common in children, hypertension occurs as a secondary phenomenon in a variety of relatively rare conditions which are mostly related to renal and adrenal diseases.

Hypertension is defined as the arterial blood pressure above the 90th percentile for the age (Table 10.3).

Blood Pressure Measurement

Blood pressure should be measured when child is relaxed because anxiety, apprehension and agitation may effect recording of blood pressure. Appropriate cuff size should be taken, ideally which should cover about two-thirds the length of upper arm and around it entirely.

Blood pressure should be measured in both the limbs; upper limb and lower limb. It can be measured by following methods:

a. Palpation
b. Auscultation
c. Flush method
d. Visual oscillometry

Visual oscillometry, flush methods are not used nowadays because of advent of sophisticated ultrasound sphygmomanometry.

Table 10.3: Blood pressure at different ages

| Age | BP in mm of Hg | |
	Systolic	Diastolic
Newborn	86	60
1 year	86	60
6 years	90	60
8 years	96	64
10 years	100	64
12 years	110	70

Classification and Etiology

Hypertension may be essential or secondary. In infancy and childhood, hypertension is usually secondary. Essential hypertension is rare.

Secondary hypertension in children may be temporary (transient) or may be chronic (persistent).

Persistent hypertension (causes)

1. Renal: Chronic renal parenchymal disease, congenital renal malformation, collagen vascular disorder.
2. Vascular: Congenital vascular malformations such as coarctation of thoracic or abdominal aorta, vasculitis, renal vein thrombosis.
3. Endocrine: Hyperthyroidism, primary hyperaldosteronism, pheochromocytoma.
4. Central nervous system: Intracerebral tumors, intracerebral hemorrhage, raised intracranial pressure secondary to trauma.
5. Essential hypertension

Transient: There are innumerable causes of transient hypertension, main conditions are grouped as follows:

1. Renal: Acute glomerulonephritis, acute tubular necrosis, pyelonephritis, obstructive uropathy.
2. Drugs: Corticosteroids, amphetamines, vitamin D intoxication and sympathomimetic drugs.

3. Central and autonomic nervous system: Raised intracranial pressure due to any cause such as meningitis, encephalitis.
4. Miscellaneous: Hyperclcaemia, post-coarctation repair, chronic airway obstruction.

Clinical Features

Hypertension may be asymptomatic, headache, nausea, vomiting, dizziness and irritability are common presenting features. Clinical signs depend on underlying illness, organic lesion.

If hypertensive encephalopathy is impending or present, vomiting, hyperreflexia, ataxia and other neurologic signs such as seizures, stupor or even coma may be prominent. Prolonged hypertension leads to congestive cardiac failure and hypertensive retinopathy.

Diagnosis and Investigations

1. Clinical features.
2. Skiagram of chest: Notching of ribs (coarctation of aorta)
3. Urine: For sugar and protein, proteinuria and hematuria in absence of renal disease suggests malignant hypertension. Urine culture for urinary tract infection.
4. Ultrasonogram: For diagnosis of obstructive uropathy, size of kidney (ulteration in size of kidney) anomalies of calysis, pelvis and ureters.
5. Intravenous urogram: For renal artery stenosis
6. Blood: Serum potassium—for diagnosis of primary aldosteronism, urea, creatinine raised in renal parenchymal disease.
7. Serum catecholamine and urinary catecholamine in pheochromocytoma.
8. Abdominal scan: Diagnosis of pheochromocytoma, suprarenal glands.
9. CT scan head: Intracranial causes.
10. Plasma renin activity: PRA in venous blood increased in renal disease.

Incurable Forms of Hypertension

Chronic glomerulonephritis, bilateral pyelo-nephritis, congenital dysphasic kidney, medullary cystic disease, unremediable renal artery diseases, post-lead intoxication, post-irradiation.

Curable Forms of Hypertension

Coarctation of aorta, remediable forms of renovascular disease, traumatic lesion of kidney, unilateral renal parenchymal disease, neuroblastoma, renal tumors, pheochromo-cytoma, Cushing disease and primary aldosteronism.

Course and Prognosis

The outcome of essential hypertension in adolescents is not yet evident. The prognosis after surgical correction in coarctation of aorta is variable. Prognosis is good in renal artery stenosis, pheochromocytoma after surgical correction. In chronic renal parenchymal disease, the prognosis depends on many factors including acceptance of dialysis and transplanted organs.

Management

The management may be both by non-pharmacological and pharmacological measures. In adolescents non-pharmacological measure must first be tried.

Non-pharmacological Measures

1. Reduction of excess weight: Every effort should be made to reduce obesity by diet and activity.
2. Reduction of excess salt intake: Severe salt restriction is very difficult to implement in children. During summer when salt is lost in sweat salt restriction is not desirable except in cardiac failure.

Pharmacological Measures

Pharmacological measures are not very often used in children. These are required in secondary hypertension and in selected cases of essential hypertension. Drugs used are:

1. Thiazide diuretics.
2. Beta blockers like atenolol.
3. Alpha blockers: Such as prazosin.
4. Alpha and beta blockers such as labetalol.
5. Calcium channel blockers like nifedipine and diltiazem.
6. Angiotensin converting enzyme inhibitors like enalapril, lisinopril.
7. Centrally acting drugs like methyldopa and clonidine.
8. Vasodilators like diazoxide hydralazine and nitroprusside.

Always avoid centrally acting drugs in children. Emergency reduction in blood pressure is required in malignant hypertension (diastolic pressure more than 130 mm Hg with retinal hemorrhage or exudate with or without papilledema).

Indications for parenteral drugs are as follows:

1. Gross ventricular failure due to hyper-tension.
2. Encephalopathy with fits or fluctuating neurological signs. Parenteral drugs used are as follows:
   a. Labetalol: 4–8 mg per hour by infusion.
   b. Nitroprusside: 0.5–8.0 mg per kg per minute by infusion.
   c. Diazoxide: 2–5 mg per kg per dose, maximum 100 mg.
   d. Hydralazine: 0.4–0.8 mg per kg per dose increased to a maximum of 200 mg per 24 hours.

Malignant hypertension without heart failure or encephalopathy is managed by (1) beta blockers (including labetalol), (2) nifedipine, (3) methyldopa, and (4) hydralazine. Avoid prazosin and angiotensin converting enzyme inhibitors.

For patient with heart failure

Nitroprusside initially followed by diuretics calcium antagonist, and prazosin is better choice.

Special circumstances: If hypertension is associated with other illness, drug of choice is as follows (Table 10.4).

Table 10.4: Drug of choice in the special circumstances

Name of drugs	Diabetes mellitus	Heart failure	Obstructive airway disease	Renal failure
Angiotensin converting enzyme inhibitors	+	+	+	–
Diuretics	–	+	+	Loop diuretics except Ethacrynic acid
Calcium antagonist		+	+	+
Parzosin	+	+		+
Hydralazine	+		+	
Beta blockers	–	–	–	+

(+ means drug of choice, – means drugs avoided)

Surgery—may be required in coarctation of arota, renal artery stenosis, pheochromocytoma, primary hyperaldosteronism.

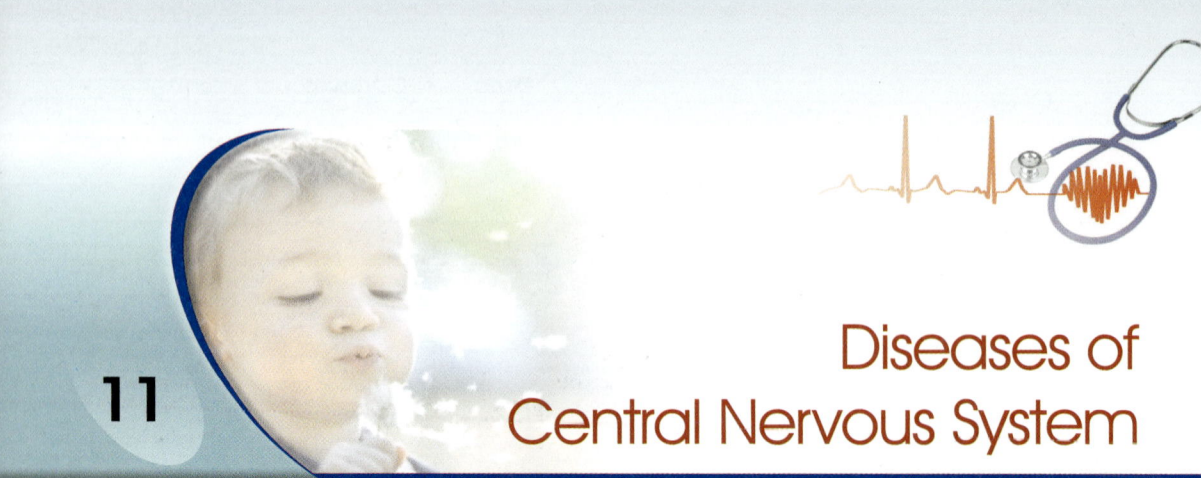

11

Diseases of Central Nervous System

Infections of central nervous system are more common during infancy and childhood, because immune mechanism and phagocytic functions are not fully mature.

MENINGITIS

Inflammation of meninges covering brain and spinal cord is known as meningitis. This is of two types: (i) Bacterial or pyogenic—meningococcal, pneumococcal, *H. influenzae,* streptococcal, staphylococcal, *E, coli,* Listeria. (ii) Aseptic—tuberculous, viral, fungal, protozoal (toxoplasmosis, amebic). This variety is characterized by absence of organism in CSF on Gram's staining and on routine culture.

Central nervous system infection is not specific, so there is always involvement of brain tissue in meningitis and meningo-encephalitis is proper term to it.

PYOGENIC MENINGITIS
(ACUTE BACTERIAL MENINGITIS)

Epidemiology

1. Acute bacterial meningitis is common in neonates and infants due to poor immunity and phagocytic functions.
2. Infants and children who are imnunodeficient, have underlying fever, renal, pulmonary or cardiac disease, have high incidence of bacterial meningitis.

Bacterial Pathogens

0–1 month—*E. coli, Streptococcus pneumoniae, Salmonella* species, *Pseudomonas aeruginosa, Streptococcus faecalis, Staphylococcus aureus.*

3 months to 3 years—*Haemophilus influenzae, S. pneumoniae,* meningococci *(Neisseria meningitis).*

Beyond 3 years—*Streptococcus pneumoniae.*

Routes of Infection

i. Infection reaches meninges through hematogenous spread from distant foci of sepsis in the body, e.g. pneumonia, infective endocarditis.
ii. Rarely spread from nearby septic foci, e.g. infected paranasal sinus, mastoiditis, osteomyelitis of skull.
iii. Through fracture of skull at its base
iv. Direct invasion of the central nervous system also may occur from dermoid sinus tracts or meningomyelocele due to direct contact of skin and meninges.

Decreased host resistance due to congenital or acquired conditions predispose to bacterial meningitis.

Pathology

- Leptomeninges are infiltrated with inflammatory cells.
- Cortex of brain—edema, exudates, proliferation of microglia.
- Ependymal cells—destroyed
- Purulent exudate—at base of brain which may block to foramen of Luschka and Magendie resulting hydrocephalus.
- Death occurs due to endotoxic shock.

Clinical Features

History of preceding respiratory or gastrointestinal tract infection is often obtained before the onset of meningitis. Onset is sudden, common symptoms are fever, vomiting, restlessness, irritability, headache and convulsions.

In infants, refusal to take feed, fever, irritability with bulging fontanelle are presenting manifestations.

Signs are neck rigidity, bulging fontanelle (if open) with diastasis of sutures. Kernig and Brudzinski sign positive. Papilledema and hemiplegia are seen in few cases.

Seizures occur in about 30% of cases, stupor, coma and focal meningeal sign noticed. Cranial nerve palsy (6th cranial nerve palsy common), blindness and deafness, squint or vestibular dysfunction are due to cranial nerve involvement (Fig. 11.1).

Characteristic signs peculiar to meningococcal infections are generalized purpuric rash found in majority of cases (difficult to see in dark skinned child) or signs of adrenal insufficiency (hypotension, shock, coma).

Collection of fluid in the subdural space is seen in 50% cases of infants. It gives focal neurological signs as in cerebral compression.

Diagnosis

1. CSF examination is essential for diagnosis. Pressure raised. On gross examination—turbid or cloudy (little opalescent). Cell count increased, mainly polymorph. Proteins increased. Sugar remarkably

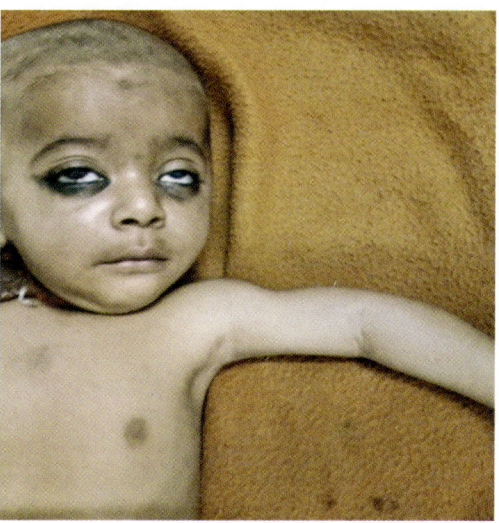

Fig. 11.1: Pyogenic meningitis.

reduced. Culture and sensitivity done for identification of organism.
2. Quellung and agglutination reactions for identification of organism.
3. Investigations for the search of foci. Blood culture is obtained in every patient.
4. CT scan—ventricular dilatation, subdural effusion, decrease in brain mass, vascular lesion and cerebral infarcts.
5. Rapid diagnostic test—may be used to distinguish between viral, bacterial and tubercular meningitis based on antigen and antibody reaction.

For example, countercurrent immunoelectrophoreses, latex particle agglutination coagulation—ELISA.

Management

Initial emperic therapy

a. *Antibiotic therapy*—third generation cephalosporin such as ceftriaxone or cefotaxime. A combination of ampicillin (200 mg/kg) and chloramphenicol (100 mg/kg/24 hr) for 10–14 days is also effective.

All antibiotics are administered intravenously.

After sensitivity report choice of antibiotic is given.

Specific antimicrobial therapy

Meningococcal or *pneumococcal*

Penicillin 400–50000 units/kg/day q 4 hr.
Cefotaxime 150–200 mg/kg/day q 8 hr.
Ceftriaxone 100–150 mg/kg/day q 12 hr.

N. influenzae

Ceftriaxone, cefotaxime, combination of ampicillin and chloramphenicol (less preferred).

Staphylococcal

Vancomyin if methicillin, or penicillin resistance.

Rifampicin

Listeria: Ampicillin and aminoglycoside, gentamicin, amikacin, netilmicin.

Gram-negative bacilli

Cefotaxime, ceftazidime, ceftriaxone or combination of ampicillin and aminoglycoside.

Pseudomonas

Combination of ceftazidime and an aminoglycoside, ticarcillin, meropenem or cefepime.

Duration of therapy

Average duration of treatment is 10–14 days except for staphylococcal and gram-negative infection where 3 weeks treatment is required.

Therapy is stopped when child becomes afebrile, CSF—sugar and protein normal, cell count less than $30/mm^3$.

Corticosteroids

Corticosteroids given with antibiotics— dexamethasone at a dose of 0.15 mg/kg/IV q 6 hr to 2–4 days given before or along with the first dose of antibiotic, it reduces hearing loss, hydrocephalus, behavioral disturbances.

This is especially useful in *Haemophilus influenzae* meningitis. No role of steroids in neonates and other meningitis.

Supportive Therapy

Increased intracranial pressure.

Osmotic diuretic—0.5 g/kg mannitol 20% solution intravenously every 4–6 hours to maximum 6 days.

Convulsions are treated as follows:

* Diazepam 0.3 mg/kg (maximum 5 mg) followed by phenytoin 15–20 mg/kg/24 hr intravenously in two divided doses and continued at a dose of 5 mg /kg/day PO or IV.
* Antiepileptic drugs can be stopped after 3 months.

Hypotension: Treated with vasopressors such as dopamine and dobutamine.

Subdural effusion or empyema managed by subdural paracentesis if signs of compression develop.

To detect it, head circumference should be measured daily and transillumination test done. Subdural effusion generally resolves spontaneously.

Hydrocephalus: Generally require ventriatrial, ventriculoperitoneal shunt is rarely needed.

Steroid has no significant effect on the course or outcome of bacterial meningitis.

Fluids: Better given intravenously to prevent risk of aspiration in orally. Requirement 1000 ml per m^2 per 24 hr per day. Diet rich in protein, calories, vitamins given by nasogastric tube.

Nursing care: Care of bladder, bowel and prevention of bedsores.

Prognosis

With proper treatment, mortality is reduced but worse in neonatal meningitis. Among survivors, half suffer from sequelae.

Complications and Sequelae

1. Cranial nerves involvement.
2. Hydrocephalus.
3. Mental retardation.
4. Language and hearing disabilities.

5. Hemi- or quadriparesis.

6. Subdural empyema.

Prevention

1. Meningococcal vaccine: Prevents *Neisseria meningitidis* infection.

2. HIB vaccine (pentavalent): Prevents *H. influenzae* infection.

TUBERCULOUS MENINGITIS

This is a complication of childhood tuberculosis. This occurs within a year of primary infection with tuberculosis, common in 1–4 years of age, rare before 6 months of age.

Pathogenesis

i. Infection is transmitted to meninges by hematogenous spread.

ii. Submeningeal tuberculoma on any part of CNS discharges the tubercular bacilli into subarachnoid space and disseminated through by way of CSF.

Picture of encephalitis is due to as follows: Inflammatory activity progress up to cortex of brain and also there is endarteritis of blood vessels embedded in inflammatory exudate, which may cause obstruction of blood supply to brain, resulting infarction of brain tissue.

Clinical Features

Clinical course of tuberculous meningitis is described in three stages.

1. **Stage 1: Prodromal stage** *(stage of invasion)*: At this stage symptoms are vague such as apathy, mood changes and decreasing school performances, increasing anorexia, vomiting, constipation, headache, child becomes irritable, restless and resents exposure to bright sunlight due to photophobia. Loss of weight and growth failure are other features.

2. **Stage 2** *[appearance of neurological sign and symptoms (stage of meningitis)]*: Irritability is increased, headache is common, neck rigidity, Kernig's and Brudzinski signs may be present. Cranial nerve palsies (III, IV/VI) are common:

- Ocular—pupillary abnormalities, diplopia and decreased visual activity.
- Facial palsy common, deafness may occur.
- Uncommon features include aphonia, slurred speech, disorientation, hemiplegia, ataxia, involuntary movements. Convulsions, hemiplegia, monoplegia may occur.

Due to increased intracranial tension—enlarging head circumference, tense anterior fontanelle and in elder child, papilledema are features.

Pyrexia may be intermittent or remittent.

3. **Stage 3** *[an alteration in the level of consciousness proceeding from stupor to coma (stage of coma)]*: Signs of diffuse cerebral dysfunction are found at the advanced stage of disease; stupor, coma, decerebrate and decorticate postures are common (Fig. 11.2).

Respiration becomes irregular. Pupils become fixed and dilated. Each stage lasts for about a week and clinical features overlap each other.

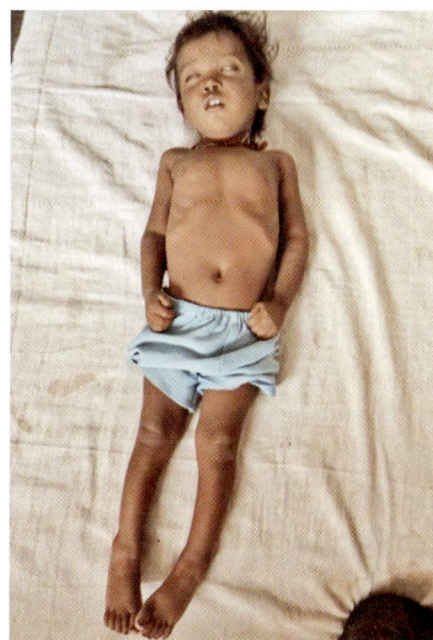

Fig. 11.2: Tuberculous meningitis.

Diagnosis

1. History of contact with case of tuberculosis give high index of suspicion.
2. Tuberculin test (or BCG test) positive, but negative does not rule out disease.
3. CSF examination:
   a. Clear, colorless fluid with increased pressure.
   b. On standing for 24 hours, surface layer forms, known as cobweb.
   c. Protein is normal or slightly elevated. 100–300 mg/dl in initial stage but exceeds 1000 mg/dl later on.
   d. Glucose reduced (but not much as in pyogenic miningitis).
   e. Chloride less
   f. Microscopic—cell count elevated, rarely more than 5000/cubic mm, mainly lymphocytes but may be polymorph also.
   g. Staining with Ziehl-Neelsen stain—30% cases show bacilli. Bacilli better seen in cobweb.
   h. Culture—best done after centrifugation.
4. *Blood:* Anemia and increased ESR hypochloremia, hyponatremia.
5. *Skiagram skull:* Normal or due to increased pressure 'spit sutures'.
6. *Skiagram chest:* Hilar adenopathy, infiltration, calcified tuberculoma, etc.
7. *CT scan:* Periventricular widening, Lucentis, edema, infarction and hydrocephalus. Serological tests

Bactec and **PCR** for tuberculosis are better sensitive and specific.

Test for HIV should be done for each suspected individual.

Differential Diagnosis

- **Purulent meningitis**
  1. Onset is acute and rapid
  2. CSF (Table 11.1)
- **Partially treated meningitis**
  1. Similar to TBM
  2. CSF picture
  3. PCR
- **Encephalitis**
  Onset acute with fever, seizures, disturbance of sensorium and diffuse and focal sign.
  CSF picture
  MRI
- **Typhoid encephalopathy**
  Toxemia high grade, drowsiness
  No meningeal sign
  CSF normal, widal positive
  Culture for *S. typhi*
- **Brain abscess**
  Irregular low grade fever
  Focal sign

Table 11.1: CSF profile in various types of meningitis

Type	WBC count/cu mm	Protein	Glucose	Gram stain, culture and other definitive test
Acute bacterial	100–50,000 polymorph	High	Low	Positive culture and Gram's stain
Partially treated bacterial	1000–10,000 mono	Normal to high	Low normal	Negative culture and usually negative Gram's stain
Viral	10–1,000 polymorphs early then mono + lympho HSV may show RBC	Normal to high	Normal	Enterovirus may be recovered after culture
Fungal	25–500 lympho	Normal to high	Low	Urine may be positive
Brain abscess	10–200 poly or mono	High	Normal	Negative culture

CSF normal

CT scan is diagnostic

- **Brain tumour**

  Onset slow

  History of headache, vomiting, disturbance of vision and localizing neurological sign.

  CT scan, MRI is diagnostic

- **Chronic subdural hematoma**

  History of trauma

  Headache, vomiting, localizing neurological sign.

  Sign of increased intracranial tension

  CSF—normal

  CT scan, ultrasound helpful

  Subdural tap—fluid with high protein concentration.

- **Amebic meningoencephalitis**

  Free living ameba is causative organism

  If no response to antibacterial antipyogenic

  CSF—motile ameba seen

  Culture confirms the diagnosis.

Treatment

1. *Antitubercular therapy:* Four antitubercular drugs are used for 2 months.

   - Isoniazid   15 mg/kg/day maximum 300 mg/day
   - Rifampicin   10 mg/kg/day maximum 600 mg/day
   - Ethambutol   15–20 mg/kg/day
   - Pyrazinamide 30 mg/kg/day PO

   Streptomycin may be used for 2–3 weeks. Its prolong use is not recommended due to ototoxicity.

   Intrathecal administration of streptomycin or rifampicin is not recommended.

   After 2 months two following drugs are continued to 10 months to complete one year of therapy

   - Isoniazid
   - Rifamipicin

2. **Corticosteroids:** Parenteral dexamethasone (0.15 mg/kg/dose q 6 hr) for early phase of treatment. Afterward oral prednisolone 2–4 mg/kg/day may be continued for 6 weeks. It is gradually tapered over 2 weeks.

   Steroids reduce cerebral edema, risk of development of arachnoiditis, fibrosis and spinal block.

3. Symptomatic therapy
   - Raised intracranial tension is treated by mannitol, lumbar puncture.
   - Seizures are controlled by anticonvulsants.
   - Dyselectrolytemia corrected.
   - Observe papilledema by regular fundus examination.
   - Increasing head circumference suggests development of hydrocephalus, which may require ventriculocaval shunt in advanced cases.

Sequelae: Developmental retardation, hydrocephalus, optic atrophy, deafness, cranial nerve palsies, paralysis, convulsions, coma and pituitary disturbances.

ENCEPHALITIS AND ENCEPHALOPATHY

Encephalitis is inflammation of brain tissue. Encephalopathy, when neurological manifestations suggesting encephalitis occur but inflammation of the brain has not occurred. This is due to circulating toxins or abnormal metabolic function of neurons (Fig. 11.3).

Etiology

1. *Infections*

   Viral—mumps, measles, rubella, enterovirus, herpes, vaccinia, variola, parvovirus, influenza A and B, arthropod-borne (Japanese B, Russian spring), rabies, lymphocytic choriomeningitis, herpes.

   Non-viral
   - Rickettsial
   - Mycoplasma
   - Bacterial tuberculosis, typhoid encephalopathy

2. Parainfectious (non-infectious)
   - *Allergic:* Post-exanthematous or postvaccinal encephalopathies

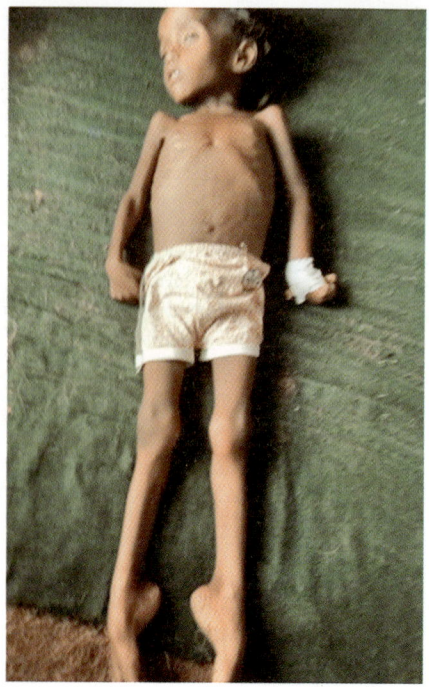

Fig. 11.3: Encephalitis.

- *Physical:* Heat stroke
- *Electrolyte imbalance:* Hyper- or hypo-natremia, acidosis, alkalosis
- Toxic, heavy metals, insecticide
- Malignancy
- Metabolic, diabetic acidosis, hypoglycemia, hyperbilirubinemia, uremia.
3. Human slow virus disease, e.g. SSPE, measles, rubella.
4. Unknown complex group: Constitute about 2/3rds of the cases. Majority are probably enterovirus or arbovirus.

Clinical Features

There is wide range of severity of clinical features but clinical picture of viral encephalitis is similar irrespective of causative organism.

There may be acute or gradual onset with fever of high grade; sensorium varies from lethargy to deep coma. Headache, abdominal distress, nausea and vomiting are common initial symptoms. Irregular involuntary move-ments, convulsions or signs of meningeal irritation appear late. Focal signs may be associated with it. Loss of bladder and bowel control may occur.

Diagnosis

1. Diagnosis mainly depends on history and clinical features and exclusion of other diseases.
2. *Lumbar puncture:* Pressure raised but biochemistry normal. Protein and sugar normal or slightly raised in CSF.
3. Identification of virus in spinal fluid, blood, faeces, throat swab.
   Diagnosis of possible cause
   For example, serum electrolyte, blood sugar, urea, blood ammonia, metabolic, screening, serum lactate, urinary ketones, urinary analysis, blood for malaria parasite, widal, etc.
4. CT scan, MRI, ECG

Management

No **specific treatment** available for viral origin.

Symptomatic treatment
   i. Hyperpyrexia is managed by cold sponging, paracetamol.
   ii. Intravenous fluid by drip, fluid is also given by feeding tube.
   iii. Antibiotics for superadded bacterial infection.
   iv. Anticonvulsants for convulsions.
   v. Reduction of intracranial pressure by lumbar puncture and mannitol.
   vi. Airway maintenance by suction or tracheostomy.

Shock: Managed by fluids and dopamine or dobutamine to maintain blood pressure.

Corticosteroids: Use of steroids is controversial but use is recommended in disseminated encephalomyelitis and autoimmune encephalitis.

In herpes simplex encephalitis: Drug of choice acyclovir (20 mg/kg/dose every 8 hourly).

CEREBRAL PALSY (LITTLE'S DISEASE)

Definition

Cerebral palsy is a non-progressive neuro-muscular disorder of cerebral origin. This is most common cause of crippling in children. This is a result of brain damage of the fetus, during birth, in immediate postnatal period. Mental retardation is associated in 25% of cases.

Etiology

This may be result of prenatal, natal or postnatal causes.

- *Prenatal:* Cerebral anoxia, maternal toxemia, maternal infections (e.g. rubella), congenital malformation of brain, cerebrovascular occlusion.
- *Natal:* Anoxia (most important), birth trauma, asphyxia, cerebral hemorrhage, prematurity.
- *Postnatal:* Kernicterus, trauma, infections (meningitis and encephalitis), vascular (hemorrhagic thrombosis and embolism).

Clinilcal Features

Classification based on motor deficit:

1. **Spastic** (most common)
2. **Atonic**
3. **Athetoid**
4. **Ataxic**
5. **Chorioathetoid or mixed.**

Spastic Cerebral Palsy

Spastic variety is the most frequent variety, characterized by spasticity of both upper as well as lower limbs. Legs are severely affected than arms or picture of hemiplegia, mono-plegia or paraplegia seen.

In severe cases, arching of back and scissoring of lower limbs at rest is seen. Tendon reflexes are brisk with clonus. Plantar may be extensor. Rigidity and spasticity leads to abnormal posture of limbs and contractures.

Heel cord contractures, limitation in abduction and external rotation of the hips and limitation in extension and supination of forearms are common.

Pseudobulbar palsy leads to swallowing difficulty and drooling of saliva.

Sudden lifting of child may produce visible adductor spasm and even crossing of the legs (scissoring), a characteristic feature (Fig. 11.4).

In infancy delayed milestones and persistence of Moro, grasp, tonic neck and other primitive reflexes after the age of 3 months are indications of cerebral palsy.

a. *Spastic diplegia:* Weakness involves lower extremities more than upper extremities or face.

Clinical examination shows history of early rolling over, increased muscle tone (spasticity) and 'scissoring' (extension and crossing of lower extremities with standing or vertical suspension).

It is a sign of spasticity.

b. *Spastic hemiplegia:* Unilateral spastic motor weakness. Clinical examination shows

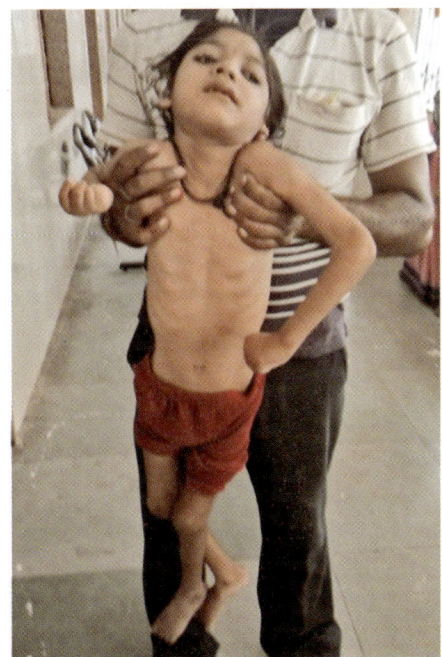

Fig. 11.4: Spastic cerebral palsy.

upper extremities involvement is typically greater than lower extremities. Early hand preferences and attempts at grasping on the same side and fisting or absent pincer on one side.

c. *Spastic quadriplegia:* Involvement of head, neck and all four limbs.

Clinical manifestations include seizures, scoliosis, weakness of face and pharyngeal muscles, dysphagia, failure to thrive.

It is associated with speech problems and sensory impairments.

Extrapyramidal (Nonspecific) Cerebral Palsy

Involvement of extrapyramidal motor system, resulting in **athetoid** movements. Main problems are related in modulating control of face, neck, trunk, and limbs. Arms are usually more affected than legs. Oral motor involvement may be more prominent.

On examination, marked hypotonia of neck and trunk, limiting child's ability to explore the environment.

Intermittent posturing or movement of head, neck and limbs. Feeding, speech and drooling problems because motor function is impaired.

Hypotonic (Atonic) Cerebral Palsy

Hypotonic cerebral palsy clinically manifests on atonic or hypotonic. Child tendon reflexes are normal or brisk and Babinski sign is positive, they are often mentally retarded.

Mixed type: These patients have clinical features of diffuse neurological involvement of mixed type.

Evaluation

- Eyes: Strabismus, paralysis of gaze, cataract, retrolental fibroplasia, refractive error.
- Mental retardation: Borderline.
- Ears: Partial or complete loss of hearing.
- Speech: Aphasia, dysarthria, dyslalia.

- Sensory defects: Astereognosis and spatial disorientation
- Seizures: Focal or generalized seizures
- Miscellaneous: Problems of social or emotional adjustment.

History and clinical examination, CT scan and MRI delineate the extent of cerebral damage.

Management

Symptomatic

1. Seizures—anticonvulsants
2. Behavioral disorder—tranquillizers
3. Muscle relaxant
4. Spasticiy—baclofen, tizanidine
5. Athetosis and spasticity—diazepam
6. Muscle relaxants—dantrolene sodium
7. Contracture—nerve block with phenol injection
8. Surgical procedures for spasticity and contractures.

Occupational Therapy

Begin with simple movements such as self feeding and dressing and progress delicately for delicate work.

Education: Speech, vision, learning is managed by proper education.

Physiotherapy to improve mobility.

Orthopedic Support

- Surgery for tendon, muscle and bone required.
- Splints may be required for tendo Achillis.

Social: Family and child should be given social and emotional support.

Rehabilitation: In severe case: Child should be given institutional care. Training given so the child adjust in society.

Prevention: Antenatal, natal, and perinatal care is required to prevent CP.

MENTAL RETARDATION
(INTELLECTUAL IMPAIRMENT)

Definition

Infants and children with subaverage general intelligence, diminished learning capacity and inadequate social adjustment are grouped under this term.

Classification

	IQ	Intellectual impairment
Borderline	70–79	20%
Mild	50–69	59%
Moderate	35–49	75%
Severe	20–34	90%
Profound	IQ below 20	100%

Etiology (Causes)

I. *Organic prenatal*
 1. **Metabolic:** Aminoacidurias, galactosemia, mucopolysaccharidosis, inherited degenerative disorders of CNS.
 2. **Chromosomal:** Down syndrome, Turner's syndrome, Klinefelter's syndrome.
 3. **Developmental deficit:** Microcephaly, craniostenosis, cretinism, porencephaly, hydrocephalus.
 4. **Maternal infections:** Rubella, toxoplasmosis, cytomegalic inclusion disease, syphilis, chickenpox, herpes.
 Maternal disease: Toxemia of pregnancy, antepartum hemorrhage, radiation during pregnancy.
 Perinatal: Birth trauma, cerebral anoxia, cerebral hemorrhage, prematurity, small for date infant.
 Postnatal: Infections of CNS, head injury, encephalopathy (whooping cough, toxic), kernicterus, cerebrovascular episode (thrombosis of cerebral vessels), hypoglycemia, hypoxia.

II. *Nonorganic:* Sociocultural factors
 Emotional disturbances
III. *Progressive encephalopathies:* Examples, metabolic effects of infections (e.g. kuru, subacute sclerosing panencephalitis).

Paraplegia

Types

1. Spastic or upper motor neuron lesion.
2. Flaccid or lower motor neuron lesion.

Spastic paraplegia causes

A. Intracranial
 i. Cerebral palsy
 ii. Hydrocephalus
 iii. Thrombosis of superior sagittal sinus
 iv. Tumors of meninges
B. In the spinal cord
 i. Cerebral palsy
 ii. Transverse myelitis
 iii. Spinal cord compression
  a. Extradural
   • Tuberculosis of spine
   • Epidural abscess
   • Achondroplasia
   • Secondary metastatic deposits from neuroblastoma, leukemia, lymphoma
  b. Intradural—neurofibroma, dermoid cyst
  c. Extramedullary—glioma, ependymoma, hematohydromyelia
C. Toxin—lathyrism
D. Trauma—fracture, dislocation.

Common causes: Transverse myelitis, cerebral palsy, spinal cord compression (tuberculosis of spine), trauma.

Flaccid Paraplegia

Causes

1. Poliomyelitis
2. Peripheral neuritis
3. Acute infective polyneuritis (Guillain-Barré syndrome)

4. Spinal shock—during initial stage of shock after injury, tumor, myelopathy.
5. Riley-Day syndrome (familial dysauto-nomia) characterized by areflexia, in diffe-rence to pain, absence of sweating and tears, recurrent pneumonia.
6. Adie's syndrome—areflexia, large pupils which react to accommodation but not to light.
7. Myopathies.

Hemiplegia

Acute hemiplegia of childhood—causes are:
1. Idiopathic
2. *Lesions in carotid artery:* Thrombosis: Following trauma, throat and ear infec-tions.
3. *Cerebrovascular disease:* Blood diseases—sickle cell disease, polycythemia, vascu-litis leading to thrombosis of venous sinuses and superficial veins of cerebral cortex.
4. *Congenital cyanotic heart disease:* Due to thrombosis.
5. *Emboli in the brain*, e.g. rheumatic heart disease, bacterial endocarditis.
6. *Intracranial bleeding:* Following leukemia, subdural hemorrhage.
7. Migraine.
8. Residual defect after encephalitis or meningitis.
9. Intracranial space occupying lesion.
10. Todd's paralysis.

DOWN SYNDROME (21 TRISOMY)

This is most frequent human chromosomal disorder. Presence of an extra chromosome in pair No. 21 is characteristic feature. So, such patient has 47 chromosomes, instead of normal 46, or one chromosome may be long (translocation) or mixed (mosaic) form seen.

Down syndrome is most common cause of mental retardation in children.

Incidence

1 in 600

Etiology

Etiology is not known but higher incidence is seen in advanced maternal age.

Clinical Features

Face: Facial appearance resembles Mongolian races like Chinese, Tibetan, Japanese, etc. That is why its name is Mongolism. This name is objected by these races, because this condition is associated with severe mental retardation.

This appearance is due to maldevelopment of basilar skull bones. Characteristic features are as follows (Fig. 11.5):
a. Eyes having upward slant, epicanthal folds confined to the inner angle. Eyes appear small.
b. Tongue protruded from small buccal cavity and may be furrowed (scrotal tongue) (Fig. 11.6).
c. Nose is flat. Sunken nasal bridge.
d. Depressed nasal bridge and epicanthal folds give impression that distance between the eyes increased (pseudohypertelorism).

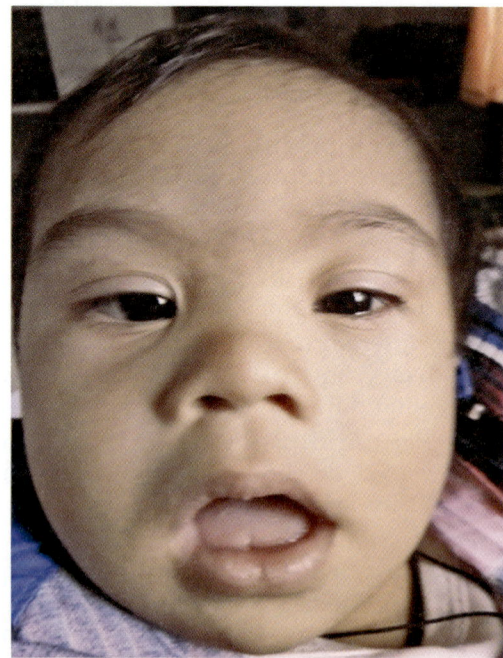
Fig. 11.5: Down syndrome.

e. Ears are low set, deformed, ear lobes may be small or absent.

f. High arched palate and malocclusion of teeth (teeth small).

g. Cataract and brushfield's spots in iris may be present.

General Features

1. *Mental retardation:* Mental retardation is most constant characteristic of the disease. All the developmental milestones are delayed, both physical and mental. Unlike other mentally defective children, Mongols are affectionate, friendly, fond of music, that is why described as 'Cheerful Idiot' (Table 11.2).

2. *Hypotonia* is a prominent feature. Hypermotility of joints enables them to place the limbs in abnormal positions (Fig. 11.7).

3. *Craniotabes:* Flat occiput, brachycephalic skull, head smaller than average.

4. *Neck is short and broad*, seems resting on lower hairline.

5. *Hands and feet:* Simian crease at palm (Fig. 11.8A and B), broad hands, hypoplasia of middle phalanx of 5th finger (Fig. 11.9), gap between 1st and 2nd toes at feet, (Fig. 11.10) deep crease starting between the sole.

6. *Thorax:* Congenital heart disease mainly septal defects are associated with it.

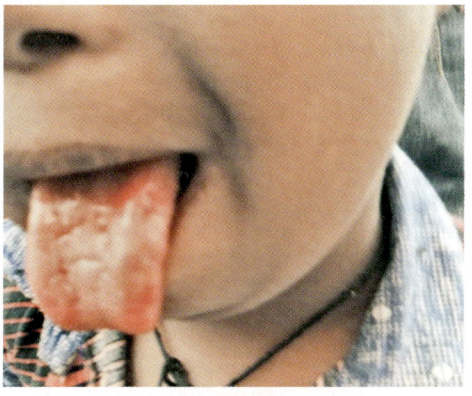

Fig. 11.6: Scrotal tongue.

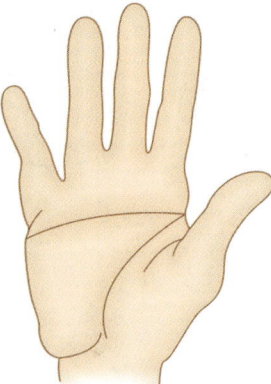

Fig. 11.8A: Simian crease of Down's syndrome.

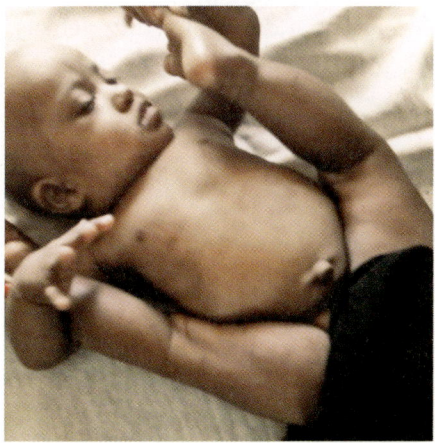

Fig. 11.7: Down syndrome showing hypotonia.

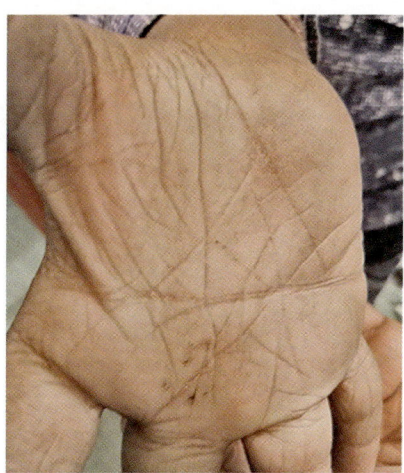

Fig. 11.8B: Simian crease.

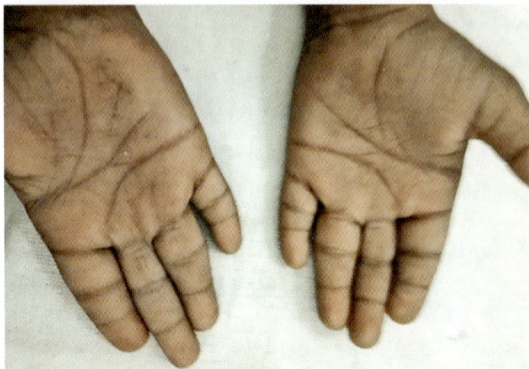

Fig. 11.9: Hypoplasia of middle phalanx of little fingers.

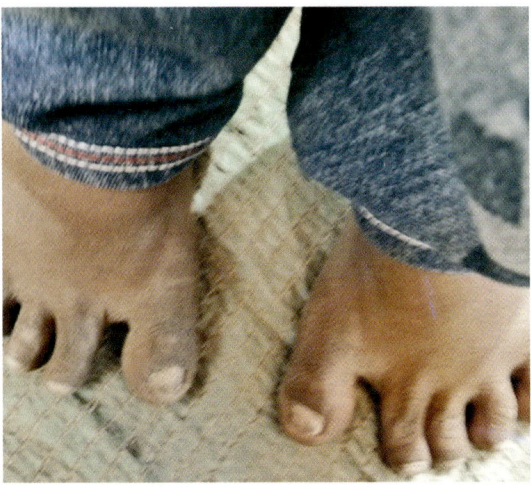

Fig. 11.10: Wide gap between toe and finger.

7. *Abdomen and pelvis:* Decreased acetabular and iliac angles. Small penis, cryptorchidism.
8. Mongols are most susceptible to recurrent respiratory tract infections.
9. Hirschsprung's disease occurs more often in Mongols.

Diagnosis

Diagnosis depends on:
   i. Clinical features
   ii. Chromosomal studies (Figs 11.11 and 11.12)
   iii. *Skiagram skull:* Hypoplasia of skull bones and nasal bones.
   iv. *Skiagram hands:* Dysplasia and hypoplasia of phalanges, accessory epiphysis at the base of metacarpals.
   v. *Skiagram chest:* 11 ribs, 2–3 ossification centres at manubrium.
   vi. Coxa valga
   vii. *X-ray pelvis:* Ilia are broad and flared, low iliac index.
   viii. *Dermatographic findings:* Characteristic.

Associated Abnormalities

- Congenital heart disease (about 40% children)
- Gastrointestinal malformation, e.g. duodenal disease, annular pancreas and Hirschsprung disease.
- Ophthalmic problems—cataract, nystagmus, squint and visual acuity defects.

Table 11.2: Differences between Down syndrome and cretinism

Down syndrome	Cretinism
1. Cheerful, active	1. Repulsive, lethargic
2. Small-for-date	2. Large-for-date
3. Epicanthal folds present	3. Absent
4. Upward stant of eye present	4. Absent
5. Skin fine tender	5. Rough skin, shallow complexion
6. Flat occiput	6. Absent
7. Simian crease	7. Absent
8. Chromosomal defect	8. Absent
9. No treatment	9. Replacement therapy results are good

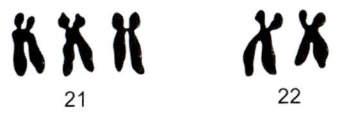

Fig. 11.11: Chromosomes in Down syndrome (21 trisomy).

21   22

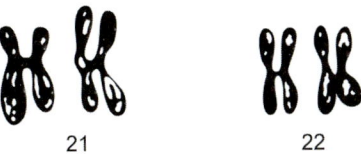

Fig. 11.12: Chromosomes in Down syndrome (translocation).

21   22

- Hearing defects—40–60%
- Hypothyroidism.
- Atlanto-occipital subluxation
- Physical growth—linear growth retardation.
- Malignancies—more prone is lymphoproliferative disorders.

Prenatal Diagnosis

Prenatal diagnosis of Down syndrome is done to detect 21 trisomy (karyotyping). It is done by:

a. *Noninvasive prenatal screening (NIPS):* In this method 21 trisomy is detected in mother's blood. It is sensitive and correct method done in 10 to 24 weeks of pregnancy.

b. *Invasive testing:* In this method 21 trisomy is detected in cells of amniotic fluid or chorionic villi. Amniocentesis is done at 16 to 18 weeks of pregnancy, about 20 ml of fluid is aspirated and cells are detected for 21 trisomy. It is a safe and simple method.

c. Chorionic villi biopsy is done at 10–12 weeks of pregnancy under supervision of sonography. Cells are detected for 21 trisomy. It should be done by skilled person.

If antenatal diagnosis of Down syndrome is confirmed, decision of abortion should be left on parent.

Management

No specific therapy. Training and rehabilitation improve living standard for some degree. Genetic counseling of parents—who have mongol child and have risk of another also.

CONVULSIVE DISORDERS IN CHILDREN

Seizures (Convulsions)

Definition

- Seizures are transient, involuntary alternation of consciousness, behavior, motor activity, sensation, or autonomic function caused by abnormal electrical discharges from neurons.
- Epilepsy is occurrence of two or more spontaneous seizures (fits) without an obvious precipitating cause.
- Status epilepticus is a seizure that lasts >30 minutes during which patient does not regain consciousness.

Epidemiology: About 5% children suffers from convulsions during first 5 years of age.

Etiology

1. The seizures are caused by imbalances between excitatory and inhibitory input within the brain or abnormality in membrane of neurons.
2. 60–70% of cases, the cause is unknown only in some children cause is known.

Causes of Convulsions (Depending on Age of Onset)

Neonatal Convulsions

First day

i. Birth asphyxia
ii. Intraventricular hemorrhage
iii. First day hypocalcemia
iv. Inborn errors of metabolism
v. Narcotic withdrawal syndrome (babies born to addicted mother to narcotic get convulsions after delivery)

vi. Pyridoxine deficiency

vii. Accidental injection of local anesthetic in fetal scalp (e.g. during paracervical block during delivery).

Second day

Cerebral contusion, intracranial hemorrhage.

Third day

Hypoglycemia.

Fourth to seventh days

i. Tetany

ii. Kernicterus

iii. Developmental malformation

iv. Meningitis

Spasm in tetanus is mistaken for convulsions. But presence of trismus, purely tonic nature of spasm, with no loss of consciousness differentiate to convulsion.

One month to 3 years

1. Febrile convulsions
2. Epilepsy
3. *Infections of CNS:* Meningitis, encephalitis, brain abscess.
4. *Post-infectious or post-vaccinal encephalopathy.*
   a. Post-measles encephalopathy
   b. Post-chickenpox encephalopathy
   c. Subacute sclerosing panencephalitis
   d. Following pertussis vaccination
   e. Following smallpox vaccination.
5. *Metabolic causes*
   a. Hypoglycemia
   b. Hypocalcemia and hypomagnesemia
   c. Renal failure
   d. Water intoxication
   e. Inborn error of metabolism
   f. Dehydration and electrolyte imbalance
6. Space occupying lesion in brain, cerebral neoplasm, brain abscess, tuberculoma, cysticercosis.
7. Cerebrovascular disorders
   Arteriovenous malformations, cortical vein thrombosis, cerebral artery thrombosis or embolism, vasculitis.
8. *Cerebral trauma:* Subdural hematoma, cerebral contusions or hemorrhage.
9. *Nutritional disorders:* Pyridoxine deficiency.
10. Poisoning
    a. Lead encephalopathy.
    b. Drug intoxication (phenothiazine, xanthine, amphetamine).
11. *Atrophic brain lesion:* Post-anoxic, post-traumatic, post-infectious.
12. Degenerative brain disease.
13. Neurocutaneous syndrome.

Classification

1. Febrile
   • Simple
   • Complex
2. Afebrile
   a. Partial (one hemisphere is involved)
      • Simple—consciousness is not impaired.
      • Complex—consciousness is impaired.
   b. Generalized (both hemispheres involved)
      • Tonic clonic
      • Tonic
      • Clonic
      • Myoclonic
      • Absence
      • Atonic

Diagnosis and Investigation of Convulsive Disorders

Clinical diagnosis of convulsive disorders can be made by history, physical examination and investigations.

Case History

A complete history, particularly stressing following points, should be obtained.

a. **Antenatal**
   i. Toxemia of pregnancy.
   ii. Infection (toxoplasmosis) of mother may cause convulsion in newborn.

b. **Natal**

i. Birth injuries or trauma such as intracranial hemorrhage, cerebral contusion, laceration of brain, focal or generalized edema may cause convulsions.

ii. History of difficult labor, prolonged delivery and forceps or vacuum application.

c. **Immediate postnatal:** Cyanosis, jaundice of newborn (kernicterus)

d. **Recurrent or non-recurrent:** Whether convulsions are:

i. Acute or non-recurrent—febrile convulsion, intracranial infection, intracranial hemorrhage, toxicity of drugs, tetanus, lead encephalopathy, anoxic, metabolic causes.

ii. Chronic or recurrent

• Epilepsy (idiopathic)

• Organic due to focal or diffuse injuries to the brain such as post-traumatic, post-hemorrhagic, post-anoxic, post-infectious, post-toxic, degenerative disorders, congenital anomalous, post-hypoglycemic, parasitic.

e. History of umbilical sepsis should be taken, because it may cause generalized septicemia.

f. Cutting of cord with unclean, old, unsterilized blade or scissors, etc. may cause tetanus neonatorum.

g. History of infectious disease such as measles, mumps, chickenpox, whooping cough taken. They may cause encephalopathy.

h. History of vaccination, e.g. DPT (pertussis), anti-rabies vaccine may lead to post-vaccinal encephalopathy.

i. Pica, e.g. lead encephalopathy.

j. Worms infestations, e.g. ascariasis encephalopathy.

k. Family history in epilepsy, febrile convulsion, metabolic disorders are often found.

l. History of drugs and poisons taken—penicillin, atropine, arsenic, phenothiazines, caffline, camphor, carbon monoxide, strychnine, salicylate poisoning, analeptics (e.g. coramine).

m. Infections (fever)—intracranial or extracranial cause.

n. Age at newborn period causes are different. See day of onset of convulsions, especially in newborn.

Physical Examination

i. *Types of convulsions:* Generalized tonic or clonic (grand mal) or focal, transient loss of consciousness (petit mal) salaam type, or myoclonic seizures.

ii. *Head circumference:* Microcephaly, hydrocephalus.

iii. *Bulging of fontanelle:* In meningitis, subdural hematoma.

iv. *Depressed fontanelle:* In dehydration encephalopathy.

v. *Fever:* Look for cause of fever.

vi. *Other features* of disease causing convulsions.

CNS

i. *Loss of consciousness:* Absent in tetanus, tetany, strychnine poisoning.

ii. *Coma:* Acute infantile hemiplegia, intracranial hemorrhage, bleeding diathesis, intracranial infections and brain tumor.

iii. *Postconvulsive coma:* Epilepsy, hypoglycemia, poisoning.

iv. *Higher function:* Look for mental retardation (microcephaly, Sturge-Weber's syndrome, tuberous sclerosis, metabolic disorders).

v. *Cranial nerves involvement:* Head injury, brain tumor pressing nerve, hydrocephalus, meningitis, encephalitis. Isolated sixth nerve palsy is known as false localizing sign, because its paralysis can occur in any condition leading to increased intracranial tension.

vi. Hemiparesis: For example, meningitis, encephalitis.

vii. Hypotonia: Cerebellar degenerative disorders.

viii. Hypertonia: Rest in all conditions.

ix. Signs of meningeal irritation are suggestive of meningitis.

CVS: Cyanotic heart disease.

Respiratory system: Tuberculosis.

GIT: Hepatosplenomegaly seen in malaria, metabolic disorders.

Fundus: Changes in retina and disc in uremia, cerebral tumor and tuberous sclerosis.

Investigations

  i. Lumbar puncture and CSF examination for diagnosis of meningitis, encephalitis.
 ii. Urine examination to exclude renal disorders.
iii. Blood examination: Serum calcium, serum magnesium, blood glucose, blood urea. Total and differential WBCs count for diagnosis of infection.
 iv. Plain X-ray skull: May suggest signs of increased intracranial tension, abnormality of bony structure, fracture and abnormal calcification.
  v. Pneumoencephalography: To detect any abnormality in basal cistern, space occupying lesion.
 vi. Ventriculography
vii. EEG: Any abnormality to diagnose cause.
viii. CAT scan: For diagnosis of tumor or cerebrovascular malformation.
 ix. Investigations to detect the cause.

FEBRILE CONVULSIONS

Definition

Febrile convulsions are generalized tonic, clonic seizures due to fever seen in childhood having following diagnostic criteria.

Diagnostic Criteria

  i. Occurrence in age of 6 months to 5 years.
 ii. Fever at the time of the attack, usually above 38°C.
iii. Convulsions last for brief duration (always less than 15 minutes).
 iv. Absence of CNS infection.
  v. Absence of neurological abnormality in the interictal period.

Pathophysiology and Etiology

a. Fever from any cause increases metabolic rate of cerebral neurons, which lower seizure threshold.
b. Genetic susceptibility is seen. 60–70% cases have history in parents.
c. Incidence: About 5% of children suffers from this. 50% of these, having more that one attack. But more than 5–6 attacks are rare. Incidence is more in boys than girls.

Clinical Features

Child suffers from febrile illness such as otitis media, roseola, URI, etc. During the period of rapid rise of fever convulsions occur.

Simple seizures are characteristically generalized (never focal), tonic and clonic or ataxic, they do not last more than 15 minutes.

Febrile convulsions generally occur at the onset of the illness, when temperature rises rapidly. The rate of the rise of temperature is important, not the degree of temperature achieved.

Rarely there is marked disturbance of respiration. Stupor after convulsions is for brief period and child becomes normal after short period.

CNS causes of convulsions should be excluded for the diagnosis of febrile convulsions.

Investigations

1. CSF: Normal picture
2. Electroencephalography: Normal.

Another type (atypical) of febrile convulsions is seen in 20% of all cases. Fever is not high. Seizures are focal and last >20 minutes show persistent EEG changes up to 2 weeks. They are basically predisposed to idiopathic epilepsy.

Treatment

1. Reduction of body temperature by cold sponging, paracetamol or by other antipyretics such as acetaminophen. Salicylates are not given in influenza due to risk of Rey's syndrome.

2. Put the child to side to prevent aspiration; tight clothing should be lessened. Put mouth gag or some object to prevent tongue injury during convulsions.
3. Intravenous:
   a. Diazepam 0.1 to 0.2 mg/kg is given. It may be given per rectal solution used for intravenous injection. Effective blood level reaches in about 10 minutes or less in a dose 0.5 mg per kg. Parents can be taught the procedure and advised to do at home, if there is recurrence on an emergency.
   b. Phenobarbitone may also be given as anticonvulsant to control convulsions.
   c. Injection of midazolam is given for control of convulsions.
4. Treatment of cause of febrile illness.
5. Subsequent use of anticonvulsant is controversial
   a. Phenobarbitone is given in a dose of 3 mg/kg/day. It decreases the number of subsequent febrile convulsions but does not eliminate. According to some authority, it is not advocated for single episode but given if there is recurrence and if convulsions are triggered only in moderate rise of temperature or 2nd type (atypical) convulsions.
   b. Acetazolamide and sodium valproate are other drugs used for continuous therapy.
   c. The use of intermittent anticonvulsants given during each episode of fever has no role because seizures generally occur during rapid rise of temperature.

Prophylaxis

1. Intermittent
2. Continuous

1. **Intermittent:** Intermittent prophylaxis is indicated if
   a. 3 or more attacks of febrile seizures in 6 months.
   b. 6 or more attacks of seizures in 1 year.

c. Febrile seizures lasting >15 minutes.
   d. Require drugs to control seizures.
   Oral clobazam (0.75–1 mg/kg/day): It is given for 3 days during fever.
2. **Continuous prophylaxis:** Indicated in failure of intermittent therapy, recurrent atypical seizures and when parents are unable to recognize fever early and promptly.
   Antiepileptic drugs: Sodium valproate (10–20 mg/kg/day) and phenobarbitone (3–5 mg/kg/day) are effective drugs. Carbamazepine and phenytoin are ineffective drugs to be used for prophylaxis. Duration of therapy is about 1–2 years or until 5 years of age.

Prognosis

- Recurrence of febrile convulsions in about 30–50%.
- Risk of developing epilepsy is higher in complex (atypical febrile convulsions).

Risk of Recurrence

The overall recurrence rate varies between 25 and 30%. The risk is greater in the younger child, especially in females. A positive family history of febrile convulsions also increases the risk of recurrence.

Risk of Subsequent Epilepsy

Risk of epilepsy is about 3% with one risk factor (abnormal neurological status prior to first seizure, family history of epilepsy, or a complex seizure) and 13% with two or more risk factors. Hence, presence of neurological abnormality greatly increases the risk of subsequent epilepsy.

EPILEPSY

Definition

This is a condition of recurrent episodes, primarily of cerebral origin in which there is disturbance of movement, sensation, behavior or consciousness.

IDIOPATHIC EPILEPSY

Definition

This is a group of conditions in which recurrent seizures occur without definable cause, diagnosis is made after exclusion of known causes of seizures.

Pathophysiology

Seizures reflect abnormal electrical activity in cerebral neurons. A balance between inhibiting and exciting influences on the activity of nerve cells is probably disturbed. Gamma aminobutyric acid (GABA), a neurotransmitter for inhibitory influences is supposed to be implicated. But it is not applicable for all cases of seizures.

Incidence: 2–6 per 1000.

Clinical Features

Classification of epilepsy

1. *Generalized seizures*
   a. Tonic clonic: Grand mal
   b. Tonic
   c. Clonic
   d. Absence
   e. Atonic
   f. Myoclonus
   g. Akinetic seizures
2. *Partial seizures*
   a. *Simple partial*
      i. Focal motor seizures, jacksonian seizures
      ii. Sensory seizures
      iii. Abdominal epilepsy
   b. *Complex partial seizures:* Psychomotor or temporal lobe seizures.

Seizures in general classified as generalized, partial/focal/local, and unclassifiable.

Generalised seizures may be primary generalized if there is no focal or partial onset. While they may be secondary generalized it associated with focal or partial onset.

Partial (focal) seizures may be simple when sensorium is absolutely normal or complex when sensorium is altered. Simple or complex partial seizures may be secondary generalized.

Partial seizure—partial seizures account for 60% of seizures in childhood.

Causes

- Inflammatory granuloma
- Atrophic lesion
- Vascular insults
- Birth asphyxia
- Head trauma
- Neoplasm

Classification

1. Simple partial
2. Complex partial

1. Simple Partial

Seizures without loss of consciousness. There is motor, sensory, autonomic or mixed symptoms.

Symptoms: Visual, olfactory, auditory or taste, hallucination.

When simple seizures spreads unilatetrally as per motor cortex. It is termed jacksonian march.

2. Complex Partial

Symptoms are variable. Brief visceral olfactory or visual aura is followed by peculiar posture, tonic jerks of face and limbs or one-sided dystonia.

It manifests as lip smacking chewing or complex automatism, vasomotor changes are often present.

Symptoms: Seizures originating from temporal lobe (psychomotor epilepsy).

Benign childhood epilepsy: It is self-limiting seizure occurs in sleep and is partial, generally occurs at sleep. There is no neurological or intellectual defect. Children 2–13 years are effected.

TONIC AND CLONIC SEIZURES
(GRAND MAL EPILEPSY)

Grand mal epilepsy may have onset in any age, from infancy to early adult life. Frequency of attacks varies from several per week to less than one per year.

Factors which trigger the attacks, may be fever in some cases, while in others, non-specific factors such as reading or to exposure to specific sound pattern. Before the period of menses in girls, fatigue, emotional upheaval are other non-specific factors implicated as precipitating factors. But in general it is not always to identify such factors.

Characteristically grand mal has four phases:

a. Aura
b. Tonic phase
c. Clonic phase
d. Postictal phase

a. **The aura:** Aura occurs before convulsions. It may be psychological, e.g. feeling of unreality or sensory, e.g. numbness or tingling, visceral, motor or autonomic. Aura is not properly described by each case.

b. **Tonic phase:** During this phase, skeletal muscles go into sustained spasm. Spasm of muscle fixes limbs. Head and eyes turn to one side. Child falls to ground or conciousness is lost. Conjugate deviation of eyes and head to one side occurs, the pupils dilate. Tongue may be bitten. Respiration temporarily ceases and child becomes cyanosed. There may be frothing from mouth. Urine and stool are passed involuntarily.

c. **Clonic phase:** It consists of series of sharp jerks due to rhythmic alternating contractions of muscles. It persists for few minutes to few hours.

d. **Postictal phase:** In this phase, after the fits, child goes into sleep for 2–3 hours. Plantar response becomes temporarily extensor. After awakening, headache and temporary confusion is common. Rarely, transient hemiplegia (Todd's palsy) or aphasia may occur. Sequellae include intellectul impairment, behavioral disorders, motor deficit, ataxia and spasticity.

MYOCLONIC
(MINOR MOTOR EPILEPSY)

This consists of sudden, brief shock like involuntary jerks (contractions) of a single muscle group. They often involve flexor muscles bilaterally, resulting massive flexon of neck, trunk and legs. In older children, myoclonic seizures often result in fall. Mental retardation is associated in majority of cases.

ATONIC SEIZURES
(AKINETIC)

Atonic seizures consist of sudden loss of postural tone and consciousness. During this period there may be sudden drop of head; or fall may be only feature.

PSYCHOMOTOR

This consists of about 5% of all epileptics. Brief visceral symptoms like nausea, vomiting, epigastric sensations, etc. are followed by short periods of increased muscular tonicity. Inappropriate purposeful movements such as lip smacking, chewing, swallowing occur during the period of impaired consciousness or amnesia.

JACKSONIAN

Seizures starting from one part and spreading to other parts in fixed pattern until an entire body is involved (jacksonian march). The patient remains alert unless seizures activity spreads to other cerebral hemisphere.

STATUS EPILEPTICUS

This is a condition in which repeated tonic and clonic seizures occur without intervening recovery of consciousness. This is a medical emergency and mortility is high and also results permanent anoxic brain damage as sequelae.

Approach to a Child with Convulsions

1. History and accurate observation and description about symptoms and convulsions are great importance in diagnosis than physical and neurological examination and laboratory tests.
2. Family history, perinatal history and developmental history should be taken in each case.
3. Search is done for any detectable cause of convulsions.
4. Neurological examination is normal in children with idiopathic epilepsy except in few exceptions. Neurological signs such as positive Babinski sign, enhanced tendon reflexes are for short period after the seizures.
5. EEG: It may confirm type of abnormality and may detect locality, extent of affection. But limitation is that EEG may be falsely normal in confirmed epilepsy in up to 40% cases. About 1% normal person has abnormal EEG.
6. CT scan of head
   a. Helps in diagnosis of tumor or cerebrovascular malformations.
   b. Differentiate idiopathic epilepsy from other conditions.
   c. It is normal in idiopathic epilepsy except as cerebral atrophy due to hypoxia or low density on CT scan occurs as a transient abnormality after prolonged seizures.
7. Blood studies: Blood glucose, calcium and lead and amino acid in serum, to exclude metabolic causes.
8. Convulsions should be excluded from:
   a. Pseudoseizures of hysteria, malingering.
   b. Benign paroxysmal vertigo
   c. Breath holding attacks
   d. Migraine
   e. Vasovagal and cardiac forms of syncope
   f. Narcolepsy.

Management

At Convulsions

i. Obtain free airway by suction, mouth gag, rubber airway or padded tongue blade or rarely by endotracheal tube.
ii. Restraints and padding are used to prevent injury; clothes are loosened.
iii. Suction of oropharynx to prevent aspiration. The patient is placed on his side or her side rather than supine to minimize the risk of aspiration.
iv. Oxygen is given.
v. Anticonvulsants are administered intravenously (Table 11.3)
   a. Diazepam is drug of choice. Dose 0.3 mg/kg; a total dose 10 mg may be given over a period of 2–3 minutes. Safe and effective, or
   b. Phenobarbital 10–20 mg per kg, injected intravenously in 2–3 minutes, for longer duration of action. May be repeated.
   c. Phenytoin 20 mg per kg; given slowly over a period of 15–20 minutes.
vi. Rapid infusion of 20% dextrose 2 ml/kg is given, if hypoglycemia is cause of convulsions.

Anticonvulsant therapy: Aim of anticonvulsant in termination of seizure activity.

Table 11.3: Anticonvulsant drugs		
Drug	*Route*	*Initial dose mg/kg*
Diazepam	IV, rectal	0.1–0.3
Lorazepam	IV	0.2–0.5
Midazolam	IV	0.05–0.2
	IM	0.05–0.2
	Buccal	0.1–0.2
	Nasal	0.1–0.2
Valproic acid	IV	20
Phenytoin	IV	15–20
Fosphenytoin	IV, IM	15-20 PE/kg
Levetiracetam	IV	20

Hospital Management

Management of acute convulsions must be energetic IV diazepam or lorazepam infusion given at the rate of 1 mg/min.

Lorazepam has longer duration of action and less respiratory depression than diazepam. Diazepam should be repeated two times at 5–10 minutes interval if convulsion persists (maximum 10 mg).

In status epilepticus along with diazepam other anticonvulsant phenytoin must be added along with it to prevent recurrence.

Paraldehyde in given with glass syringe.

Phenytoin should be mixed in normal saline, not in dextrose because it may precipitate. Phenytoin has lower duration of action.

Fosphenytoin has less phlebitis, it can be given IM, but costly.

If raised intracranial tension—if convulsions are due to raised intracranial tension IV mannitol (20%) at a dose of 5 ml/kg is given intravenously.

Status Epilepticus

Prolong single seizures or multiple episodes of seizures which last more than 30 minutes during which patient does not regain consciousness.

Convulsions are tonic clonic, clonic tonic or myoclonic. This is most medical emergency, also results permanent brain damage due to anoxia, it has high mortality and sequelae.

Management of Status Epilepticus

Proposed management of control of seizure is as follows for status epilepticus (Flowchart 11.1).

Midazolam infusion—dose 0.15 mg/kg is given as bolus dose followed by continuous infusion at the rate of 1 µg/kg/min every 15 min increasing by 1 µg/min every 15 min until 18 µg/kg/min or seizure controlled.

Rate of infusion in which seizure control is maintained at the period of 48 hours. Afterward infusion rate is gradually reduced 1 µg/kg/min every 3 hours.

Flowchart 11.1

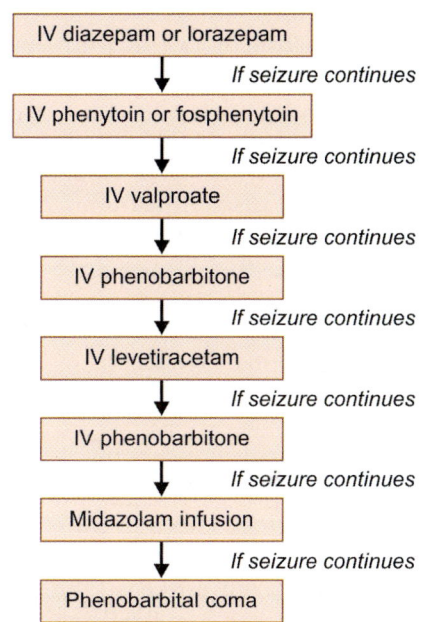

If recurrence occurs then immediately infusion restarted and maintained up to seizure-free period of 48 hours.

If not responding pentobarbital or thiopental has been used for barbiturate coma.

Refractory status epilepticus: If seizures are not controlled with two doses of benzodiazepines followed by phenytoin/valproate and phenobarbitone or midazolam infusion beyond 60 minutes are termed refractory epilepticus.

After Convulsions (Long-term Treatment)

Principles of treatment:

a. Chemotherapy of epilepsy depends on type of epilepsy. Drug is selected on the basis of best effects and least side effects. Start the drug with single drug (first order monothreapy).

b. Most of the anticonvulsants when given, steady level as reached on blood slowly, so in initial days of anticonvulsant therapy seizures may be noticed. It does not mean that drug is not effective.

c. If one drug fails to control, the other drug can be combined with it. It is not clear that control is better or not, if four or more drugs are combined. Drug of first choice (Table 11.4).

In West syndrome ACTH 20–40 units per day given intramuscularly for 4–6 weeks. If no response discontinue after 2 weeks. Prednisolone 2 mg/kg/day in 2 divided doses may be used. Nitrazepam 5–10 mg/kg/day in 2 divided doses may be given. But its use is limited due to its toxicity.

For carbamazepine the oral drug is started from low dose and gradually increased to usual daily dose. In case of inadequate control of seizures, increase the dose of the drug to the maximum daily dose, if seizures are still uncontrolled and/or side effects of the drugs appear and increase the dose or add the next drug, increase the dose to maximum and then stop the first drug after tapering over a month or so.

Unsatisfactory control of seizures despite optimum plasma concentration and/or occurrence of adverse reactions should be pre-requisite for switching to another drug also used in monotherapy.

If still uncontrolled, add previous drug with slight lowering of dose of both. Also serum level of drug may of help in this situation also. If facility is not available, clinical monitoring is sufficient for proper management. All anticonvulsants have narrow therapeutic range. It means that the difference between lowest therapeutic serum level and toxic levels is very small. So, correct dose of anticonvulsants should be known to pediatrician dealing a case of convulsions. The steady state concentration is achieved after 5 half lives of the durg if maintenance therapy is started (Table 11.5).

d. Consider following factors for selection of drug

Sex—adolescent females preferably should avoid using phenytoin because of cosmetic reasons (coarsening of face).

Economy of parents—carbamazepine is the drug of choice in complex partial or focal seizures but in poor patient cheaper alternative, e.g. phenytion should be prescribed, valproate is also costlier.

Education—if patient is studying or doing intellectual work drugs like phenytion and probably phenobarbitone are to be avoided.

Table 11.4: Antiepileptic drugs	
Type of seizures	*Drug of choice*
Tonic clonic seizures	• Carbamazepine
Partial	• Phenobarbitone below 1 year • Phenytoin
Complex partial seizures	• Carbamazepine • Oxcarbazepine
Absence seizures	• Ethosuximide • Sodium valproate • Lamotrigine • Benzodiazepine
Myoclonic and atonic seizures	• Sodium valproate • Levetiracetam • Benzodiazepine (clonazepam, nitrozepam or clobazam)
Infantile spasm	• ACTH in West syndrome 40–60 unit/day for 4–6 weeks • Prednisolone 2 mg/kg/day in 2 diveded doses • Vigabatrin
Partial epilepsies	• Oxcarbazepine

Table 11.5: Commonly used anticonvulsant

Drug	Dose (mg/kg/day)	Daily dose	Side effects
Phenobarbital	2–3	1–2	Hyperkinesis, drowsiness, Stevens-Johnson syndrome
Primidone	5	2–3	— Same —
Phenytoin	5–7	2	Hirsutism, gingival hyperplasia, Stevens-Johnson syndrome (rare) Hepatic necrosis (rare) Blood dyscrasia (rare)
Carbamazepine	10–15	2–3	Leukopenia, thrombocytopenia, aplastic anemia, (rare) drowsiness, abdominal distension
Valproic acid	10–20	3–4	Acute hepatic failure, hyperammonemia, drowsiness, alopecia, abdominal discomfort
Ethosuximide	10–20	2	Blood dyscrasia (rare), drowsiness
Clonazepam	0.04–0.05	2	Blood dyscrasia, drowsiness
Acetazolamide	10–20	2–3	Blood dyscrasia, metabolic acidosis, paresthesia

Facility for investigations, e.g. CT scan if available then one must be liberal regarding these investigations. If not available then we have to put our discretion about its indication.

Pediatrician treating epilepsy must stick to a single standard preparation, change of one standard preparation to another standard preparation brought on recurrence due to different bioavailability due to changed base.

Role of society—epilepsy is a stigma in the society, superstition and wrong customs about it should be removed.

Residence of the patient and distance to reach up to pediatrician should also be considered for decision about treating simple seizures and also change in drug if made.

When to increase the dose—if the seizures are recurring enquire about non-compliance, change of formulation and risk factors like fever, systemic illness which may worsen seizures control. Decide now to increase the dose of anticonvulsant drug modest at a time within the therapeutic range. Wait for new steady state concentration to be achieved.

Surgical Treatment

Medically resistant cases of epilepsy should be treated surgically—resection of epileptic areas, resection of corpus collosum and focal resection of part of cerebral cortex.

Duration of Treatment

Drug withdrawal is indicated after a seizure free period of two years. The drug in tapered gradually over a period of 3 months.

Treatment of juvenile myoclonic epilepsy is lifelong.

Social Aspects

Encourage full participation in educational and extracurricular activities except sports, swimming, riding bicycle in traffic.

Monitoring: Monitoring of effects and toxicity of drugs is essential, which can be done by direct methods serum drug level or by indirect method by clinical examination for side effects and laboratory examination.

Prognosis: Prognosis of seizure depends on age of onset, duration and frequency, underline cause, underline condition of brain, type of seizures.

Prognosis is better in generalized tonic clonic, typical absence seizure than other type except the benign form. Simple partial seizure has better prognosis than complex seizure. Idiopathic West syndrome, juvenile myoclonic responds better to treatment. Lennox-Gastaut's syndrome has worse prognosis.

Single seizure: Initiation of treatment, the recurrence rate following a single seizure is variable. Factors which increase the risk of recurrence are as follows:

1. History of prior neurological insult.
2. Family history of epilepsy.
3. Single seizure presenting as status epi-lepticus.
4. Todd's palsy or focal abnormality.
5. Gross EEC abnormality.
6. Focal abnormality on imaging study.

If anyone of them risk factor is present anticonvulsant therapy following single seizure may be started. Also consider the distance of medical facility for starting the anticonvulsant therapy.

In absence of above risk factors general consensus is that one should not put the patient on long-term anticonvulsant therapy but to keep under close observation and keep all seizure prophylaxis.

Prophylactic anticonvulsant: Following head injury craniotomy, brain surgery or brain abscess, anticonvulsant therapy is controversial in absence of seizure and duration of therapy is also even more controversial. But consensus is to put on phenytoin or carbamazepine for 1–2 weeks in case of severe cortical damage. Because it complicates management and definite anticovulsant actions of such durgs are not definitely proved.

Neonatal seizures: Refer to page 66.

CRANIOSTENOSIS

This is a condition caused by premature closure of skull sutures. Brain cannot grow due to stiff skull vault. Signs of intracranial tension develop. On examination, micro-cephaly with united sutures are present. A ridge is felt on palpation. Skiagram skull confirms the closure of sutures and silver beaten appearance is seen. Mental retardation is an important feature (Fig. 11.13).

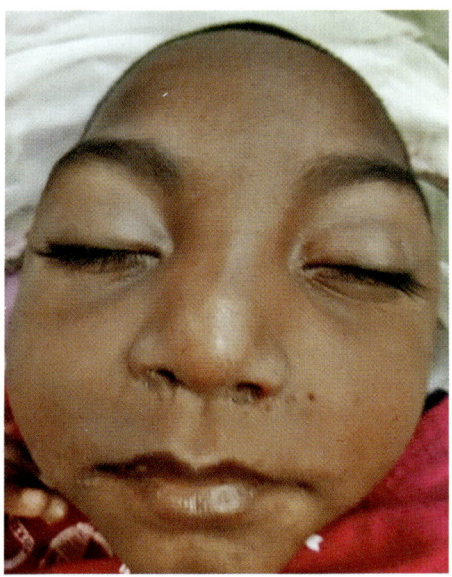

Fig. 11.13: Craniostenosis.

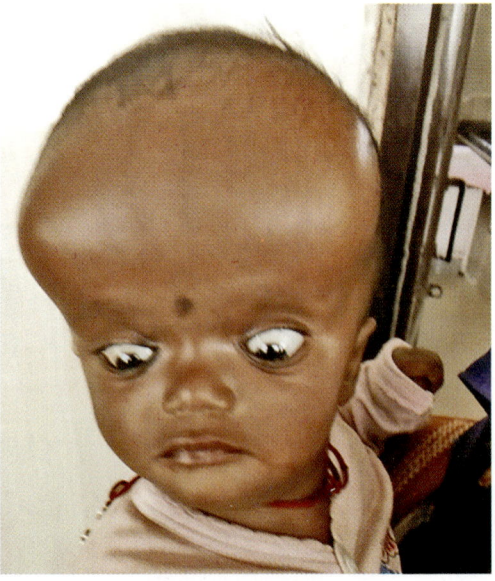

Fig. 11.14: Hydrocephalus.

Surgical correction is done as earliest as possible to prevent mental retardation.

HYDROCEPHALUS

Enlargement of head due to abnormally high accumulation of CSF in the intracranial spaces. It may be due to increased production obstruction to flow or interference with absorption. Causes may be congenital or acquire characteristic features are large head, wide, bulging fontanelle, open suture. Sunset sign, cracked pot sign and positive transillumination. Diagnosed by clinical sign, ventriculography and CT scan (Fig. 11.14).

Medical management is aimed to reduce intracranial tension. Hypertonic solution, acetazolamide or diuretics, surgical treatment is shunt operation. Prognosis is not good.

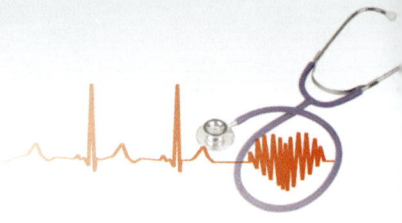

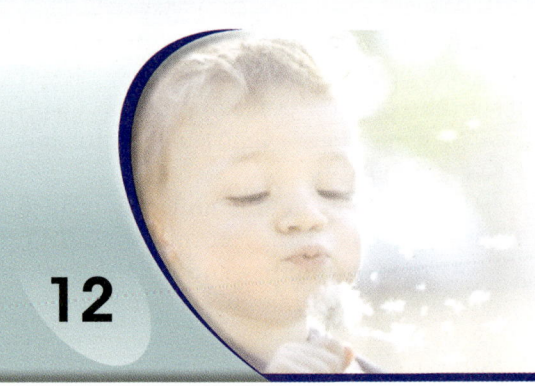

12

Bacterial Diseases

WHOOPING COUGH

This is a highly communicable disease, characterized by paroxysm of cough (Fig. 12.1).

Etiology

This is caused by *Haemophilus pertussis* bacteria. Transmission is by droplet method. Infection reaches at healthy child by air, due to sneezing, coughing of sick person, specially during catarrhal or paroxysmal stage of the disease.

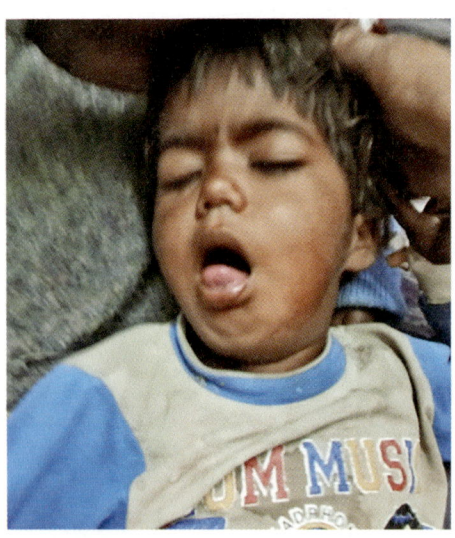

Fig. 12.1: Whooping cough.

Clinical Features

Whooping cough is common in children below 10 years of age (peak incidence is at about 4 years of age).

Incubation period is 7–14 days. Disease occurs in three stages. Every stage is of about two weeks duration.

i. *Catarrhal stage:* At this stage, symptoms are mild cough, running of nose and mild fever. Cough is mainly in night initially, but later on it occurs in day also.

ii. *Paroxysmal or spasmodic stage:* After 10–14 days of catarrhal symptoms, cough becomes explosive and markedly aggravated.

Rapidly successive bouts of cough, as many as 10–20 or more may occur, followed by hurried deep inspiration, which causes the typical 'whoop' due to entry of air through partially closed larynx.

Face becomes flushed, sometimes vomiting occurs.

Child usually sleeps after the paroxysm because of exhaustion. Convulsions, puffiness of face and subconjunctival hemorrhage may also occur at this stage. Child is afebrile during this stage. Such attacks occur many times in a day.

iii. *Convalescent stage:* At this stage, bouts of cough ceases. Appetite is regained and cough becomes less.

Diagnosis

a. Mainly depends on clinical features.
b. *Blood examination:* WBC count is increased, especially lymphocytes 50–90%.
c. ESR is less (1–2 only)
d. Positive culture or immunofluorescence of nasopharyngeal secretions for *Bordetella pertussis,* bacteria identification.
e. *Serology:* Detection of increased antibodies against pertussis.

Complications

a. *Respiratory system:* Pneumonia, collapse, emphysema, bronchiectasis, pneumothorax.
b. Nervous system: Convulsions, paralysis, mental retardation.
c. Epistaxis due to increased pressure during cough.
d. Tuberculosis focus may flared up.

Treatment

General treatment
a. Patient should be kept in ventilated room.
b. Diet should be light, frequent and small.
c. During attack of spasmodic cough, child should be kept upside down to prevent inhalation of secretions.
d. Oxygen—in case of respiratory distress.
e. Throat suction, when necessary.

Drugs

a. *Sedative:* Such as phenergan, chloral hydrate.
b. *Antibiotics:* Antibiotics are given for 5–7 days. Chloromycetin is drug of choice, given in dose 50–100 mg/kg/day orally or intramuscularly.
Apart from it erythromycin or ampicillin may be given.
Antibiotics do not shorten duration of paroxysmal stage of the disease but shorten period of communicability.

c. Antispasmodics such as ephedrine hydrochloride is given for symptomatic relief of spasm.
d. Isonex is also recommended to patient of whooping cough for 1 month, to prevent flaring up of tubercular focus.

Prevention

a. By the active immunization (DPT vaccination or pentavalent)
b. By gamma globulins given below 2 years may perhaps have beneficial effects on children, but not recommended.

DIPHTHERIA

This is an acute infectious disease, characterized by formation of membrane in upper respiratory tract and production of toxin causing different clinical manifestations.

Diphtheria is common in 2–5 years age group, but adult is not spared.

Etiology

This is caused by bacteria, *Corynebacterium diphtheriae.* Transmission is by coughing, sneezing (droplet infection). Acuteness of disease is due to toxins liberated by bacteria, which is also responsible for variable symptoms.

Clinical Features

Incubation period of the disease is about 3 days (1–7 days). Disease occurs in following groups.

Respiratory Group

1. *Tonsillar diphtheria (faucial diphtheria):* Frequent than other groups characterized by following symptoms:
   • Mild fever, sore throat, difficulty in deglutition. Sometimes fever reaches 101–103°F.
   • Bodyache, drowsiness and restlessness increases.

MEMBRANE

The exuding lymph coagulates and forms a membrane containing many bacilli, the toxins of which produced at the site of exudate are absorbed into blood stream (toxemia).

- *Membrane:* A thin white brown membrane is seen at tonsils may extend to pharynx, uvula, soft or hard palate and up to larynx which is difficult to remove and attempt to remove is followed by bleeding. It is characteristic feature and differentiated from membrane of fungal infection, which is easy to remove (Figs 12.2 and 12.3).
- Neck glands are swollen. They may be severe by enlarge which give appearance of 'bull neck'.
- Edema may be present at neck, which is brown, pitting, warm and tender. It may obliterate border of sternocleidomastoid.
- Pulse rate is disproportionately increased in comparison to temperature.

2. *Laryngeal diphtheria:* This is most severe form, turn out to be fatal. Features are as follows:
   - Voice is barking or there may be aphasia.

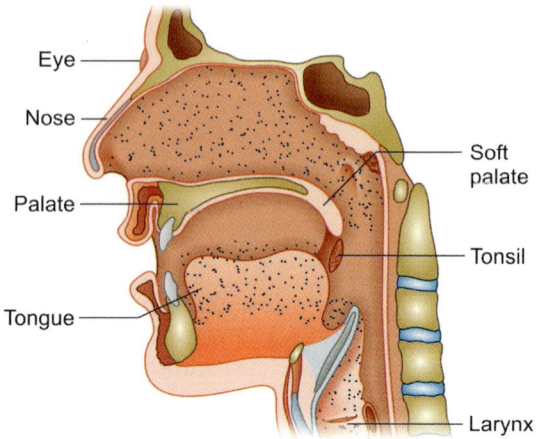

Fig. 12.3: Common sites for diphtheric membrane (dotted area)

- Patient may have dyspnea, hoarseness and stridor. Increasing dyspnea causes restlessness, cyanosis and prostration. If unrelieved, may lead to death due to exhaustion, suffocation and heart failure.
- Membrane at larynx is seen by laryngoscope.

3. *Nasal diphtheria:* Patient may suffer from mild fever, running of nose, nasal obstruction or epistaxis; membrane can be identified within nose.

Non-respiratory Group

Sometimes diphtheria can affect tongue, skin, ears, external genital organs or wounds.

Complications

1. Bronchopneumonia
2. Nephritis
3. Myocarditis and peripheral circulatory failure
4. Paralysis
   a. Paralysis of soft palate (at the end of 1st or 2nd weeks) — Nasal twang of speech dysphasia, regurgitation of food from nose
   b. Eye muscles (3–4 weeks) Muscles of accommodation — Squint, ptosis, diplopia

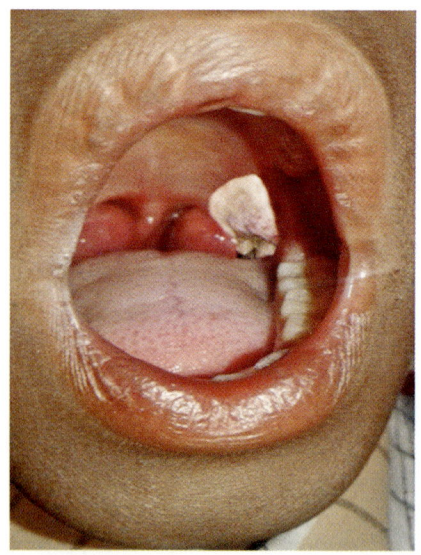

Fig. 12.2: Diphtheric membrane

c. General paralysis (3–6 weeks)
- Inability to lift head due to paralysis of neck muscles.
- Paralysis of limbs.
- Paralysis of phrenic nerves, respiratory embarrassment after 4 weeks.

Diagnosis

i. *Depends on clinical features:* Membrane is characteristic of the disease.
ii. *Throat swab:* For identification of organism diphtheria bacilli and culture. Precaution during swab taking swab is taken systematically from both tonsils, the pillars, fauces, back of throat. Take care to catch up exudate and membrane. Swab should be rubbed deep because diphtheria bacilli are deeply located and only staphylococci are found on surface.
iii. Identification of organism by fluorescent antibody technique.
    Diagnosis should be made promptly on clinical ground, any delay in therapy poses a serious risk to patient.

Treatment

a. *Antitoxin (ADS):* Antitoxin is the only specific treatment used to neutralize free toxin and should be given as early as possible by intravenous route after the sensitivity test.
   Dose: 40,000 units for mild cases, 80,000 units for moderate cases and 1,20,000 units for severe cases (symptoms with browny edema or disease of longer duration than 48 hours)
b. *Antibiotics*
   - Procaine penicillin 6 lakh units intramuscularly for 7 days.
   - If patient is sensitive to penicillin— Erythromycin is the drug of choice 40 mg/kg/24 hours daily in divided doses for 7–10 days. Antibiotics are given up to the period when three consecutive cultures become negative.

Other effective antibiotics are amoxycillin, rifampicin and cleidomycin. Carriers are treated by benzathine penicillin or oral erythromycin.
- Immune human globulin (Dipglob) is recent introduction for treatment of diphtheria.

General Measures

1. Hospitalization and absolute bedrest is essential for 2 weeks.
2. Diet must be liquid or semiliquid initially.
3. Fever is treated with paracetamol.
4. If child is toxic, intravenous glucose or tube feeding may be required.
5. Secretions of throat must be sucked frequently.
6. If respiratory distress is severe, suffocation is dealt with oxygen inhalation, tracheostomy or respirator.

Prevention

Immunization (DPT or pentavalent vaccination).

Prognosis

Prognosis is worse, 50% of all cases die.

Test for Sensitivity of ADS

0.1 ml of 1:1000 dilution of antitoxin in isotonic saline is given intracutaneous or placed on conjunctival sac. A positive reaction is formation of erythema more than 10 mm within 20 minutes or development of conjunctivitis with tearing.

Sensitive individual should be desensitized.

TYPHOID FEVER

This is an acute illness of children caused by *Salmonella typhi*, characterized by prolonged fever, splenomegaly and lymphadenitis.

Agent: Causative agent is gram-negative bacillus *Salmonella typhi*. This consists of three antigen structures:

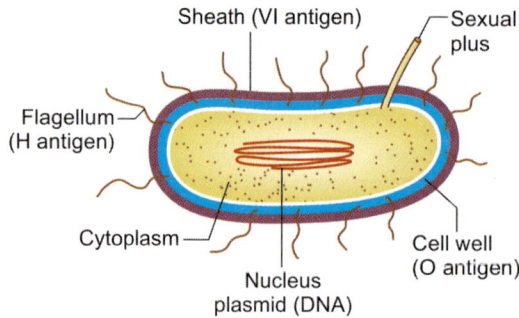

Fig. 12.4: Structure of *Salmonella typhi.*

1. Somatic antigen (O) corresponding to endotoxin.
2. Flagellar antigen (H) proteinic structure
3. Capsular antigen also called V antigen, is the polysaccharide responsible for virulence.

The VI antigen is not found in *Salmonella paratyphi A* and *paratyphi B,* agents responsible for paratyphoid fevers. A and B which are less frequent and less serious for virulence. Septicemia is linked to the VI antigen (marker of severe form) (Fig. 12.4).

Mode of Infection

The reservoir of bacteria is strictly human, the agent responsible can however survive several months in soil or water. In 90% cases, infection is indirect by ingestion of water or food soiled with excrement from infected subjects. Housefly also acts as passive vector due to contact with their legs, commute between latrine and kitchens.

Transmission also occurs in the family or contact of a patient or a chronic carrier.

Epidemiology

This is quite common in India, and developing countries because of poor sanitation and unhygienic condition. Disease is common in infants and young children. High incidence is in summer and rainy seasons due to increased number of housefly in these seasons, which spread disease.

Pathogenesis

Infection reaches within body orally by ingestion of contaminated food. Bacilli invade the blood stream generally in upper small bowel and reaches mesenteric lymph nodes and other portions of reticuloendothelial system, where they multiply and produce inflammation in lymph nodes, liver, spleen. Peyer's patches are gut become swollen, necrosed and later on form ulcer, which may potentially lead to hemorrhage or perforation.

The bacteria then re-enters the blood stream from these sites. Thus, secondary septicemia is of long duration and many organs are seeded with bacilli, especially gall bladder. In gall bladder organism multiply and discharged at intestines.

Outer portion of cell wall of bacteria may act as pyrogenic endotoxin, which produce symptoms. Immunity is cell mediated which protects humans.

Typhoid fever—septicemia of lymphatic origin is shown in Fig. 12.5.

Clinical Features of Typhoid Fever

Typhoid fever often presents atypical clinical pictures (clinical polymorphism) which hinder its diagnosis.

Classical form: This is only seen in 50% of cases:

   i. *Incubation period:* Incubation period is asymptomatic and its duration depends on the quantity of bacteria ingested (from 7–21 days).

  ii. The 7-day invasive phase is characterized by varied and insidious disturbances oscillating continuous fever, dissociated pulse, persistent headache, asthenia, abdominal distension and discomfort. Diarrhea is common than constipation as an associated symptom. Other associated features are dizziness, nausea and epistaxis.

At this stage hemoculture is the only biological test permitting the isolation of

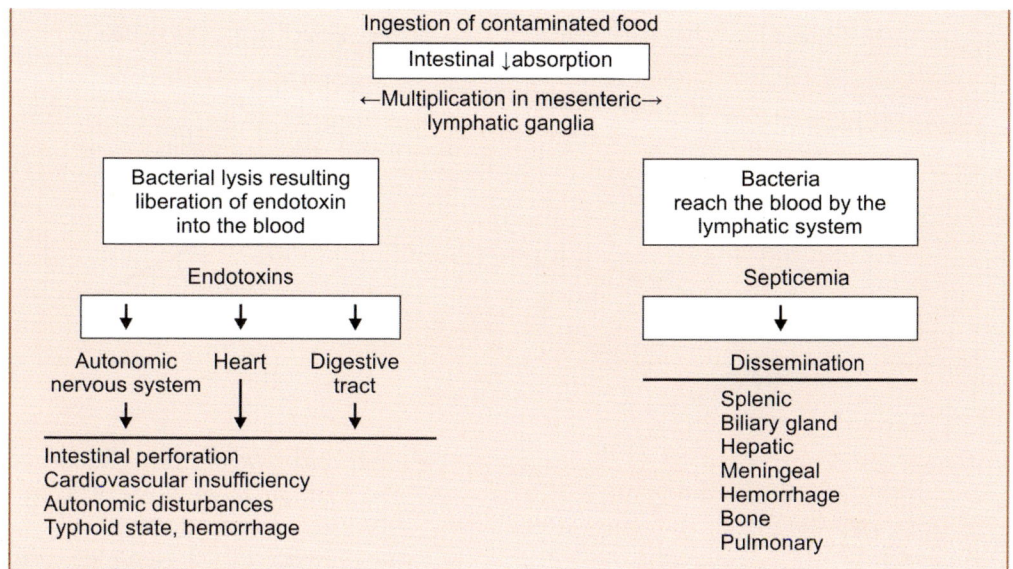

Fig. 12.5: Typhoid fever—septicemia of lymphatic origin.

the bacterium. This test is positive in 45–70% cases and must be repeated if negative.

iii. *Status period:* During the two weeks of status period, the clinical signs are continuous high fever 39–40°C, a typhoid state of prostration of the patient, indifference and inversion of the nyctohemeral cycle and a 'melon juice' diarrhea, sometimes preceded by constipation.

As in adults relationship between rise of fever and low pulse rate (bradycardia) is not a feature in children. Moderate splenomegaly or a hepatosplenomegaly is seen. Abdomen is distended and tender. Classically inconstant but suggestive signs are described pinkish ventricular abdominal marks, superficial ulceration of the soft palate. Spots (rose spots) rash is seen in chest and abdomen; although uncommon in our country.

Chest signs (creptations) are found, sometimes, convulsions may occur. Anemia is also associated feature.

Coproculture is positive in 30% cases. The widal and felix serodiagnosis test measures antibodies against (O) and (H) antigen of the *Salmonella typhi* titre greater than 1/100 or 1/200 for O and H antibodies respectively are indicative, diagnostic reliability depends on the isolation of the bacterium in hemoculture.

iv. *The evolution:* The evolution phase which is favorable given suitable antibiotic treatment, requires a long period of convalescence.

Complications are frequent and sometimes serious. Relapses are seen in 10–20% of patients. In 3–5% cases, the patient remains chronic carrier despite antibiotic therapy.

In uncomplicated case, physical findings resolve within 2–4 weeks malaise and lethargy may last for 1–2 months.

Diagnosis depends on: (a) Clinical features, (b) blood examination—absolute absence of eosinophils or reduction in number is a reliable sign of

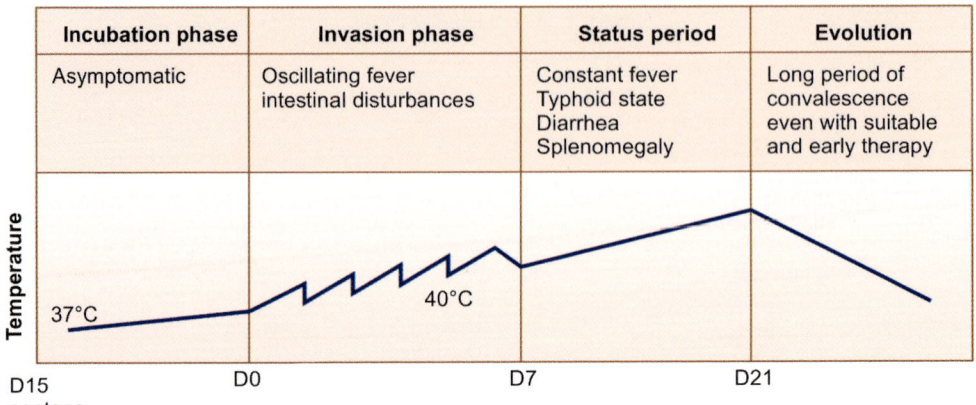

Incubation phase	Invasion phase	Status period	Evolution
Asymptomatic	Oscillating fever intestinal disturbances	Constant fever Typhoid state Diarrhea Splenomegaly	Long period of convalescence even with suitable and early therapy

typhoid fever, (c) Widal test—positive after 10th day. 'O' antibody titre 1 in 250 or more is diagnostic (positive) after one week.

It detects IgG, IgM antibodies to H flagger antigen of *S. typhi*. Four times rise in antibody titre in two samples taken in 10 days interval.

A single titre in first week and specificity is low owing to amnestic reaction.

- Blood—SGPT and SGOT elevated.
- Molecular diagnosis—C-reactive protein is high.
- Microbiological test—blood culture-diagnostic. It has greater sensitivity but may be low in endemic area with high rates of antibiotic use.
  First week—sensitivity 90%
  Second week—sensitivity 40%

- Bone marrow culture—greater sensitivity but due to invasive procedure, it has limited clinical value.
v. *Urine and stool culture:* Generally positive at third week but they are not of much value as blood culture because of the delay in their appearance.
vi. *Blood culture:* Blood culture is positive during first week.

Biological diagnosis of typhoid fever is given in Table 12.1.

COMPLICATIONS OF TYPHOID FEVER

Complications due to unsuitable or delayed antibiotic treatment are frequent. Digestive complications are most common, hemorrhage and intestinal perforations are seen in 5–10% of cases. In developing countries, 12–32% of cases of typhoid fever have a fatal outcome.

Table 12.1: Biological diagnosis of typhoid

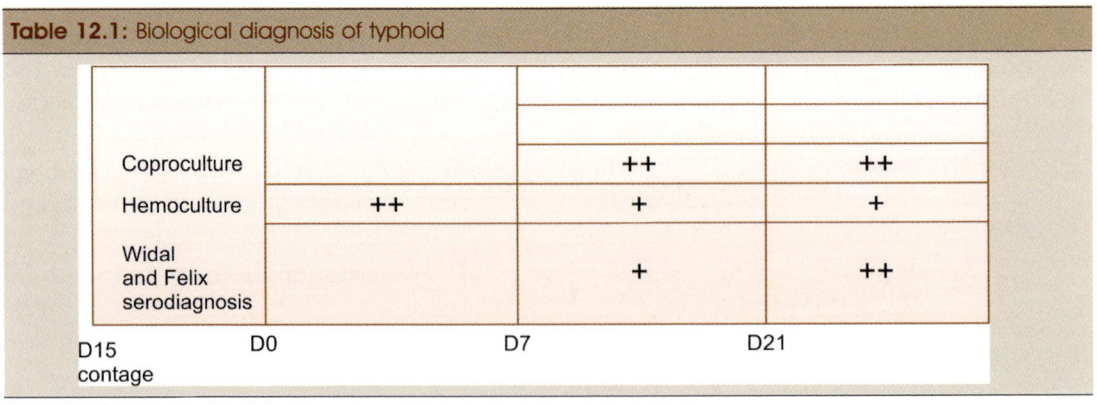

	D0	D7	D21
Coproculture		++	++
Hemoculture	++	+	+
Widal and Felix serodiagnosis		+	++

D15 contage

Table 12.2: Complications of typhoid fever

Origin of complications	Nature of complications
Toxin	• Digestive hemorrhage and intestinal perforation
	• Cardiovascular – Cardiovascular insufficiency
	– Myocarditis
	• Neurologic encephalitis
Septicemia	Hepatic involvement
	Cholecystitis, phlebitis and arteritis, meningitis, myositis, pleuropulmonary involvement, osteitis, thyroiditis

Complications of typhoid fever are shown in Table 12.2.

Treatment

Owing to emergence of resistance to previously used antibiotics following drugs are used as empirical therapy.

a. Cefixime (oral)—20 mg/kg/day is the drug of choice.
b. Fluoroquinolones
c. Azithromycin (10–20 mg/kg/day) is second choice drug.
d. Chloramphenicol (50 mg/kg/day), amoxicillin and cotrimoxazole are alternate second line drugs.

Severe illness

a. Ceftriaxone or cefotaxime are drugs given intravenously.
b. Patient allergic to penicillin or cephalosporin—aztreonam, chloramphenicol in higher doses.
c. Parenteral treatment is indicated until oral intake is permitted and complication resolved. Switch to oral antibiotics. Cefixime for 14 days to complete the course.

Other oral drugs are:
• Cefpodoxime
• Amoxicillin
• Azithromycin
• Cotrimoxazole

If sensitivity to drug is found, drug is switched to another drug according to sensitivity.

Therapy of relapse—fluocinolone is used for relapse cases.

Therapy of carrier—treatment is done by:
1. Amoxicillin 100 mg/kg/day with probenecid
2. Cotrimoxazole 10 mg/kg/day for 6–12 weeks
3. Nalidixic acid

General treatment

a. Bedrest.
b. Care of oral hygiene.
c. Diet: Liquid diet such as milk, fruit juices should be given initially, followed by semiliquid diet later on. Vitamins and iron must be sufficient in diet.
d. Blood transfusion is indicated for anemia and excessive hemorrhage.
e. Fever is treated with cold sponging, avoid aspirin-like drugs.
f. Toxemia is treated by steroids, such as dexamethasone or prednisolone. Dose is tapered gradually.
g. Abdominal distension is managed by omission of sugar in diet, less milk intake and turpentine snipping.
h. Surgery is indicated in perforation of typhoid ulcer.

Prophylaxis

Typhoid fever is not a disease which induce immunity, although high level of antibodies (anti-H, anti O, anti-Vi) are detected during fever, which decreases on recovery.

Only vaccination can produce high and lasting level of antibody. Vaccination is done by TAB vaccine. Recently Typhim Vi vaccine has been introduced. It is given in dose 0.5 ml as a single injection, subcutaneous or intramuscular ensure protection, which is rapid (15 days to 3 weeks) and lasting for at least 3 years. It acts against VI antigen, which is responsible for septicemia. Vaccine does not act against paratyphoid fever and antibody response below 2 years age is poor.

Care of personal hygiene and sanitation is essential for prophylaxis of typhoid fever.

TETANUS

This is an acute toxemic illness, caused by soluble exotoxin of bacterium *Clostridium tetani,* characterized by increased nervous irritability and muscular spasms.

Etiology

Tetanus bacillus is a gram-positive, anaerobic spore-bearing bacillus with characteristic drumstick appearance. Actively motile. Spores are resistant to boiling but destroyed in autoclaving and survive in soil for years if not exposed to sunlight, found in house dust, soil, water and faeces of many animals; vegetative form is susceptible to heat.

Modes of Introduction into Body

a. Commonly occurs through the infected wounds.
b. Organism can contaminate umbilical stump in neonate, when delivery is conducted by untrained dais; dirty sharp weapon is used to cut the umbilical cord or paint the stump with cow dung due to misbelief.
c. Site of infection may be gastrointestinal tract, tonsillar crypts, contaminated sera vaccine and suture material.

Pathogenesis

Bacteria (spores) are converted into vegetative forms in the wound, which release powerful toxin (tetanospasmin). Bacteria remain at the site and tetanospasmin is responsible for various clinical manifestations.

Tetanospasmin reaches the central nervous system from two routes:

i. By absorption at myoneural junction, followed by migration through perineural tissue space of nerve, or
ii. By transfer to the blood by lymphocytes and then to the central nervous system:
   a. Tetanospasmin acts on spinal cord, lead to disturb function of polysynaptic reflexes.
   b. It becomes bound to gangliosides and suppress inhibitory effect on motor neuron and interneuron.
   c. The antidromic inhibition of evolved cortical activity is reduced.
   d. Toxin inhibits release of acetylcholine transmission from nerve ending at muscle.

These actions are responsible for hypertonicity, spasm and seizures.

Tetanospasmin also acts at sympathetic nervous system, producing hypertension, cardiac arrhythmia, vasoconstriction, sweating.

Once toxin is bound to the tissue, it cannot be dissociated or neutralized by tetanus antitoxin. Antitoxin can only prevent binding, if it has not reached up to central nervous system.

Muscles supplied by short nerves are first effected, e.g. face, jaw stiffness. It is followed by spinal muscles and muscles of limbs clenching of fist, extension of lower extremities.

Clinical Features

Incubation period is 3–14 days after the injury but may be short as 1 day, as long as several months.

Disease can manifest in 3 forms:
   1. Localized tetanus.
   2. Generalized tetanus.
   3. Cephalic tetanus.

Localized Tetanus

This produce pain, continuous rigidity and spasm of muscle around the wound. Sometimes this is followed by generalized tetanus.

Generalized Tetanus

This is most common form, trismus is common presenting symptom, there is gradually increasing jaw stiffness resulting difficulty in opening mouth.

Restlessness, irritability and headache are early findings. Spasm of muscles of face produces a fixed sardonic face (risus sardonicus). Spasm of the muscles of neck, difficulty in swallowing. Later on stiffness and rigidity of the back and abdominal muscles develop, as the back muscles are more powerful, ophisthotonus occurs (Fig. 12.6).

Lastly limbs are involved. Other features are as follows:

a. Seizures are characteristically sudden, tonic contractions of various muscles group producing flexon and adduction of arm, clenching of fist, extension of lower extremities.

b. Initially seizures last for seconds to several minutes, followed by relaxation period of variable interval, later on they becomes more powerful and exhausting. They may be introduced on touching the patient, sudden light or noise. They are very painful, because prime movers and antagonist muscles contract at the same time.

Patient remains conscious during course of the disease up to the end. It is most characteristic of tetanus.

c. Rigidity present all the times which is different from stychnine poisoning in which there is period of relaxation.

d. Dysuria or retention of urine due to spasm of bladder sphincter or involuntary defecation and urination.

e. Powerful and forceful contractions of muscles may cause fracture of spine and hemorrhage into muscles.

f. Elevation of temperature, mild, to 40°C, may be noted due to production of heat during seizures. Tachycardia, hypertension, cardiac arrhythmias and hyperhidrosis may be seen.

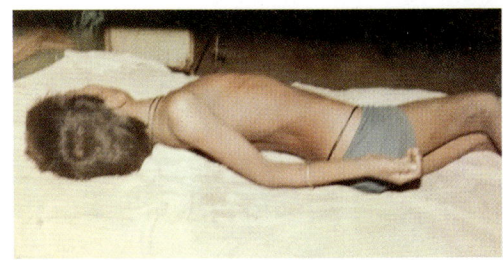

Fig. 12.6: Opisthotonus.

Course

Up to 3–7 days, there is increase in signs and symptoms, then they abate gradually; complete recovery occurs in 2–6 weeks.

Cephalic Tetanus

This is unusual form results after otitis media, head or nose injury. Cranial nerves III, IV, VII, IX, X are involved. Facial nerve is affected most commonly. Cephalic tetanus is followed by generalized form in some cases.

Tetanus Neonatorum

Majority of cases, age of onset of disease is 5–15 days newborn cry excessively initially, followed by refusal of feeds and apathy. Newborn keeps mouth slightly open due to pull of neck muscles. There is dysphagia and choking during feeds (Fig. 12.7).

Lock jaw or reflex trismus is followed by spasm of limbs. Opisthotonus may be extreme or absent in newborn.

There is fever, tachypnea, tachycardia and constipation. Secondary infection, dehydration and acidosis may be seen later on. Cyanosis or apnea may be present due to spasm of larynx and respiratoiy muscles.

Spasms are more severe in newborn than adult due to lack of inhibitory impulses from higher center in newborn, resulting anterior horn cell excitation powerful. Spasms are feeble in premature.

Prognosis

Depends on:

a. Amount of tetanospasmin absorbed.

b. Site of wound—more dangerous near face.

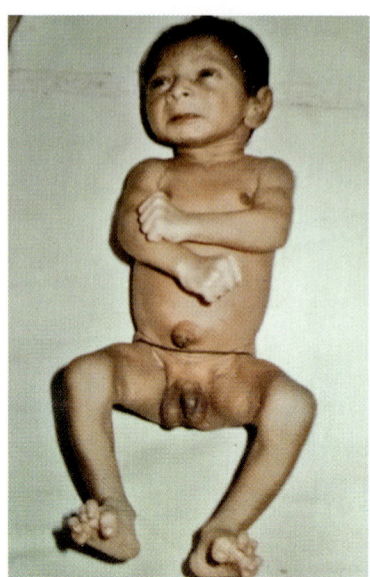

Fig. 12.7: Tetanus neonatorum.

c. Length of incubation period, if short prognosis is worse.

d. Interval between first symptom and fresh seizure. If period is less than 24 hours. Prognosis is worse.

e. Severity of spasm—specially in larynx muscle.

f. High frequency of convulsions worse prognosis.

g. (i) Tetanus neonatorum: Worse prognosis, (ii) old age worse prognosis.

Diagnosis

a. Clinically

b. Culture from wound site and identification of bacteria.

Management

i. Tetanus immunoglobulin (TIG) of human origin 3000–6000 units is given intramuscularly as a single dose (newborn or children). No need of sensitivity test. It has no effect on fixed toxin and also does not cross blood–brain barrier, but neutralize circulatory and uncombined tetanospasmin.

ii. Tetanus antitoxin (TAT) is given in dose of 50,000–100,000 units, half intramuscular and half intravenous as a single dose, after sensitivity test, if TIG is not available.

iii. *Wound:* Wound should be cleaned and foreign body removed. Surgical efforts are done after giving TAT and sedation.

iv. *Antibiotics:* Penicillin 2 lac units/kg/24 hours given intravenously in six divided doses for 10 days, if sensitive to penicillin, tetracycline 30–40 mg/kg/24 hours (not more than 2 gm) in divided doses.

v. *General nursing*
  - Patient is kept in quite room, eliminate noise and light stimuli.
  - Oxygen inhalation
  - Tracheostomy and IPPR, if needed
  - Feeding with nasogastric tube or intravenous fluid
  - Child turned frequently at interval
  - Care of the bowel and bladder.

Control of spasm

1. Spasms are precipitated by stimulus therefore avoid bright lights, pain, and loud noises, keep the patient in dark, minimum handling, avoid intramuscular injection.

2. Temperature should be maintained normal

3. Adequate hydration

4. The spasms are controlled by *benzodiazepines*—diazepam is used to control spasm. It also reduces anxiety and promotes muscle relaxation.
Suction of oropharyngeal secretions.

5. IV line is maintained for fluid, calories and for medication.

6. Afterward feeding is started with nasogastric tube.

7. α- and β-adrenergic blockers used to control autonomic instability, muscle spasm (propranolol and labetalol).

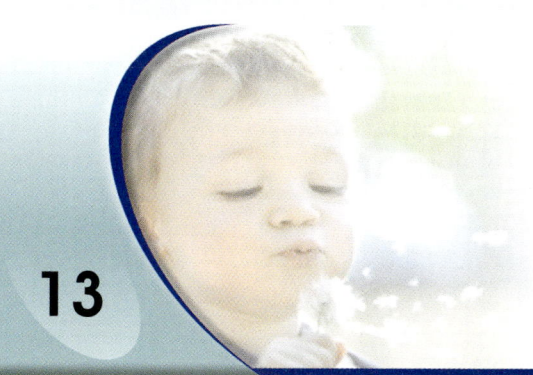

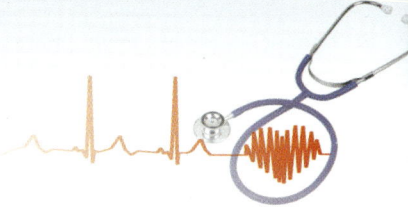

13

Viral Infections

CHICKENPOX

This is caused by virus varicella zoster. Virus enters in the body through droplet infections via respiratory tract and causes various clinical manifestations in the body.

Etiopathogenesis

Chickenpox is caused by the varicella zoster virus (VZV). It is a DNA virus of herpesvirus family. Virus enters in the body through droplets infection via respiratory tract.

The period of infectivity lasts from 24 to 48 hours before the rash until all the vesicles are crusted.

It is a highly contagious disease. Varicella virus may result lifelong latent infection in sensory ganglia.

Chickenpox is transmitted by

- Direct contact with the blisters of someone who have the varicella zoster virus.
- Breathing on the virus particles from someone blisters.
- Breathing in small particles from the mouth of someone talking or coughing.

Clinical Features

i. Incubation period is about 15 days. Early features are pyrexia, bodyache, headache and cold, which last about 24 hours.

ii. Rashes appear on body after general symptoms. They are macule, papule, vesicles and pustules and scab formation. It takes about 4–7 days.

Characteristically appears in 2–4 crops. Different types of rashes can be seen in one time. Site of rash is trunk. They do not appear on palm and soles. Itching is common.

The classic lesion is described as a dew drop on a rose petal or a vesicle on a red background (Fig. 13.1).

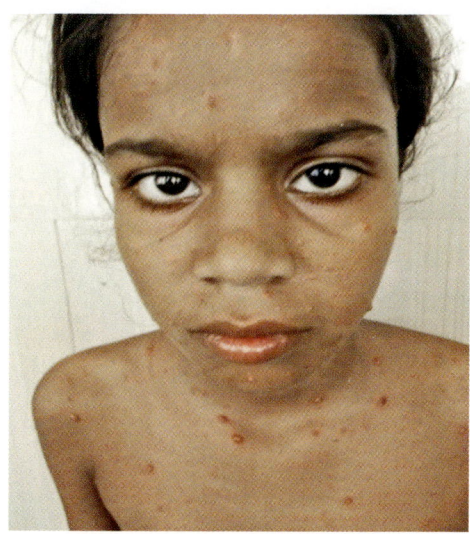

Fig. 13.1: Chickenpox

Rash appears 24–48 hours after the prodromal symptoms. Intensely pruritic erythematous macules first seen on trunk which spreads to face and extremities.

Multiple crops of lesion are present at a time (*polymorphic rash*). It is characteristic of varicella infection. Baby who develops symptoms can get 250–500 itchy blisters (Fig. 13.2).

Diagnosis

Depends on:
1. Clinical presentation is generally diagnostic.
2. Tzanck smear of lesion which shows multinucleated cells.
3. Demonstration of IgM antibody to varicella.

Complications

1. Bacterial superinfections
2. Nacrotising fasciitis
3. Septicemia
4. Arthritis
5. Bronchopneumonia
6. Encephalitis
7. Acute cerebellar ataxia
8. Reye's syndrome (associated with ingestion of salicylates)
9. Infection during pregnancy.

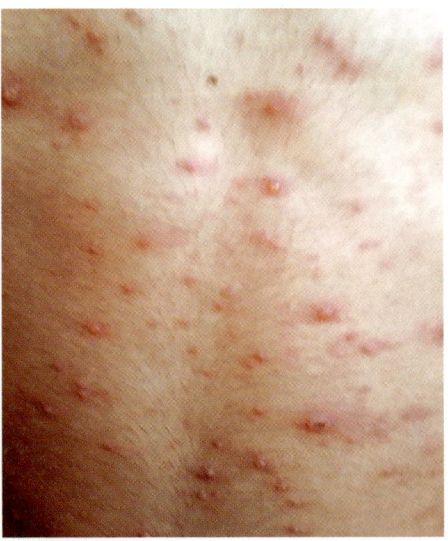

Fig. 13.2: Polymorphic rash.

Teratogenic effects (*congenital varicella syndrome*): Neonate suffers zigzag scarring of skin, shortened or malformed extremities, central nervous system damage, eye abnormalities such as cataracts or chorioretinitis.

Neonate may develop if mother acquires chickenpox within one week of delivery.

10. Risk to develop herpes zoster.

Treatment

No specific treatment is available. Treatment is symptomatic and care of feeding. Steroids are contraindicated.

1. Symptomatic
   - *Antipyretic paracetamol.* Aspirin is contraindicated due to risk of Rey syndrome.
   - *Antipruritic* for relief of itching.
   - Proper hygiene.
2. Oral aciclovir—20 mg/kg/dose four times a day to 5 days. It is given within 24 hours of onset of rash. It reduces duration of rash by one day.

Intravenous aciclovir administered to patients with varicella pneumonia and encephalitis and in neonates, immunocompromised children, pregnant women.

Topical aciclovir—if ophthalmic involvement.

Prevention

a. *Varicella vaccine:* Two doses: 12–16 months and 4–5 years of age.
b. Varicella zoster immune globulin (VZIG) to post-exposure prophylaxis.

MEASLES (RUBEOLA)

This is most common communicable viral infection during childhood and most common cause of mortality due to infectious disease in children (Fig. 13.3).

Morbidity, malnutrition and chances of tubeculosis are common after this illness.

of March to June. This can occur at any age in India, but this is mostly seen before the third birthday of child.

Etiology

This is caused by measles RNA virus (rubeola), spread is by means of droplet infections from the patient with active disease or by means of indirect contact from fomites or by air-borne route.

Portal of entry is respiratory tract, where virus multiply in respiratory epithelium. Infection of reticuloendothelial system results in primary viremia, which is followed by secondary viremia which is responsible for systemic symptoms.

This is common before 3 years age of the child. It is highly infectious disease spreads easily among susceptible unvaccinated individuals in households and schools.

Owing to measles vaccination incidence and severity of measles declined.

Clinical Features

Disease is common in preschool children but can occur at any age. Transplacental antibodies protect the child at about 9 months of age so measles vaccine is given after age of 9 months.

The three 'Cs'—cough, coryza, conjunctivitis and with rash in mnemonic to help to remember to diagnose classic syndrome.

Measles is almost always symptomatic. Incubation period is about 10 days (8–14 days). This occurs in three stages:

1. **Prodromal phase** (catarrhal phase)
   - This remains first 3–4 days. Common cold, fever, conjunctivitis and photophobia are characteristic features.
   - Most important and diagnostic feature of this stage is Koplik's spots. These are tiny white papules, surrounded by an inflammatory red areola, comparable to grains of salt on red base, appears on buccal mucosa near first molar teeth first.

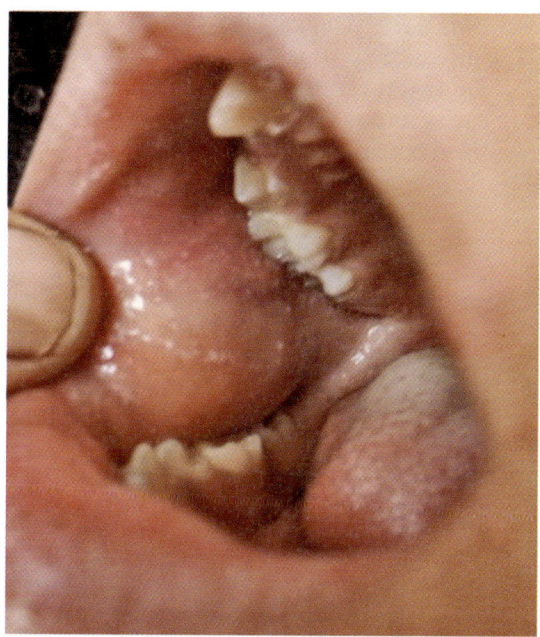

Fig. 13.3A: Koplik's spots on buccal mucosa

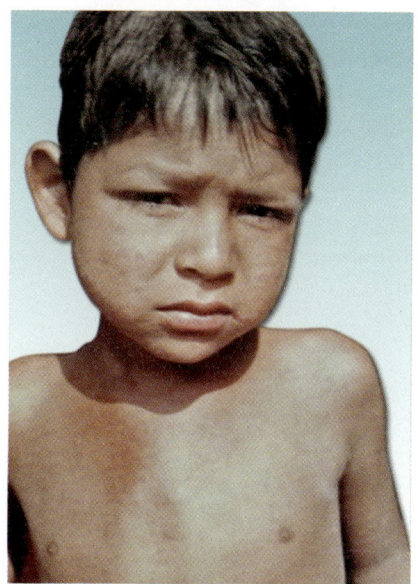

Fig. 13.3B: Measles

Incidence

Common all over the world, seasonal variation is seen, higher incidence during period

Then spread on whole mucosa. They fade away by the time the rash makes its appearance (about 5th day) (Fig. 13.3A).

2. **Eruptive phase:** Rash appears on skin after 3–5 days of onset of illness. These are irregular maculopapular rash appears first on face and neck behind ear at the hairline and gradually spread in a downward directions to involve the extremities and trunk within a day or two. Earlier rash may coalesce, while later on may remain discrete. Rash disappears in same pattern, as of the evolution of rash (Fig. 13.3B).

The rash commences to fade in 3–4 days leaving a light brown color at its site, known as postmeasles staining.

In this phase, temperature is high, hacking cough, itching and lymphadenopathy may occur.

3. **Convalescent phase:** In this phase, fever, rash and other symptoms disappear.

Diagnosis

1. *Clinical:* Three C+ rash
2. IgM antimeasles antibody estimation— present 3 days after rash and persist to 1 month.
3. Isolation of virus from nasopharynx or blood during acute stage.

Complications

i. *Ear:* Otitis media (2% cases).
ii. *Respiratory system:* Tracheobronchitis, laryngobronchitis, bronchopneumonia (4% case).
iii. *Gastrointestinal system:* Stomatitis, enteritis, dysentery, diarrhea, appendicitis
iv. *Eye:* Corneal ulcer
v. *Black measles:* High fever, convulsions, unconsciousness and extensive hemorrhage are its manifestation; outcome is fatal.
vi. *Encephalitis:* Most serious complications leading to death. Those who survive are prone to permanent mental retardation.
vii. *Heart:* Myocarditis

viii. *Subacute panencephalitis:* This occurs after many years of measles infection, characterized by mental changes, myoclonic jerks. Grand mal seizures may also occur. Child dies within 7 years.
ix. *Vitamin A deficiency:* Many children develop deficiency of vitamin A (acute), leading to keratomalacia and blindness.

Differential Diagnosis

i. Exanthema subitum
ii. Rubella
iii. Infections due to echo, coxsachie, adenoviral, infectious mononucleosis, toxoplasmosis, meningococcus, scarlet fever.

Measles should be differentiated from other exanthematous illnesses.

- *Rubella: Enteroviral and adenoviral infection.* Rash is milder and fever is less prominent.
- *Roseola infantum:* Rash appears once when fever disappears. In measles, fever increases with rash.
- *Rickettsial infections:* Face spared from rash but in measles face always involved.
- *Meningococcemia:* Upper respiratory tract symptoms, e.g. cough, corryza absent.
- *Drug rash:* History of drug intake.
- *Kawasaki disease:* Glossitis, cervical lymphadenopathy.

Death

In India, 2–3% children die generally following measles but in epidemic, case fatality is as high as 30%.

Treatment

No specific treatment is available. Symptomatic treatment is as follows:
a. Isolation of patient.
b. If fever, give paracetamol.
c. During cough—cough sedative mixture and for cold-nasal drops.
d. During itching—calamine lotion, antihistaminics.

e. Care of oral hygiene.

f. Superadded infection—antibiotics.

g. Eyes conjunctivitis—antibiotic drops.

h. Feeding—sufficient fluid intake. Diet must be light, milk, fruit juices.

Feeding should never be stopped. Measles is an important cause of malnutrition.

i. Vitamin A should be given to all children suffering from measles.

Vitamin A supplements: Vitamin A should be given to every patient of measles. 100000 units below 1 year age and 200000 units over 1 year age. Two doses of vitamin A supplements are given 24 hours apart.

Vitamin A is shown to reduce number of death from measles by 50%.

Rehydration: If child is having dehydration.

Prevention

1. **Measles vaccine:** Two doses of vaccine are recommended to ensure immunity and prevent outbreaks, as about 15% of vaccinated children fail to develop immunity from the first dose.

Person in contact with infected measles patient should receive measles vaccine within 72 hours of contact to prevent measles.

2. **MMR vaccine:** It prevents measles, mumps and rubella.

3. **Gamma globulins** are indicated to prevent measles.

Period of Infectivity

Maximum dissemination of virus takes place by droplet infection during prodromal or catarrhal stage. Isolation and precaution is maintained from the 7th day after exposure, until 5th day after the rash has appeared.

So, isolation of patient, when he is on rash stage, is of no relevance in the control of disease.

GERMAN MEASLES (RUBELLA)

This is less infectious in comparison to measles. Important features are lymphadenitis behind the ear, fever and rash. Rash disappears after 3 days. If pregnant woman suffers from German measles during its first or second months of pregnancy, infant suffers from various congenital anomalies, which are called congenital rubella syndrome. No specific treatment is avialable.

POLIOMYELITIS

This is an acute viral infection characterized by clinical manifestations of varying degree of paralysis from nil to rapid paralysis and even death. This is a disease which occurs only in human.

Definition

A case of poliomyelitis is defined as any patient of acute flaccid paralysis (including any child less than 15 years of age, diagnosed to have Guillain-Barré syndrome) for which no, other cause can be identified.

Etiopathogenesis

Poliomyelitis is caused by poliovirus (strain 1, 2, 3) transmission is mainly by oral or respiratory route. Implantation occurs in pharynx and lower alimentary tract and within 1 day the infection reaches regional lymph nodes and reticuloendothelial structure. On about 3rd day minor viremia occurs involving various sites in the body. Multiplication

Flowchart 13.1: Pathogenesis of poliomyelitis

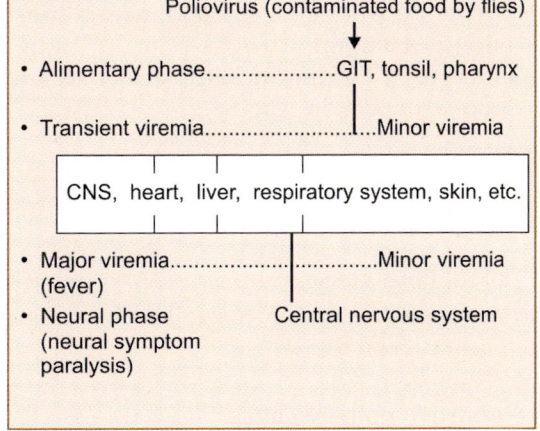

of virus in these sites coincides with the onset of clinical symptoms. Major viremia occurs during period of multiplication of virus in these secondary sites, usually lasting 3rd to 7th days of infection.

If antibody formation fails to neutralize virus particles, there results proliferation of virus and invasion of nerve structures. Nerve system may also be affected directly by invasion of virus, e.g. subcuteneously injected virus, during tonsillectomy virus may enter through severed cranial nerves. Neuronal lesions occur in the: (i) *Spinal cord:* Anterior horn cells, mainly and to a lesser degree, the intermediate and dorsal horn and dorsal root ganglion; (ii) *Medulla:* Vesicular nuclei, cranial nerve nuclei and reticular formation, which contain vital centers; (iii) *Cerebellum:* Nuclei in the roof and vermis only; (iv) *Midbrain:* Grey matter, substantia nigra, sometimes red nucleus; (v) Thalamus and hypothalamus; (vi) Pallidium; (vii) Cerebral cortex (motor cortex).

Following areas are spared:
1. Entire cerebral cortex except motor area.
2. The cerebellum except vermis and deep line nuclei.
3. The white matter of spinal cord.

In majority of cases, infection is silent. Only in minority of cases, virus passes in through all phases as above.

Epidemiology

Worldwide prevalence. Incidence is high where vaccination status is poor. In India, summer and autumn months are epidemic period with peak in August.

Age

Majority of cases below 3 years of age, peak is 2 years age. Rare after 8 years.

Clinical Features

Poliomyelitis occurs in the following stages (clinical types):
a. Asymptomatic
b. Abortive poliomyelitis

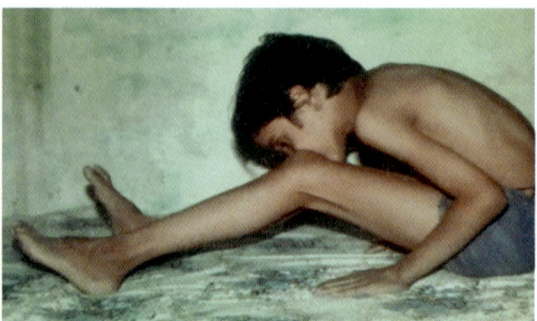

Fig. 13.4: Kiss the knee test in poliomyelitis.

c. Non-paralytic
d. Paralytic

a. **Asymptomatic (silent):** Child has no complaints. Virus can be identified in stool; this consists of 90–95% of those infected.
b. **Abortive:** Fever, malaise, bodyache, cough, coryza, vomiting and diarrhea are features of this stage. Fever subside within 36–48 hr. This stage corresponds to viremia but not affects central nervous system.
c. **Non-paralytic:** Virus have entered in central nervous system but cells are not destroyed. Following are clinical features.
   1. Fever 101–102°F, bodyache, muscle pain at back.
   2. No loss of consciousness or paralysis.
   3. Nuchal and spinal rigidity is present, which is detected by following ways.
      - **Kiss the knee test:** Direct the child to sit up and kiss his knee. Test is positive, if he fails to do so without bending the knees (Fig. 13.4).
      - **Tripod sign:** Ask the child to sit up. He assumes a tripod position, while doing so. Test is said to be positive.
      - **Kernig and Brudzinski signs** are elicited. Gentle forward flexon of occiput and neck will elicit nuchal rigidity.
      - **Head drop:** Place the hands under the patient shoulders and raise the trunk. Normally, head follows in the plane of trunk but in poliomyelitis, it often falls backward limply.

- In uncooperative patient, place the shoulders at the edge of the table supporting the occiput manually, flex anteriorly. Only true involuntary rigidity persists.

Reflexes: Reflexes are either decreased or increased. Sensory defects do not occur in poliomyelitis.

Paralytic: Paralysis is feature of this stage; paralysis due to polio has following characteristics:

1. It occurs within 1–3 days of illness and increases for 1–3 days.
2. Paralysis is flaccid, which is maximum at onset, remain stationary for about one week and then improve gradually.
3. Paralysis is asymmetrical. A large muscle groups are often involved than small muscles.
4. No loss of sensations is associated with it.
5. Paralysis is lower motor neuron type (flaccid, absent reflexes, etc.)
6. Paralysis of abdominal wall musculature produces a bulge when infant cries 'phantom hernia'. (Fig. 13.5) This is very useful sign. Paralysis occurs in following forms:

   a. **Spinal form:** Characterized by bodyache, paralysis of muscles of extremities; lower limbs are more affected than upper limbs. There may be monoplegia, diplegia, paraplegia or quadriplegia. Apart from extremities there is involvement of groups of muscles of neck, abdomen, diaphragm and intercostats'.

   Retention of urine may occur due to bladder paralysis and constipation due to paralysis of bowel.

   b. **Bulbar form:** Paralysis of cranial nerves causes difficulty in deglutition, nasal twang of speech, facial paralysis and difficulty in breathing, circulatory system and heart is affected.

   c. **Bulbospinal form:** Features of bulbar and spinal form are seen.

   d. **Encephalitic form:** Mood changes such as irritability, apathy or loss of consciousness.

Cause of death is respiratory failure due to effect on respiratory center and paralysis of diaphragm and intercostal muscles.

Complications

1. *Gastroentestinal tract:* Malena, perforation.
2. *Circulatory system:* Hypertension, tachycardia, heart block, congestive cardiac failure, myocarditis.
3. *Respiratory system:* Dyspnea, pneumonia, lung collapse, pulmonary edema.
4. *Urinary system:* Bladder paralysis, infection, stone formation.

Causes of respiratory insufficiency—respiratory insufficiency is detected by breathlessness and increased respiratory rate, causes are as follows:

   i. Pooling of secretions in the throat due to cranial nerves (9th–12th) involvement (bulbar polio).
   ii. Laryngeal involvement, either spasm or paralysis due to involvement of vagus nuclei.
   iii. Involvement of respiratory centre in bulbar polio.

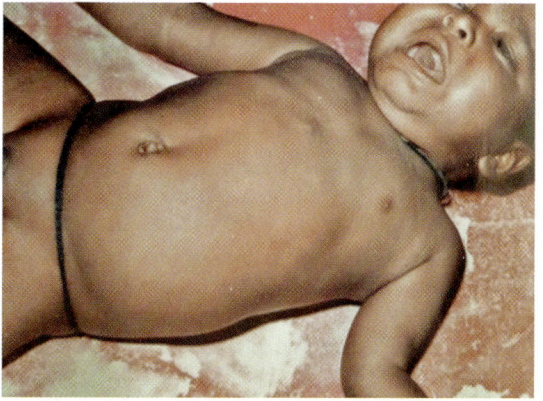

Fig. 13.5: Abdominal bulge in poliomyelitis.

Table 13.1: Differential diagnosis of poliomyelitis

Signs and symptoms	Polio	GBS	Transverse myelitis
Age of onset	less than 3 years	More than 3 years	3 years
Fever at onset	Present	Absent	Absent
Meningeal irritation	Present/absent	Absent	Absent
Muscle pain/spasm	Present	Variable	Absent
Paresthesia	No	Yes	Yes
Sensations	Normal	Diminished	Absent
Tendon reflexes	Diminished or absent	Diminished, may return in few days	Absent may return in 1–3 weeks
Paralysis	Asymmetrical	Symmetrical, ascending	Symmetrical, stationary
Progression	Less than 1 week	2 weeks	Few hours
Type	Flaccid	Flaccid	Flaccid
Residual	Yes	No	No
CSF			
Protein	Normal to slight high	High	Moderate to high
WBC	High	Normal	Normal to high

iv. Paralysis of respiratory muscles (intercostal and diaphragm) in spinal polio.

In diaphragm paralysis, there is often paradoxical movement of abdomen (during expiration abdominal wall expand) voice may be weak but not aphonic, child speaks in short jerky 'breathless'. Paralysis of diaphragm is observed better by lightly splinting the thoracic case manually and detection of effectiveness of diaphragmatic muscles. Paralysis of intercostal muscles is detected by splinting abdominal muscle manually and look for thoracic breathing.

Diagnosis

Depends on:
i. Clinical features
ii. Identification of organism in stool and throat swab and culture.
iii. *Positive serology:* Four-fold or greater rise in serum polio antibody titres. Fecal samples should be collected up to 6 weeks of onset of disease but the yield is highest in the first two weeks.

Differential Diagnosis (Table 13.1)

Acute phase (first 6 weeks)—poliomyelitis should be differentiated from Guillain-Barré syndrome, transverse myelitis and other conditions which leads to paucity of movements of affected limb(s) due to pain and, therefore, potentially be confused with poliomyelitis are trauma, sprains, septic arthritis, osteomyelitis, scurvy and rheumatic fever.

Treatment

No specific treatment is avialable.

Although poliomyelitis is usually self limiting, proper management in the early stages is important to promote recovery and to arrest progress of paralysis.

Acute Phase (First 6 Weeks)

Management in the acute phase is symptomatic. The child needs rest and care to ensure that there is no stress on affected muscles. Care is also required to see that the child does not suffer from secondary infections. Massage and injections during this period are contraindicated.

a. *Rest:* Complete bedrest is essential during acute phase, exertion should be avoided. There should be no stress on the muscles involved. The mother or attendant caring the child should be instructed to frequently change the posture of child in the bed every two to three hours. The child should be placed on the stomach for short periods each day to avoid risk of pneumonia.

b. *Positioning of limb:* The limbs should be placed in the optimum position for relaxation of paralyzed muscles with pillow, sand bags, rolled towels.

The recommended positions are—hip slight flexion; knee 5° flexion, foot 90° (support against the sole of the foot). Both the legs should be supported from lateral sides with pillows or rolled towels to prevent external rotation. Rolled towels should also be placed under the knee for positioning of hips and knees.

Passive movements of the joints: Joints of the paralyzed muscles should be moved passively, gently through their full range of motion to prevent contracture, such passive movements should be done for 10 minutes 2–3 times in a day. Such movements should involve all joints of the affected limb. The movement should be within range of pain.

Warm water fomentation: Warm water fomentation by hot packs with soaked towels wrapped around the affected parts for 10 minutes 2–3 times daily should be started as soon as possible and continued up to 6 weeks after onset.

Symptomatic treatment for fever, pain: For fever and pain, paracetamol can be given.

Diet—no restriction, normal food may be given, *constipation*—liquid paraffin given half teaspoonful under 1 year and one teaspoonful to children above one year.

For urinary retention alternate hot and cold compresses over suprapubic region may relieve transient retension. Catheterization may be needed.

Observation of progression of paralysis should be noted. Reassess after 1 week and after 6 weeks.

All the cases of upper limb paralysis and extending paralysis in a child with lower limb involvement seen in first week, should be referred to hospital. If seen later, such children can be treated at home, as the condition stabilizes after first week.

Indications for referral to hospital: Progression of paralysis, respiratory distress, bulbar involvement, paralysis of upper limbs of less than 3 days, marked drowsiness and other "complications".

Child with respiratory difficulties are hospitalized immediately. Paralysis of respiratory muscle is managed by artificial ventilation by the use of ventilator, tracheostomy is done if needed. Suction of secretions at throat is done frequently and antibiotics are given for secondary infection.

Recovery Phase (6 Weeks to 2 Years)

As the acute phase of illness subsides, the recovery of strength begins. New emphasis is shifted to active rather than passive movements and vigorous program of physical therapy is initiated to regain muscle power. It is impossible to predict about degree of recovery in the early convalescence. Maximum recovery of affected muscles takes place in the first six months. Physical therapy is necessary to prevent deformities and contractures due to muscle imbalance or improper posture.

Electrotherapy in the form of galvanic current is given to paralyzed muscles to improve circulation and prevent atrophy. Any tendency for deformity and tightening of muscles is corrected by paraffin wax baths and manipulation, stretching and use of splints.

The physiotherapy is given in intermittent courses of 2 weeks every 3 to 4 months.

Braces are used to compensate for weak muscle groups, e.g. foot drop, more severe leg weakness. Infants and young children are also given abdominal support and jackets to help in sitting in case of trunk weakness.

Physiotherapy methods

• Exercises (active and passive)
• Electrotherapy
• Hydrotherapy
• Paraffin wax baths
• Manual manipulations

Chronic Phase (Residual Paralysis after 2 Years)

Although further recovery is not expected, physiotherapy is required to prevent deformities. Children with weak and flail limbs without any fixed deformities are advised braces. But cases with contractures and fixed deformities need surgical correction before fitting callipers.

Prevention

i. Polio vaccination
ii. Gamma globulins are given to contacts to prevent attack in case of epidemic.

VACCINE DERIVED PARALYTIC POLIOMYELITIS

When a child is vaccinated, the weakened vaccine virus replicates in the intestine and enters into blood stream, triggering a protective immune response.

Child excretes the vaccine virus for a period of 6–8 weeks. As it is excreted, some of the vaccine virus may no longer be the original vaccine virus. Virus as it has genetically altered during replication this is called vaccine derived poliovirus (PDPV).

So, on very rare occasion strain of poliovirus in OPV may change and revert to that may also to cause paralysis in human it is called vaccine derived paralytic poliomyelitis (VDPP).

90% of vaccine derived polio cases are due to serotype 2 of strain of trivalent vaccine. So, to eliminate the vaccine derived polio cases this strain (type 2) is removed and bivalent polio vaccine is used. Switch over from trivalent (TOPV) to bivalent (BOPV) vaccine is done in April 2016.

Inactivated vaccine (IPV) is now included in UIP along with OPV. It gives humoral antibodies, and prevent VDPP cases.

MUMPS

This is a viral disease, characterized by swelling of parotid glands. Swelling of other salivary glands may also occur (Fig. 13.6).

This is an cosmopolitan disease. Commonly occurs in winter and spring. More common in urban than rural areas.

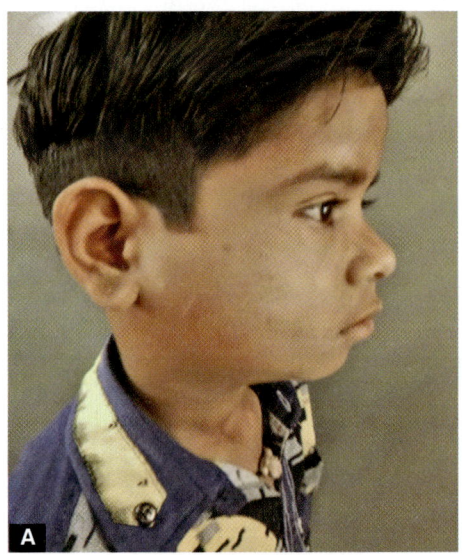

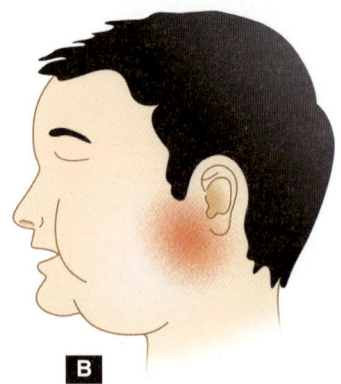

Fig. 13.6A and B: Mumps (site of swelling).

Epidemiology

Human is only reservoir of this disease. There in no carrier. Mumps is a contagious disease caused by virus that passes from one person to another through saliva, nasal secretions and contact.

Transplacental antibodies protect the infant. Mumps infection or immunization gives lifelong immunity.

Mumps mostly occurs 5–15 years of age.

Clinical Features

1. Incubation period is 17 days (12–24 days). Child suffers from bodyache, chills, pyrexia and earache. Earache is more during eating. These symptoms last for 2–3 days.
2. The swelling appears on lower and in front and behind the ear due to parotitis which is tender and painful. Pain lasts for 1–3 days but swelling takes 7–10 days to subside. Parotitis may be unilateral or bilateral.
3. This manifests as earache, jaw tenderness while chewing, dryness of mouth and swelling at the angle of jaw. The ear lobe may appear to be pushed upwards and outwards.
4. Sometimes submaxillary gland is effected, which causes swelling below jaw and sublingual gland causes swelling and pain below tongue.

Diagnosis

Depends on:
i. Clinical features
ii. Blood examination for detection of antibodies against mumps
iii. Serum amylase elevated.

Complications

i. Orchitis–epididymitis—causes pain and swelling of testis. Pyrexia and testicular atrophy, common in adolescent boys or postpubertal men.
ii. Meningitis and encephalitis may be fatal.
iii. Paralysis of cranial nerves causes facial paralysis, squint and deafness.

iv. Pancreatitis
v. Myocarditis
vi. Nephritis
vii. Thyroiditis
viii. Arthritis

Treatment

No specific treatment is available, symptomatic treatment is as follows:
1. Rest to patient for about 10 days.
2. Diet: Semisolid or liquid diet is given.
3. Care of oral hygiene is essential.
4. Pain is relieved by aspirin and fever by paracetamol.
5. Hot fomentation for swelling.
6. Orchitis is treated by bedrest. Ice is applied to testicle and support is given. Steroids are given. ACTH or in case of intolerable pain 1% Xylocaine in spermatic cord at external inguinal ring. Oxyphenbutazone for relief of pain.

Prevention

MMR vaccination—12–15 months of age
Second vaccination—4–6 years of age

HUMAN IMMUNODEFICIENCY VIRUS (HIV)
(ACQUIRED IMMUNODEFICIENCY SYNDROME: AIDS)

Epidemiology

Worldwide more than 1 million children have AIDS and as many as 10 times of this number are infected with HIV.

Transmission

a. Perinatal transmission from mother to infant accounts for more than 95% pediatric HIV.
b. Sexual contact—important mode of infection in adolescents.
c. Blood product transfusion
d. Sharing of intravenous needles

In utero intrapartum or postpartum (through breastfeeding) transmission of HIV from an infected mother to her infant takes place.

Risk Factors

- High maternal viral load
- Advanced maternal HIV infections
- Maternal genital infections
- Premature birth
- Prolonged rupture of membranes

Clinical Features

Most of the infants are asymptomatic early symptoms of HIV infection include failure to thrive, thrombocytopenia, recurrent infections, lymphadenopathy, parotitis, loss of developmental mile stone.

Diagnosis

All infants to HIV infected mothers have transplacental acquired antibody that may be detected for a long 15–24 months.

HIV specific DNA PCR: Positive in newborn who is infected. It is detected in all infants until 4 months of age. Negative result at 4 months of age means infant is not infected.

Complications

Opportunistic infections—more chances of fungal, viral, parasitic infections.

Management

Infant born to HIV infection, if positive

i. Zidovudine for 6 weeks to post-exposure prophylaxis.
ii. Trimethoprim/sulfamethoxazole prophylaxis for *Pneumocystis carinii* pneumonia, until HIV is negative at age of 4 months.
iii. No breastfeeding.

Management of HIV Infected Children

i. Antiretroviral agents
- Nucleoside reverse transcriptase inhibitors (NRTIs)
- Non-nucleoside reverse transcriptase inhibitors (NNRTIs)
- Protease inhibitors combined therapy to avoid selection of resistant virus.
ii. Prophylaxis for opportunistic infection

iii. Immunization—all routine vaccine should be given.
iv. Routine laboratory tests—HIV, RNA, PCR to assess viral load.
v. Ophthalmic examination to assess cytomegalovirus retinitis.
vi. Urine culture for cytomegalovirus to detect coinfections.

CHIKUNGUNYA

It is an acute viral disease characterized by fever, arthritis and skin rash.

Epidemiology: Chikungunya fever is an acute viral disease transmitted by the bite of infected *Aedes aegypti* mosquito.

The term is derived from *kungunyala* meaning to become contorted or more specifically as 'that what bands up' this refer to the stooped posture adopted by the patient as a result of arthritic symptoms.

This is a self-limiting disease and rarely fatal, maximum cases occur in rainy season (mosquito's season of breeding).

Clinical Features

Incubation period is usually 3–12 days. There is sudden onset of symptoms flues like such as severe headache, chills, fever of high grade, arthralgia, or arthritis. Conjunctival suffusion, mild photophobia, nausea and vomiting are usually associated.

Joints of extremities are swollen painful to touch which in some cases last to longer time.

Maculopapular or patechial rash may be seen on skin of limb. Fever lasts for few days.

Enephalopathy is also rare manifestation.

Fatality is due to thrombocytopenia or shock.

Diagnosis

1. Clinical features
2. Detection of virus specific IgM and antibody in blood detected by ELISA test and hemagglutination inhibition assays.
3. Polymerase chain reaction to confirm the disease.

Treatment

No specific treatment.

Symptomatic

1. Rest
2. Fluid
3. Analgesic—ibuprofen, acetaminophen or paracetamol. Aspirin should be avoided.

Acute Flaccid Paralysis

Acute flaccid paralysis (AFP) is defined as a sudden onset of paralysis weakness of the body of a child less than 15 years of age. WHO launched AFP surveillance program of all AFP cases to detect AFP is due to polio or not. Two sample of stool is taken at 24 hours interval and identified for presence of virus.

Causes of AFP

Peripheral neuropathy
1. Gullain-Barré syndrome
2. Acute axonal neuropathy
3. Neuropathies of infectious disease (diphtheria, Lyme disease)
4. Arthropod bite
5. Focal mononeuropathy

Anterior horn cell disease
1. Acute anterior poliomyelitis
2. Vaccine associated paralytic polio
3. Other neurotropic virus (anteroviruses and herpesviruses)

Muscle Disorders

- Polymyositis
- Dermatomyositis
- Periodic paralysis
- Corticosteroids and blocking agents
- Post-viral myositis

Disorders of neuromuscular transmission
- Myasthenia gravis
- Botulism
- Insecticide—organophosphorus poisoning
- Tick bite paralysis
- Snakebite

Systemic disease
- Porphyrias
- Critical illness neuropathy
- Acute myopathy in ICU patient

Acute myopathy
Cord compression.

Demyelinating diseases
- Multiple sclerosis
- Transverse myelitis
- Acute disseminated encephalomyelitis (ADEM)
- Ischemic cord damage.

DENGUE INFECTION

This is an acute viral infection characterized by fever, myalgia, arthralgia and rash.

Epidemiology

1. It is transmitted by mosquito vector *Aedes aegypti* by the bite of mosquito.
2. Dengue viruses (4 serotypes) are arbovirus.
3. Incubation period is 8–10 days. The virus circulate in the blood of infected person for two to seven days. Person suffers from fever. Aedes mosquito may acquire infection when they suck the blood of person in this time.

Pathophysiology

Person suffering from acute dengue infection causes abnormal hemostasis, thrombocytopenia, there is generation of antibodies against dengue virus protein (especially NSI) which react platelets and cause thrombocytopenia. Disseminated intravascular coagulation, liver injury and thrombocytopenia, all together results hemorrhagic tendency. Central nervous system is attributed to direct neurotropic effect of dengue virus.

Virus causes hemodynamic alteration, generalized vascular congestion and increased permeability, and mast cell recruitment in lungs. No gross or microscopic lesion is detected causing death. Only gastrointestinal and intracranial bleeding is attributed.

Clinical Manifestations

Incubation period is 4–10 days. Most infections are subclinical. Febrile illness is only presenting clinical manifestations in young children.

In older children and adult clinical manifestations are divided in three phases.

1. Febrile Phase

Fever lasts for 2–7 days, headache, retro-orbital pain, muscle and joint pain, rash and hemorrhagic manifestations.

2. Critical Phase

Bleeding and shock may occur. Some patients develop nephritis, encephalitis or myocarditis. Severe bleeding may lead to shock, platelet count is low, increase in hematocrit on blood examination.

3. Recovery Phase

After 24–48 hours of critical phase child improves, appetite recurs. Gastrointestinal symptoms subside, some patient may have rash.

Bradycardia, pruritus, respiratory distress due to pulmonary edema may develop. Blood picture shows increasing while blood cell count, platelets count increase take long time.

Differential Diagnosis

Dengue should be differentiated from influenza, malaria, enteric fever, leptospirosis, hemorrhagic fevers, meningococcemia, rickettsial infection.

Clinical Criteria for Diagnosis

1. High grade fever
2. Hemorrhagic manifestations (at least one positive torniquet test)
3. Hepatomegaly—tender
4. Effusion—pleural, peritoneal, shock.

Laboratory Criteria

1. Thrombocytopenia (<100000 cells/cumm or 1–2 platelets per oil immersion field)
2. Hematocrit—elevated

Others

3. Leucocyte count—low
4. Total serum—low
5. Transaminase protein—increase
6. SGPT, SGOT—raised
7. Serum sodium—raised

X-ray chest and USG

For detection of pleural effusion and ascites.

Confirmations of dengue

1. Direct method
   - Isolation of virus by culture
   - Genome detection by PCR
   - NSI antigen detection
2. Indirect method
   - IgM detection
   - IgG detection

Management

No specific treatment for dengue fever exists. Patient of dengue is treated as per following guidelines:

1. Undifferentiated fever—give paracetamol
2. Without warning signs:
   a. Fever and body aches are treated with paracetamol. Salicylates and other non-steroidal drugs should be avoided, these may lead to bleeding tendency.
   b. Plenty of fluids—orally
   c. Monitor any warning signs
3. With warning signs: Patient if have one of the warning signs such as:
   a. Abdominal pain or tenderness
   b. Persistent vomiting
   c. Clinical fluid accumulation
   d. Bleeding from mucosal sites
   e. Restlessness
   f. Lethargy
   g. Liver enlargements—more than 2 cm

h. Laboratory findings
- Increase in packed cell count (hematocrit)
- Decrease in platelet count: If child has above warning signs. Treat as follows:
  - Fluids

    Intravenous fluids—Ringer lactate at rate of 7 ml/kg over one hour. If child improves, rate is reduced 5 ml/kg over next hour and then 3 ml/kg for 24–48 hours. Monitor blood pressure, oral intake, blood examination (hematocrit).

If no improvement
- Fluid rate increased 10 ml/kg over next hour then 15 ml/kg.
- Colloid and plasma infusion (10 ml/kg) is administered.

If improves

Fluid rate reduced to 10 ml/kg

Severe dengue

If child is having following signs:
1. Shock
2. Respiratory distress
3. Severe organ involvement—liver, CNS, heart.

Management

A. Normal saline or Ringer lactate 10–20 ml/kg infused over 1 hour or as bolus.
B. IV 5% dextrose and potassium is introduced in second, IV line.

If no improvement
1. Colloid 10 ml/kg is introduced. Blood transfusion should be done with care (decrease infusion rate).

2. Oxygen is introduced to all patient with shock.
3. Management of bleeding:
   a. Mild bleeding stable patient—rest, maintenance of hydration. Do not give intramuscular injection.
   b. Severe bleeding unstable patient
      - Blood transfusion
      - Platelets rich plasma
   c. Fluid overload, stable patient, reduce IV fluids, avoid diuretics, introduce blood transfusion carefully.

Supporting care
1. Organ dysfunction (liver, kidney) should be treated.
2. No use of corticosteroids, immunoglobulins or recombinant activated factor seventh.
3. Antibiotics are introduced in superadded bacterial infection.
4. Blood transfusion is indicated if hematocrit is not improving.
5. Oxygen—in all cases of shock

Monitoring

Heart rate, blood pressure, respiratory rate should be monitored in every 30 min. Urine output assessed.

Prognosis: It is a self-limiting disease but mortality is 20–30% in untreated cases.

Prevention

Elimination of mosquito and larvae specially in rainy season. Mesocyclops, selfish are executed to eat and eliminate larvae of *Aedes aegypti*.

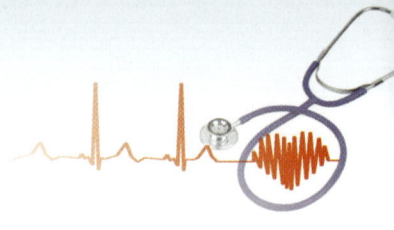

14

Parasitic Diseases

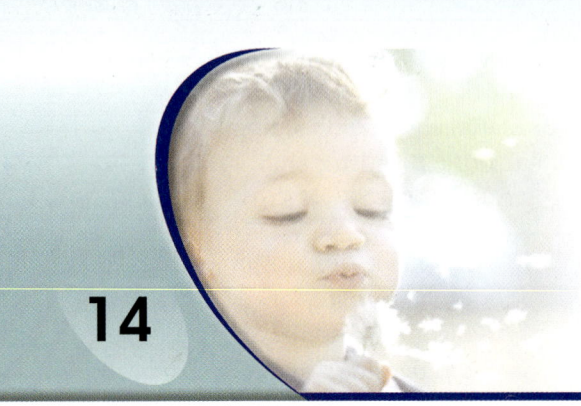

WORM INFESTATIONS

Worm infestations are quite common in India, where sanitary and hygienic conditions are not good and common in children. Generally, infestation is by many worms simultaneously, it is called polyparasitism.

ENTEROBIASIS
(OXYURIASIS, THREADWORM, PINWORM)

This is most common worm infestation caused by *Enterobius vermicularis*. Male is 2–5 mm long, curved; female is 8–13 mm long. Common site is caecum or appendix into intestine.

Clinical Features

Worms are seen mixed in stool of the patient. Itching is common around anus, especially at night. Skin becomes red due to itching. Some patients are irritable, not having proper sleep at night. Loss of appetite and abdominal pain is common. Bruxism and eneuresis are often clinical features may be associated with pinworm infestation.

Vulvovaginitis may occur in girls due to its entrance through genitals.

Diagnosis

Perianal swab: Eggs can be demonstrated in perianal swab taken early in the morning before defecation.

Treatment

1. Albendazole—400 mg once (oral) repeat after 2 weeks.
2. Mebendazole—100 mg once repeat after 2 weeks.
3. Pyrantel pamoate—11 mg/kg (max 1 gm) repeat after 2 weeks.

General Treatment

a. Nails should be cut and cleaned with brush because ova scratched due to itching remains in them and ingested during taking feed.
b. Itching is treated by ammoniated mercury ointment locally.

ASCARIASIS (ROUNDWORMS)

Ascaris lumbricoides is common worm found in children. This is 20 cm long and shape is like earthworm.

Clinical Features

Pain and distension of abdomen are common symptoms. Growth failure, anemia, pica may be associated with it.

In some patients itching, irritability and diarrhea may be seen. Obstruction is due to collection of worms in intestine. Worms pass through stool or in vomitus sometimes.

Larva in lungs may cause pneumonia. Liver enlargement and convulsions also seen in a few cases.

Diagnosis

Stool examination: Presence of eggs in the stool sometimes adult worms are seen in stool or vomitus.

Treatment

1. Albendazole
   Dose: 400 mg once (oral)
2. Mebendazole
   Dose: 100 mg two times in a day for 3 days or 500 mg once (oral)
3. Ivermectin
   Dose: 150–200 mg/kg once (oral)
4. Nitazoxamide
   Dose: 1–3 years 100 mg q 12 hr
   4–11 years 200 mg q 12 hr
   >11 years 500 mg q 12 hr

HOOKWORMS (ANKYLOSTOMIASIS)

This is caused by *Ancylostoma duodenale.* Common in barefooted children. Hookworm infestation is common cause of anemia in children.

Clinical Manifestations

Loss of appetite and pain in abdomen are common symptoms. Anemia gradually increases and child becomes malnourished. Pica is also a feature of hookworm infestation. Anemia causes edema in different parts of body then afterward resulting into anasarca. Tachycardia and tachypnea are other symptoms due to anemia.

Itching may occur at the entry place of larva in the body.

Diagnosis

Depends on clinical features are:
   i. *Stool examination:* Identification of ova.
   ii. *Blood:* RBCs are hypochromic, microcytic.

Treatment

1. Albendazole—400 mg once (oral)
2. Mebendazole—100 mg q 12 hr in a day for 3 days
3. Pyrantel pamoate—11 mg/kg base (maximum 1 gm) daily for 3 days.

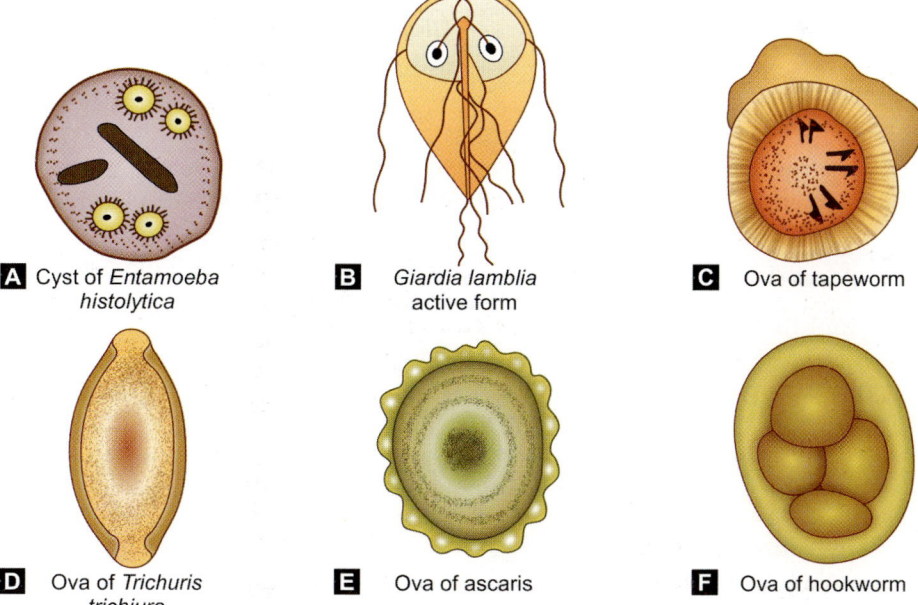

| A | Cyst of *Entamoeba histolytica* | B | *Giardia lamblia* active form | C | Ova of tapeworm |
| D | Ova of *Trichuris trichiura* | E | Ova of ascaris | F | Ova of hookworm |

Fig. 14.1A to F: Common parasites

TAPEWORM INFESTATION

Worms are like tape, which are seen sometimes in stool. Abdominal pain, loss of appetite, diarrhea and malnutrition are common clinical manifestations.

Treatment

1. Praziquantel
   Dose: 5–10 mg/kg once (drug of choice)
2. Niclosamide
   Dose: 50 mg/kg once

TRICHURIASIS

This is caused by *Trichuris trichiura.*

Clinical Features

Common symptoms are dysentery mixed with blood, abdominal cramps and anemia. Diagnosis is made by examination of stool for identification of ova.

Treatment

i. Mebendazole 100 mg in two divided doses for 3 days.
ii. Thiobendazole 200 mg in three divided doses.
iii. Ivermectin 200 mg/kg once daily for 3 days.

INTESTINAL PROTOZOA
(AMOEBIASIS)

Amoebiasis is caused by *Entamoeba histolytica;* more common in adult than children.

Clinical Features

Amoeba causes vague symptoms; mild abdominal pain, diarrhea or dysentery are common symptoms. Dysentery increases in frequency resulting passage of mucus and blood through rectum or only blood. Abdominal cramps are associated with it. Mild pyrexia is sometimes associated with it.

Complications cause liver enlargement or liver abscess which causes pyrexia, pain in abdomen on right side. Liver is tender. Sometimes, signs of intestinal perforation or obstruction are seen.

Diagnosis

- *Stool examination*
  - Presence of motile trophozoites, cysts.
  - Few leukocytes, plenty of RBCs
- *Serological tests*—ELISA, IHA and IFA. These tests are used to identify extraintestinal amoebiasis. IHA is very sensitive and specific.
- X-ray chest, ultrasound, CT, and MRI are used to localize liver abscess.

Treatment

1. Metronidazole—35–50 mg/kg/day for 7–10 days in 3 divided doses.
2. Tinidazole—50 mg/kg/day once daily for 3 days.

GIARDIASIS

Giardiasis is caused by *Giardia lamblia.* This is an important cause of morbidity in children.

Clinical Features

Mild abdominal pain and diarrhea are common features. Foul smelling stool, recurrent diarrhea is common. Loss of appetite, pica causes malnutrition.

Diagnosis

- *Stool examination*
  - Identification of *Giardia lamblia*
  - No blood in stool
- *Enzyme immunoassay* (EIA and direct fluorescent antibody test for Giardia antigens in stool have better sensitivity
- Duodenal aspirate or biopsy.
  - Presence of trophozoites is suggestive.

Treatment

- Tinidazole—50 mg/kg single dose (max 2 g)
- Metronidazole—5–10 mg/kg orally q 8 hr for 7 days (max 250 mg)
- Nitazoxanide
  Age 1–3 years 100 mg orally q 12 hr 3 days
  4–11 years 200 mg orally q 12 hr 3 days
  >11 years 500 mg orally q 12 hr 3 days

Alternative agents—albendazole, mebendazole, paromomycin, furazolidone, quinacrine.

Followed by:

Paramomycin: 25–35/kg/day for 7 days (in 3 divided doses)

Or

Diloxanide furoate: 20 mg/kg/day for 7 days (in 3 divided doses)

Or

Iodoquinol: 30–40 mg/kg/day for 20 days (in 3 divided doses)

Liver abscess

• Medical treatment with drugs—same as above.
• Aspiration is generally not required but indicated if patient is not improving by metronidazole or large abscess or when diagnosis is uncertain (pyogenic abscess or else).

MALARIA

This is common protozoal infection caused by Plasmodium, characterized by high fever, splenomegaly and anemia.

Etiology

Following species of malaria parasite causes this disease.

1. *Plasmodium vivax*
2. *Plasmodium falciparum*
3. *Plasmodium malariae*
4. *Plasmodium ovale*.

Parasites enter in the body due to bite of female Anopheles mosquito and multiply in liver and enter in red blood cells and liberate toxin after rupture of red blood cells and produce symptoms.

Clinical Features

Contrary to the adult, in children disease is not associated with rigors. Below 5 years of age high fever, irritability, headache are only symptoms. Fever is followed by sweating.

On examination, splenomegaly or hepatomegaly and anemia of various grades are found. Sometimes, pain in abdomen, vomiting, convulsion or loss of consciousness are also seen.

Child, who suffers from malaria first time, does not have immunity, resulting more serious illness. Irritability, loss of appetite, excessive crying, lack of sleep are other symptoms found. Sometime, fever is quite high (even up to 105°F or no pyrexia).

Children who suffered from malaria many times are semi-immune and have mild symptoms.

P. falciparum causes continuous fever. Other clinical features of malaria are as follows:

a. *Algid malaria:* Shock, unconsciousness and cold and calmy skin are its manifestations.
b. *Renal failure:* Anuria and retension of urine.
c. *Hyperpyrexia:* High fever causes convulsions irrelevant speech or exitation.
d. *Gastrointestinal:* Diarrhea, vomiting or dysentery.

Chronic Malaria

When child suffers from malaria many times; such child suffers from growth retardation, anemia, splenomegaly or hepatosplenomegaly. Sometimes, splenomegaly is massive.

Diagnosis
Blood Smear

Thick smear: For quick identification of malaria parasite (Fig. 14.2).

Thin smear: For identification of species.

Smear may be negative after partial treatment or sequestration of parasitized red blood cells in vascular bed. Repeat smear 6–8 hourly.

Quantitative buffy coat

• Centrifuge the blood.
• Stain compressed RBC with acridine orange
• Examine under UV light source.

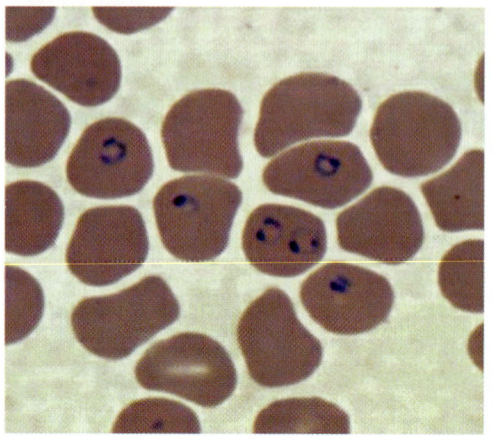

Fig. 14.2: Peripheral blood film showing malaria parasite in RBCs

Rapid diagnostic test

It detects malaria antigen from sexual or asexual forms of malaria parasite with the help of test strips as color changes on antibody coated lines on the strip. It has lower sensitivity.

Polymerase chain reaction (PCR)

Highly sensitive test but not available commercially and has limited value.

Treatment

Specific Treatment

It consists of giving chloroquine.

National Malaria Control Programme recommended following dose schedule for chloroquine.

Age (years)	Chloroquine tab 250 mg with 150 mg base	Primaquine (daily)
0–1	½ tab once	Nil
1–4	1 tab once	2.5 mg
5–8	2 tab once	5 mg
9–12	3 tab once	10 mg
12–14	4 tab once	15 mg
Adult		

If malaria parasite is found in blood smear. Primaquine is given from second day for 5 days. Drugs are given after food. They may cause gastritis, gastric ulcer, if given on empty stomach.

Oral dose: 15 mg/kg.

Parenteral Treatment

Parenteral administration of chloroquine in children should be avoided because it may cause shock, parenteral administration is indicated in following situation.

   i. If child is vomiting continuously
   ii. Unconcious patient
   iii. Child is unable to take due to bitter taste.

Dose: 5 mg/kg body weight, per day generally given intramuscularly.

Uncomplicated malaria	P. vivax malaria	
Drug of choice	**Doses**	
Chloroquine	Total	25 mg/kg (oral)
	First	10 mg/kg
	Second	5 mg/kg after 6 hours
	Third	5 mg/kg after 24 hours
	Fourth	5 mg/kg after 48 hours
Radical therapy		
Primaquine	0.25–0.3 mg/kg/day for 14 days	

Given to reduce risk of relapse. Contraindicated in infant, breastfeeding mothers and G6PD deficiency patient (should be checked before giving primaquine).

Note: Quinine and pyrimethamine–sulfadoxine do not have adequate activity.

Mixed malaria (uncomplicated)

P. falciparum malaria with artemisinin based combination therapy (ACT). Primaquine is used for radical cure as mentioned previously.

Complicated or severe malaria

Any of the following criteria is present with a sexual parasitemia with *P. falciparum* or

P. vivax is termed complicated or *severe malaria*.

- Coma or altered consciousness.
- Convulsions
- Deep breathing, respiratory distress.
- Sign of shock, circulatory collapse, cold and calmy skin
- Clinical jaundice
- Hemoglobinuria
- Prostration
- Failure to feed
- Abnormal bleeding from any site
- Pulmonary edema detected radiologically.

Laboratory Investigations

- Blood glucose <40 mg/dl, serum creatinine >265 µmol/L
- Plasma bicarbonate <15 mg/dl
- Anemia (Hb <5 g/dl, PCV <15%)
- Urine—presence of hemoglobin
- Hyperlactatemia (lactate >5 mmol/L).
  P. falciparum malaria (uncomplicated)
  Drug of choice
  (ACT: Artemisinin-based combination therapy)
- Artemether + lumefantrine (tab—20 mg artemether and lumefantrine 120 mg.

  Dose: 6 doses at 0, 8, 24, 36, 48 and 60 hr.

Child weight (in kg)	5–14	15–24	25–34	>35
Dose	1 tab	2 tab	3 tab	4 tab

Other drugs

- Mefloquine (250 mg tab) 15 mg/kg
  First dose   10 mg/kg
  Second dose   after 8 hr
- Pyrimethamine sulfadoxine 1.25 mg/kg single dose
- Doxycycline 3.5 mg/kg/day for 7 days
- Clindamycin 10 mg/kg twice daily
- Quinine 10 mg/kg thrice daily for 5–7 days

Note: Chloroquine is not used for treatment of *P. falciparum* malaria. Oral quinine, clindamycin and doxycycline can be used at the age more than 8 years.

Treatment of complicated or severe malaria

It is a medical emergency because mortality is about 20% in severe malaria. Choice of drugs is artemisinin or quinine. Drugs are given parenterally.

a. *Artemisinin-based therapy*
   1. Artesunate—2.4 mg/kg IV (as bolus) stat, repeat after 12, 24 hr and then daily for 6 days
   2. Artemether—3.2 mg/kg IM followed by 1.6 mg/kg for 6 days

b. *Quinine-based therapy:* Quinine dihydrochloride
   - 20 mg salt/kg IV (loading dose) diluted in 10 ml/kg of normal saline or dextrose over a period of 4 hours at the onset of treatment.
   - Then 10 mg salt/kg as infusing every 8 hours internal.

Intramuscular administration is also alternative if facilities for IV not available, dose is reduced to 5–7 mg salt/kg to avoid quinine toxicity. Artemisinin is very less toxic as compared to quinine, as patient improves, parasitemia abates, quinine can be given orally.

Total duration of quinine therapy is 7 days.
Side effects of quinine—prolongation of QTC interval, hypoglycemia, intravascular hemolysis, or black water fever.

Supportive Care

- Good nursing care, oxygen therapy, monitoring of TPR, assessment of improvement with laboratory finding.
  Investigation: Broad-spectrum antibiotics aminoglycosides are indicated if localized signs of bacterial infection present.
- Cold sponging for hyperpyrexia.
- Packed cell transfusion in severe anemia.
- Give 50% glucose 1 ml/kg if hypoglycemia.

- Metabolic acidosis corrected by IV soda bicarbonate.
- Shock: Blood culture done, administer broad spectrum antibiotics.
- Hemolysis: Give packed cell transfusion.
- Exchange transfusion: If hyperparasitemia.
- Anticonvulsants for treatment of convulsions.

FILARIASIS

Filariasis is caused by *Wuchereria bancrofti, Brugia malayi.* It is thread-like parasite lives in lymphatic system.

Clinical Features

Acute manifestations of filariasis are recurrent attacks of fever, lymph nodes inflammation (lymphadenitis) and lymph vessels inflammation (lymphangitis).

Recurrent attacks are common. Both lower and upper limbs are effected. Genital involvement occurs in bancroftian infection.

Chronic stage results elephantiasis (Fig. 14.3), hydrocoele, chyluria, lymphadema.

Diagnosis

- Identification of worms in the blood film, biopsy of lymph nodes.
- Lymphoscintigraphy—abnormality in lymph vessels.

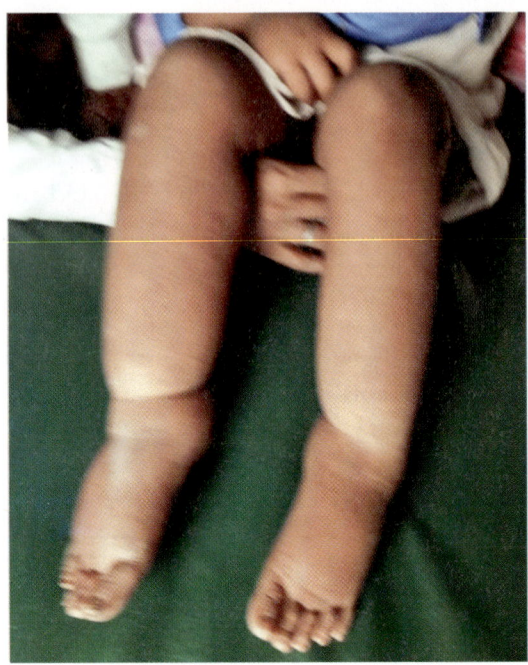

Fig. 14.3: Elephantiasis.

Treatment

1. Diethylcarbamazine
   Dose: 2 mg/kg q 8 hr (orally) for 12 days. Repeat to eradicate infection.
2. Ivermectin and albendazole combination once is also effective.

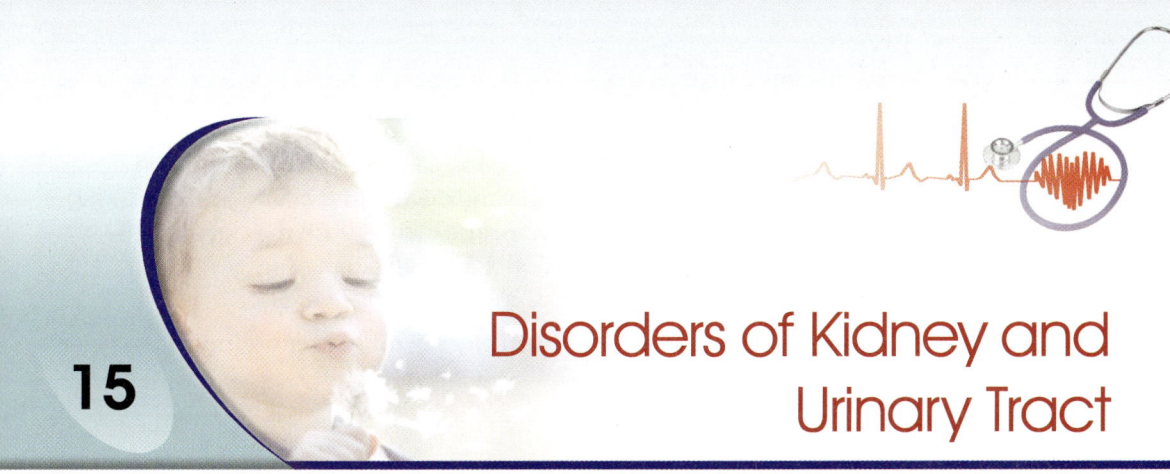

15

Disorders of Kidney and Urinary Tract

Special Points Regarding Urinary System in Children

i. Bladder is abdominal organ in infancy and early childhood, as pelvis is not enough to contain it, so it is easily palpable compared to adult.

ii. Histologically, up to 35th week, kidney of fetus appears immature.

iii. In infants, kidney works adequately for normal purpose but has very little reserve. Concentration power is small, that is why kidney requires relatively large quantity of water in order to excrete electrolytes efficiently.

URINARY TRACT INFECTIONS (UTI)

Etiology

Common in children.

UTI common in females due to short urethra. Presence of congenital anomalies, instrumentation of urinary tract predispose to UTI.

Common organsisms: E. coli, Klebsiella, Proteus, Staphylococcus and virus.

Pathogenesis

Most bacteria enter the urinary tract by ascending through urethra. Adherence of bacteria to urothelium is a bacterial property, that increases the UTI.

Clinical Features

In neonates: Symptoms are nonspecific. Neonates become lethargic, febrile, irritable, develops jaundice.

In older children: Fever, vomiting and irritability increased frequency of micturition, pain or incontinence, abdominal colic, bed wetting are common symptoms. Tenderness is present at flanks. Hematuria is occasional. Pyelonephritis (upper urinary tract infection) is associated with high fever, flank pain, vomiting and dehydration.

Diagnosis

In neonates and infants: Urine for culture must be collected suprapubic aspiration or by sterile urethral catheterization. A clean 'bagged' urine sample is adequate for urinalysis but not for culture.

In older children: Who can void on command a 'clean catch' urine sample is adequate for culture.

Culture immediately because bacteria multiply fast on room temperature or urine sample refrigerated immediately until it can be cultured.

Urinalysis

- Presence of leukocytes on microscopy (>5–10 WBC/HPF)

- Positive nitrite or leukocyte esterase on dipstick.

Urine culture: Best method to identify UTI.

Colony count: >10,000 colonies in sample obtained by sterile urethral catheterization.
>50,000–1,00000 colonies of a single organism in urine collected by clean catch technique.

Occurrence of significant bacteriuria in absence of symptoms is termed asymptomatic bacteriuria.

Imaging
- Ultrasonography: To detect structural abnormality.
- Micturating cystourethrogram: For diagnosis and grading of vesicourethral reflex and defines urethral or bladder anatomy.
- DMSA scintigraphy: For detection of cortical scars.

Treatment

Cystitis is treated for 7–10 days and pyelonephritis is treated for 14 days. Emperic antibiotic therapy should be started in symptomatic patient with uncertain urinalysis culture and sensitivity.

Infant below 3 years of age and children with complicated UTI.
- Parenteral antibiotics
  Ceftriaxone: 70–100 mg/kg/day in divided doses
  Cefotaxime: 100–150 mg/kg/day in divided doses
  Amikacin: 10–15 mg/kg/day single dose IV, IM
  Gentamicin: 5–6 mg/kg/day single dose IV, IM
  Coamoxiclav: 30–35 of amoxicillin in 2 divided doses.

Once oral intake improve usually in 48–72 hours, parenteral therapy is switched to oral therapy.

Oral
- Cifixime: 8–10 mg/kg in 2 divided doses
- Coamoxiclav (amoxicillin 35–35 mg/kg)
- Ciprofloxacin: 10–20 mg/kg
- Ofloxacin: 15–20 mg/kg
- Cephalexin: 50–70 mg/kg

Culture sensitivity report indicates specific antibiotic use.

Other measures
1. Antipyretic for pyrexia.
2. Instruct patient to take more fluid and empty bladder to prevent stasis.
3. Alkalizers of urine not routinely indicated.

Prevention

Indicated in patient with vesicoureteric reflux, single dose at bedtime.

Drug	Dose (mg/kg)
Cotrimoxazole (trimethoprim)	1–21
Nitrofurantoin	1–2
Cephalexin	10
Cefadroxil	5

Because of risk of renal scarring after pyelonephritis in infants they should receive low dose prophylactic antibiotic for at least 3 months.

ACUTE POST-STREPTOCOCCAL GLOMERULONEPHRITIS

This is a disease characterized by gross hematuria, edema, hypertension and renal insufficiency and resulting from prior beta-hemolytic streptococci infection.

Etiology

This results secondary to streptococcal infection (nephritogenic strains of group A beta-hemolytic streptococci) at throat (serotype 12) or skin (serotype 49).

Pathology

All glomeruli are large and ischemic, show mesangial cell proliferation with an increase in mesangial matrix with infiltration of leukocytes.

Immunofluorescent study shows deposition of lumps on the epithelial aspect of glomerular basement membrane.

Mechanism by which streptococci induce immune complex formation, is not yet determined.

Clinical Manifestations

Disease is rare below 3 years of age. Develops after one or two weeks of streptococcal infection. Patient may be asymptomatic with microscopic hematuria. Onset is acute with puffiness around eyes (Fig. 15.1) and edema due to salt and water retention. Hematuria gives characteristic appearance to urine, 'smoky brown' due to formation of acid hematin.

Varying degrees of oliguria and hypertension are present.

Nonspecific symptoms such as malaise, lethargy, abdominal and flank pain and pyrexia are associated features.

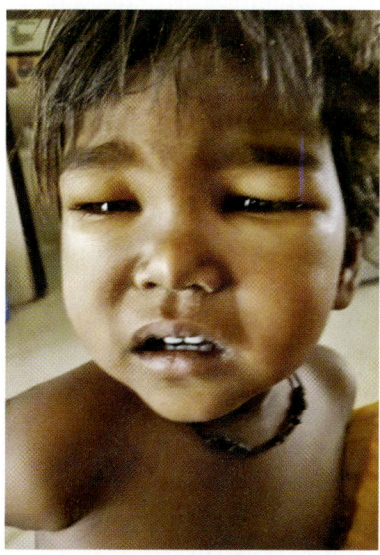

Fig. 15.1: Acute nephritis.

Acute stage subsides within 1 month but hematuria may persist for more than 1 year.

Gross hematuria

Oliguria: Urine volume less than 0.5 ml/kg/ hours

Diagnosis

 i. Clinical
 ii. *Urine examination:* Gross-smoky dirty brown urine.
Protein—one+ or two++
RBC—several RBCs/HPF
WBC and granular casts may be present
 iii. *Blood*
  1. Normocytic anemia due to hemodilution.
  2. ESR raised.
  3. Blood urea raised as per severity of illness.
  4. Serum creatinine raised.
  5. Serum potassium increased.
  6. ASO titer high, anti-DNase, anti-hyaluronidase titer high; serum complement normal within 5–6 weeks.
 iv. *X-ray chest:* Prominent vascular marking.
 v. *Throat swab culture:* Occasionally shows hemolytic streptococci.

Investigations

- Blood low serum complement (C_3), normalize by 8–12 weeks.
Persistent low C_3 indicates other forms of glomerulonephritis.
- Renal biopsy is indicated if renal impairment is severe or if serum complement (C_3) fails to normalize within 8 weeks.
Renal biopsy shows mesangial cell proliferation and increased mesangial matrix.

Complications

Acute renal failure, CCF, hypertension, hyperkalemia, hyperphosphatemia, hypocalcemia, acidosis, seizures and uremia.

Differential Diagnosis

Causes of hematuria.

Treatment

There is no specific therapy. The management is that of acute renal failure.

 i. *Bedrest:* In general, activity is not restricted, only during acute phase with renal failure, bedrest is advised.

 ii. *Antibiotics:* Systemic penicillin is given for 10 days to limit the spread of streptococci. But it does not effect nature of course of disease.

 iii. *Diet*
   • Fluid restriction: Requirement is calculated by amount of urine passed and insensible water loss, overhydration is prevented.
   • Potassium, sodium and proteins are restricted.

 iv. *Weight record:* Child weight recorded. Increase in weight suggests accumulation of fluid intake is reduced. During oliguria, child loses 0.5% weight daily.

 v. *Hypertension:* Should be controlled by antihypertensive drugs.

 vi. *Left ventricular failure:* Hypertension is controlled, diuretics given. Congestive cardiac failure is managed by adequate digitalization.
   Diuretics: Patients showing with modest edema are treated with oral frusemide 1–3 mg/kg. In pulmonary edema or left ventricular failure IV frusemide (2–4 mg/kg) is indicated.

 vii. Renal failure is treated with peritoneal dialysis, hypertonic saline and cation exchange resin.

Prognosis

Prognosis is good in 95% cases. Recurrences are infrequent. It is a self-limiting disorder.

IgA nephropathy: Cause in poorly understood. Clinical features include recurrent bouts of gross hematuria associated with respiratory infections. Diagnosis is confirmed by renal biopsy which shows mesangial proliferation and increased mesangial matrix on light microscopy. Immunofluorescent microscopy shows mesangial deposition of IgA as the dominant immunoglobulin. Management is supportive. Prognosis is variable.

Henoch-Schönlein purpura (HSP) nephritis: Characterized by nonthrombocytopenic purpura on buttocks and thigh, abdominal pain, arthritis, arthralgia and gross or microscopic hematuria. Salt limiting disorder in most of the cases.

Membranoproliferative glomerulonephritis Characterized by mesangial hypercellularity and thickening of the glomerular basement membrane. It shows clinical features as post-streptococcal GN. Treatment is supportive.

Membranous nephropathy: Rare, develop heavy proteinuria and often progress to renal failure.

Systemic lupus erythematosus nephritis: Asymptomatic proteinuria or hematuria, acute nephritic syndrome or nephritic syndrome are common. It shows clinical features as malar rash, alopecia, Raynaud's phenomenon, remission and relapses are common treatment. Corticosteroids, cytotoxic drugs and calcineurin inhibitors are indicated.

HEMATURIA

Definition: Hematuria is defined as presence of red blood cells (RBCs) in urine.

Gross hematuria means hematuria is seen on voiding urine.

Causes

 I. Glomerular diseases
   a. Recurrent gross hematuria syndrome, IgA nephropathy, idiopathic hematuria, Alport syndrome.
   b. Acute post-streptococcal glomerulonephritis
   c. Membranous glomerulopathy
   d. Systemic lupus erythematosus
   e. Membranoproliferative glomerulonephritis
   f. Chronic nephritis
   g. Rapidly progressive glomerulonephritis

h. Goodpasture's disease
i. Anaphylactoid purpura
j. Hemolytic uremic syndrome
II. Infections
a. Bacterial
b. Viral
c. Tuberculosis
III. Hematologic
a. Coagulopathies
b. Thrombocytopenia
c. Sickle cell disease
d. Renal vein thrombosis
e. Stones and hypercalciuria
f. Anatomic abnormalities.
- Congenital anomalies
- Trauma
- Polycystic kidney
- Vascular abnormalities
- Tumors
- Exercise
- *Drugs:* Sulfonamide, salicylates.

IgA nephropathy is most common cause of gross hematuria. Basic pathology is IgA as predominant immunoglobulin deposited in mesangium. No effective treatment is known. Microscopic hematuria is defined as more than five RBCs per high power field in the sediment from 10 ml of centrifuged freshly voided urine.

INVESTIGATION OF A CASE OF HEMATURIA

1. *Age*
   Newborn—hemorrrhagic disease due to deficiency of vitamin K.
   Child—acute nephritis, leukemia
   Second decade—membranous glomerulonephritis.
   Sex
   Bladder stone is almost always in males. SLE common in girls.
2. *Drugs:* History of taking sulfonamide, large doses of aspirin or anticoagulants, cyclophosphamide.
3. *Previous history:* Previous history of hematuria (recurrent gross hematuria

syndrome), renal colic (stone) suprapubic pain (bladder stone).
4. *Quantity of blood:* Gross hematuria may originate from kidney. Urine is brown or cola colored or from lower urinary tract (bladder or urethra)—urine red to pink colored contain clots.
5. *Exciting causes:* Injury, instrumentation.
6. *Color:* Bright red from lower urinary tract or dark from kidney.
7. *Relation with act of micturition:* Whether blood appears at beginning of act (urethral), towards the end (vesical) mixed throughout the flow (prerenal, renal, vesical).
8. *Relation to exercise:* Whether exercise brings the attack.
9. Diurnal (stones) or nocturnal (tuberculosis of kidney).
10. *Pain:* Colicy in stones.
    Site: Lumbar in renal, at tip of penis in irritation of trigone. Hypogastric in cystitis, flank (renal vein thrombosis).
11. *Frequency of micturition*—increased in cystitis, tuberculosis of kidney.
12. *Dysuria:* Difficulty in micturition in vesical calculus.
13. *Pyrexia:* Pyelitis, cystitis.
14. *Hemorrhagic disease:* Purpura, hemophilia
15. Course: Fast progressing in renal failure, in rapidly progressive glomerulonephritis.

Physical Examination

Edema: Acute post-streptococcal glomerulonephritis, hemolytic uremic syndrome.

Hypertension: Acute post-streptococcal glomerulonephritis, membrane proliferative glomerulonephritis, polycystic disease.

Abdominal mass—unilateral or bilateral, flank mass in Wilms' tumor, hydronephrosis.

Investigations

1. *Urine:* For the presence of blood, red cells, protein, casts, absence of red cells suggest

hemoglobinuria, such as hemolysis after ingestion of primaquine in G6PD deficiency.

Microscopic hematuria seen in only microscopic examination. Protein (e.g. in acute nephritis), pus cells (pyelonephritis), crystals of uric acid and oxalate (presence of stones).

2. *Blood:* Complete blood count.
   - Anemia may be dilutional, due to result of overload in renal failure, hemolytic as a result of blood losses.
   - Reticulocyte count increases: Hemolytic state.
   - Blood film: Bizarre-shaped fragmented RBC in hemolytic uremic syndrome.
   - Antibodies presence by Coombs test, leukopenia.
   - Sickle cell anemia.
   - *Thrombocytopenia:* Decreased platelet production (malignancy), increased platelet consumption SLE, thrombocytopenic purpura, hemolytic uremic syndrome, renal vein thrombosis.
   - *Serum C$_3$ level:* Low level—glomerulonephritis, post-streptococcal, membranoproliferative chronic infection.
   - ANA titer for lupus.
3. Plain X-ray KUB area for stone
4. Intravenous pyelography to exclude structural abnormality.
5. *Cystography:* In patient with infection or in patient, in whom a lesion of lower urinary tract is suspected.
6. *Cystoscopy:* For trauma, dysurea and in sterile urine culture.
7. *DNase:* B titer or streptozyme Q test for hematuria less than 6 months duration.
8. Skin and throat culture.
9. Renal biopsy is indicated for:
   a. Persistent high grade microscopic hematuria.
   b. Microscopic hematuria, if associated with any of the following:
      - Disturbed renal function

- Proteinuria exceeding 150 mg/ 24 hours
- Hypertension
c. Second episode of gross hematuria.

NEPHROTIC SYNDROME

Definition

Nephrotic syndrome is characterized by gross proteinuria, hypoproteinemia, edema and hyperlipidemia.

Hematuria and azotemia may or may not be. Blood pressure and blood urea are usually normal.

Pathophysiology

Proteinuria is due to increased glomerular capillary wall permeability. Protein loss (albumin) generally exceeds 2 gm/day.

Hypoproteinemia

Hypoalbuminemia is due to albumin loss.

Edema

i. Is due to fall in albumin level.
ii. Due to decrease in plasma oncotic pressure resulting in transudation of fluid from intravascular compartment to interstitial space.
iii. Reduction in intravascular volume
   a. Decrease in renal perfusion pressure activating renin angiotensin aldo-

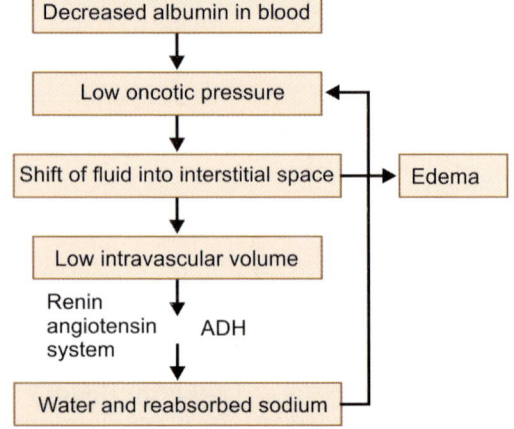

sterone system, which stimulates distal tubules reabsorption of sodium.

b. Stimulate release of antidiuretic hormone, which enhances reabsorption of water in the collecting duct; ultimately due to decreased oncotic pressure, reabsorbed sodium and water are lost in interstital space and increases the edema. Apart from above, other factors also contribute in formation of edema because patient with normal or increased intravascular volume and low renin and aldosterone, have edema. Hypothetical explanation to it is:

• In nephrotic syndrome intrarenal defect is in sodium and water, or

• Increased permeability of capillary wall throughout the body.

Hyperlipidemia

Increased triglycerides and cholesterol are due to:

i. Hypoproteinemia stimulates the generalized protein synthesis in the liver, including the lipoproteins, which is carrier to cholesterol.

ii. Lipid catabolism is reduced due to decreased level of lipoprotein lipase. It is a major enzyme that removes lipids from the plasma.

Causes

1. Idiopathic nephrotic syndrome
2. Secondary
   i. Nephritic stage of glomerulonephritis
   ii. Metabolic: Diabetes, amyloidosis
   iii. Collagen disease: SLE
   iv. Mechanical: Renal vein thrombosis
   v. Toxin: Mercury, gold, tridion
   vi. Allergy: Insect bite, snake bite
   vii. Infection: Syphilis, malaria
   viii. Anaphylactoid purpura
   ix. Congenital

Types of Lesion

i. Idiopathic—minimal change lesion in 85%.

ii. Mesangial proliferation in 5%.

iii. Focal sclerosis in 10%.

STEROID SENSITIVE NEPHROTIC SYNDROME (IDIOPATHIC NEPHROTIC SYNDROME)

Epidemiology

1. Two-thirds of cases are before the 5 years of age.
2. Ratio of boys to girls is 2:1 in young children but in adolescence both sexes are equally effected.

Etiology

Cause is unknown. Possible causes are as follows:

1. It is regarded as a sort of autoimmune disease, because it responds to immunosuppressive drugs.

   Objections are:

   i. Mechanism by which immunologic injury is produced, is not clear.

   ii. Immunosuppressive drugs have effects other than antibody formation.

2. It may be due to thymus derived (T cell) lymphocyte function probably by the production of factor that increases vascular permeability.

Pathology

Occurs in three morphologic patterns:

a. Minimal change disease—85% cases: Glomeruli normal or minimal change in mesangial cells and matrix. 95% of patients respond to corticosteroids.

Electron microscopy shows retraction (fusion) of the epithelial cell foot processes of the basement membrane, resulting in increased permeability of plasma proteins. Kidney becomes large and big on gross examination. Light microscopy shows normal picture (Figs 15.2 and 15.3).

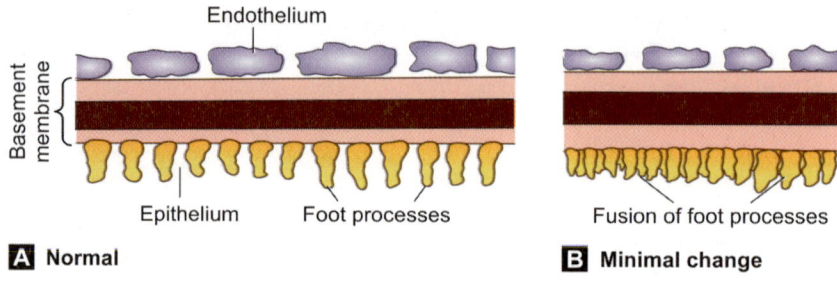

Fig. 15.2A and B: Electron microscopic picture in nephrotic syndrome.

b. Mesangial proliferative group—increase in mesangial cells and matrix. 50–60% respond to corticosteroids.
c. Focal sclerosis (10%) glomeruli near medulla show scarring in one or more lobules. About 20% responds to prednisolone and cytotoxic drugs.

Clinical Manifestations

Common in boys than girls (2:1). Common age is 2–6 years of age. There is history of upper respiratory tract infection before the initial attack.

a. *Edema:* Edema is first noticed around the eyes and subsequently on leg where it is pitting on pressure. It becomes generalized all over body. Hydrothorax, ascites and edema on dependent parts of the body resulting in weight gain (Fig. 15.3).
b. Blood pressure is normal. If elevated, it suggests glomerular lesion.
c. Infections in various parts of body are common.
d. Anorexia, abdominal pain and diarrhea are common.
e. Declining output of urine.

Laboratory Investigations

Urine: Gross proteinuria. 3+ or 4+ excretion of protein (2 gm/24 hours)

Microscopic: Hematuria may or may not be present. Hyaline and granular casts may be present.

Blood

i. Hypoalbuminemia: Serum albumin below 2.5 gm/dl.

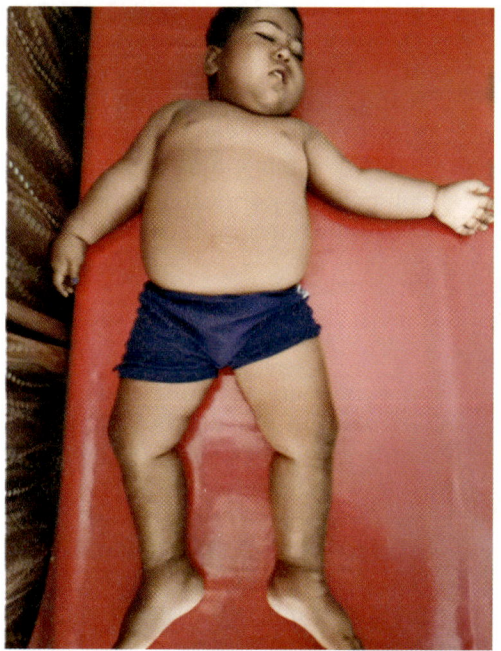

Fig. 15.3: Nephrotic syndrome.

ii. Hypogammaglobulinemia.
iii. Increase in lipoprotein α_2.
iv. Serum cholesterol is moderately or severely increased.
v. Blood urea may be raised.
vi. Total serum calcium is low.
vii. C_3 is normal
viii. Creatinine clearance is low.

Tuberculin Test

Renal ultrasound—enlarged kidney
Renal biopsy—not routinely indicated.

Indications

- If corticosteroids are ineffective
- Creatinine clearance is impaired
- Age below 12 months
- Gross or persistent microscopic hematuria
- Low C_3 level
- Hypertension or impaired renal function.

Renal biopsy is indicated to detect type of histological lesion, generally done after 8 years of age. Not routinely indicated. Mostly lesion below 8 years of age is minimal lesion and steroid dependent.

Complications

i. *Infections:* Peritonitis, sepsis, cellulitis, pneumonia, UTI.
ii. Increased tendency to arterial and venous thrombosis; so femoral vein puncture avoided.
iii. Deficiency of coagulation factors. Reduced vitamin D level.

Treatment

Child should be hospitalized for diagnosis, treatment and educational purpose to parents.

Management of initial episode

1. Diet
   - High protein diet.
   - Salt restriction by way 'no added salt diet', start giving salt when edema subsides.
   - Fluid restriction is not encouraged until unless edema is severe.
2. Physical activity is such as tolerated by patient.
3. Presence of tuberculosis should be looked for.
4. *Diuretics:* If edema is massive, significant
   - Frusemide (1–4 mg/kg in 2 divided doses)
   - Spironolactone (3–4 mg/kg/24 hours) in 4 divided doses.
5. *Antibiotics:* If infection suspected along with NS.
6. Parent education about usual outcome, no diet restriction during relapse.

Corticosteroids

Only prednisolone is proven benefit in the treatment of proteinuria.

Table 15.1: Differences between acute nephritis and nephrosis (nephrotic syndrome)

	Feature	Acute nephritis	Nephrotic syndrome
1.	Onset	Acute	Insidious
2.	History of preceding URI	Present	Absent
3.	Hematuria	Present	Absent
4.	Edema	Slight	Marked
5.	Urine		
	Albumin	+	+++
	RBC	+	–
	Casts	+	–
6.	Blood pressure	Raised	Not usually raised
7.	Blood		
	Protein	Normal	Low albumin
	Cholesterol	Normal	Elevated
	Calcium	Normal	Elevated
8.	Complications	Hypertensive, encephalopathy, CCF	Tetany, occasionally, CCF
9.	Recurrence	Infrequent	Frequent

Prednisolone

Given in dose of 2 mg/kg/day (max 60 mg) in single or divided doses for 6 weeks followed by:

- 1.5 mg/kg (max 40 mg) as a single morning dose or alternate day for next 6 weeks.
- Stop the therapy abruptly. Some experts suggest that therapy with corticosteroid should not be stopped abruptly and tapered of gradually. Benefits of prolonged therapy need to the assessed by the risk of steroid adverse effect.
- For average period, response is 10–14 days (protein-free urine).

Subsequent Course

- Majority of patient show(s) 3–4 relapses or more relapses in a year.
- Steroid dependent—15% remain on remission while on prednisolone therapy and relapse whenever dose is reduced or 2 weeks of its discontinuation.
- Steroid resistant: 10–15% of patients do not respond to initial treatment with prednisolone or respond initially later cease to respond.

Long-term alternate day prednisolone

Indicated for steroid dependent and patient with frequent relapses.

- Treatment of relapse followed by prednisolone is tapered to maintain remission with small dose on alternate day for 9–18 months. It prevents relapses in many patient.
- At the time of infection give small dose for 5–7 days from onset of infection which prevents relapse.
- If patient relapses on this therapy prednisolone 2 mg/kg/day until remission followed by prednisolone 1–5 mg/kg alternate day.
- Steroid sparing agent.

If repeated relapses occur, long-term steroid sparing agent is considered. Indications are:

1. Prednisolone dose needed to maintain remission higher than 0.5–0.7 mg/kg on alternate day.
2. Features of toxicity of corticosteroids—growth failure, hypertension, cataract appear.

Agent	Dose
Levamisole	2–2.5 mg/kg on alternate day (9–18 months)
Cyclophosphamide	2–2.5 mg/kg/day (1–2 yr)
Mycophenolate	600–1000 mg/m^2/day (1–3 yr) or 20–25 mg/kg/day
Cyclosporine A (CyA)	4–5 mg/kg/day (12–36 months)
Tacrolimus (TAc)	0.1–0.2 mg/kg/day (12–36 months)
Rituximab	375 mg/m^2 IV once a week (2–3 doses)

Management of Relapse

a. • Infections often cause relapse so infections are treated with suitable antibiotics. It results remission to low grade proteinuria 1–2+.

- Remission means urine albumin nil or trace for 3 consecutive days.
- Relapse means urine albumin 3+ or 4+ for 3 consecutive days.

b. If proteinuria is 3+ or 4+ prednisolone is given at a dose of 2 mg/kg/day until the protein is negative or traces for 3 consecutive days then prednisolone 1.5 mg/kg for 4 weeks.

Duration: This treatment of relapse usually lasts for 5–6 weeks.

About 3–4 relapses treated as above described manner, then therapy is individualized.

Frequent relapses: Frequent relapses mean two or more relapses in initial 6 months or 4 or more than 4 relapses in any 12 months.

Such patient require long-term treatment.

Thrombotic complication: Patients are at risk of thrombosis. Treated with heparin followed by oral anticoagulant.

Hypovolemia and acute renal failure

- Stop diuretics. Infuse normal saline 10–20 ml/kg over 20–30 min. If not respond, two bolus of normal saline given.
- Infuse albumin 10–15 ml/kg or 20% albumin: 0.5–1 gm/kg.

Prognosis

Children with minimum change nephrotic syndrome have excellent prognosis. Mortality rate 1–4% in steroid resistant cases due to hypovolemia or infection, thromboses which can be managed.

Relapses decrease with time.

PROTEINURIA

Definition

Presence of protein in urine. Normal protein excretion in urine is 150 mg/24 hr.

Classification

  i. Pathologic proteinuria
  ii. Non-pathologic proteinuria

Pathologic Proteinuria: Causes

1. Glomerular
   a. Nephrotic syndrome
   b. Persistent asymptomatic
2. Tubular

   Hereditary
   a. Cystinosis
   b. Wilson's disease
   c. Lowe's syndrome
   d. Proximal renal tubular acidosis
   e. Galactosemia

   Acquired
   a. Analgesic abuse
   b. Vitamin D toxicity
   c. Interstitial nephritis
   d. Acute tubular necrosis
   e. Sarcoidosis
   f. Cystic disease
   g. Homograft rejection

h. Penicillamine poisoning
i. Heavy metal poisoning
j. Hypokalemia.

Non-pathologic proteinuria

1. Postural
2. Febrile
3. Exercise.

ACUTE KIDNEY INJURY
(ACUTE RENAL FAILURE)

Acute renal failure (ARF) is a complex syndrome resulting from an acute reduction in or cessation of renal function (excretory and regulatory) and is characterized by anuria or oliguria, electrolyte and acid–base disturbance (notably hyperkalemia and metabolic acidosis), and impaired excretion substances such as creatinine, urea and phosphate.

Definition

Acute kidney injury (AKI) is diagnosed if there is abrupt onset of kidney function either

1. If patient serum creatinine increases within 48 hr more than or equal to 0.3 mg/dl or a percentage increase of more than or equal to 50% from baseline.
2. Oliguria

Anuria or severe oliguria means urine flow less than 0.5 ml/kg/hour or less than 180 ml/m^2/24 hr.

It is a life-threatening situation.

Reduction in urine flow is not always essential feature. This non-oliguric form develops after burn, trauma or exposure to nephrotoxin.

Etiology
Causes

Prerenal

1. *Dehydration:* Acute gastroenteritis, burns, heat stroke.
2. *Hypovolemia:* Hemorrhage.
3. *Shock:*
   a. Septicemic shock.
   b. Cardiogenic shock—myocarditis, arrhythmias.

4. Renal artery or vein thrombosis.
5. Coagulation disturbances:
   a. Disseminated intravascular coagulation
      • Sepsis especially gram-negative septicemia.
      • Snake bite.
      • Incompatible blood transfusion.
   b. Hemolytic uremic syndrome

Renal

1. *Acute tubular necrosis*
   a. Hemorrhage
   b. Shock
   c. Intravascular hemolysis (anti-malarial drugs in G6PD deficiency patients)
   d. Drugs and chemicals: Mercury, carbon tetrachloride, phosphorus, arsenic, lead.
   e. Burns, major surgical procedures
   f. *Antibiotics:* Aminoglycosides, cephaloridines
   g. Hepatic insufficiency
2. *Glomerulonephritis:* Post-streptococcal, membranoproliferative, SLE, Henoch-Schönlein purpura. Drug anaphylaxis, e.g. penicillin.
3. *Interstitial nephritis*
   a. Acute bacterial pyelonephritis
   b. Sulphonamides
   c. Methicillin.
4. *Hemolytic uremic syndrome:* Acute dysentery.
5. *Infections*
6. *Traumatic:* Renal parenchymal hemorrhage.

Postrenal

1. Calculus
2. Blood clots
3. Crystals of sulfonamide, uric acid.
4. Structural abnormalities.

Clinical Manifestations

The clinical manifestations of acute renel failure are often overshadowed by the manifestations of the precipitating cause. Apart from features of the precipitating cause features specific to acute renel failure are decreased urinary output (oliguria or anuria), edema, drowsiness leading to coma, irregularities of cardiac rate caused by hyperkalemia. Findings due to circulatory congestion, acidotic breathing are other common manifestations.

In acute tubular necrosis oliguric phase lasts for 3–7 days followed by diuretic phase lasting for a week during which loss of water and electrolyte results dehydration.

Investigations

Blood: Hyperkalemia, hypernatremia, metabolic acidosis, elevation of serum urea, phosphate, uric acid, creatinine, hypercalcemia and anemia.

Urine: Urine may contain RBC, protein, casts and tubular cells. Urinary sodium is low (<20 mEq/L) in prerenal failure, high (70–90 mEq/L) in tabular disorders.

ECG: ECG shows features of hyperkalemia.

Radionuclide studies: Assess about blood flow and diagnosis about renal necrosis.

Roentgenographic studies may reveal cardiomegaly, pulmonary congestion, radiopaque calculi, shruken kidney or a single enlarged kidney.

Intravenous urogram: Indicated if anuria persists after the patient is out of shock or when circulatory congestion is no longer present.

Catheterization is done to exclude any obstruction.

Ultrasonography: To determine, renal size, pelvicalyceal system, structural anomalies, calculi.

Indications of biopsy

1. Rapidly progressive or nonresolving glomerulonephritis.
2. ARF associated with underlying systemic disorder, e.g. Henoch-Schönlein purpura
3. Suspected interstitial nephritis
4. Acute tubular necrosis

Investigation to determine cause

1. Peripheral blood smear, platelet, reticulocyte count
2. C_3
3. LDH levels
4. Stool shigatoxin (suspected hemolytic uremic syndrome)
5. Blood ASO titer
6. Antinuclear antibody
7. Antineutrophil cytoplasmic antibody
8. Doppler ultrasonography (suspected arterial or venous thrombosis)
9. Biopsy

Lab findings

Prenal: BUN/creatinine ratio >20
Urine SG >1.030
Urine osmolarity >500
Urine Na^+ <20
FENa: <1% in older children
<2.5% in neonates

Renal: Damage to glomerulus
Hematuria
Proteinuria

Damage to tubules: Urinary β_2-microglobulin. FENa: >1% in children, >2.5% in neonates.

Damage to interstitium (drugs): Eosinophilia, Eosinophiluria.

Increased urinary β_2-microglobulin

Postrenal: Dilatation of renal collective system on renal ultrasound.

Vascular: Renal blood flow on nuclear scan.

Management of AKI

For successful management identify the cause, evaluate the laboratory data and take the decision about the line of treatment depending upon presence of complication.

Fluid restriction

Daily fluid requirement is restricted to insensible water losses (300–400 ml/m²/24 hr). If patient tolerate well then increase it equal to 24 hours urine output and other losses.

Fluids are given orally, intravenous fluid is not required.

Appropriate fluid is assessed by daily weight record of patient and blood sodium measurement.

If proper fluid is given then
- Loose weight 0.5–1% daily
- Normal blood sodium

If inappropriate fluid is given then
- Rapid weight loss
- Raising sodium

If excess fluid is given then
- No weight loss
- Low sodium

Identify the cause and correct underlying cause of ARF.

Fluid repletion—prerenal type of ARF is corrected by fluid replacement which is followed by giving diuretics.

1. Correction of dehydration is done by normal saline or Ringer lactate 20–30 ml/kg over 45–60 min.
2. Hemorrhage resulting shock is corrected by blood transfusion.
3. Potassium should not be given until renal function established.
   - Bladder should be catheterized to measure urine output. If urine output increased 2–4 ml/kg over 2–3 hr continue therapy.
   - If above measures fail to induce diuresis and patient is hydrated but not overhydrated—frusemide 2–3 mg/kg IV should be given.
   - If no response of fluid repletion and diuretics irreversible intrinsic failure is diagnosed.

Diet: Diet should be given which contain liberal calories and fat. Protein intake is restricted.

Protein: 1–1.2 g/kg in infant daily
0.8–1.2 g/kg in older children daily
Calories: 60–80 cal/kg daily
Vitamins and micronutrients supplemented

General measures

1. Daily intake output record maintained
2. Infections are treated with antibiotics. Avoid or give dose adjusted drugs. Aminoglycosides, indomethacin ACE inhibitors, amphotericin, radiocontrast media.

Hyperkalemia

a. Hyperkalmia is corrected by intravenous administration of glucose 0.5 gm/kg along with soluble insulin 0.1 unit/kg.
b. Calcium gluconate: 10–15 mg/kg of elemental calcium is given to correct hyperkalemia. Calcium antagonize cardiotoxicity of potassium.
c. Sodium bicarbonate given intravenously also serve to reduce hyperkalemia.
d. Ion exchange resin (e.g. kayexalate) is given orally or rectally (as rectal enema 10–20 gm disolved in 10% dextrose retained 30–60 minutes).
e. In life-threatening situation peritoneal dialysis or hemodialysis is required.
f. Salbutamol: 5–10 mg nebulized.

Metabolic Acidosis

a. Severe metabolic acidosis is corrected by providing sodium bicarbonate (IV) in the dosage of weight in kg × 0.6 × base deficit. Half of it is given over a period if 2–4 hours, the rest over the next 12–24 hours.
b. Dialysis in persistent cases.
c. General measures include correction of hypercatabolic state by:
   1. Provision of adequate calories (300 cal/m^2/dose as carbohydrate and fat)
   2. Treatment of shock, infection and hypoxia.

Pulmonary edema

- Oxygen
- Frusemide

Hypertension: Symptomatic sodium nitroprusside 0.5–8 µg/day/min infusion.

Frusemide: 2–4 mg/kg IV

Nifedipine: 0.3–0.5 mg/kg oral or sublingual

Asymptomatic nifedipine

Amlodipine

- Prazosin
- Hyponatremia—sodium <130 mEq/litre
  1. Fluid restriction
  2. If sensorium altered 3% saline 6–12 ml/kg over 30–90 min.

Anemia: Packed cell transfusion.

Hyperphosphatemia: Phosphate, calcium carbonate, acetate, aluminum hydroxide.

Dialysis: Indication

1. Persistent hyperkalemia (>6.5 mEq/L)
2. Fluid overload (pulmonary edema, hypertension)
3. Uremic encephalopathy
4. Severe metabolic acidosis
5. Hyponatremia

Dopamine: Recent trials do not support the low dose dopamine in severely ill patient at the risk of ARF.

Prognosis

If well treated, acute renal failure caused by post-streptocaccal glomerulonephritis recovery is the rule. In other cases it is life-threatening and worse. In prerenal type recovery is best.

Complication: Control
Fluid overload controlled by:

- Fluid restriction (400 ml/m^2/day + urine output + other losses)
- 5% dextrose for insensible losses
- N/S saline for urine output.

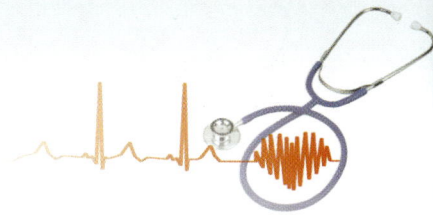

16

Hematological Disorders

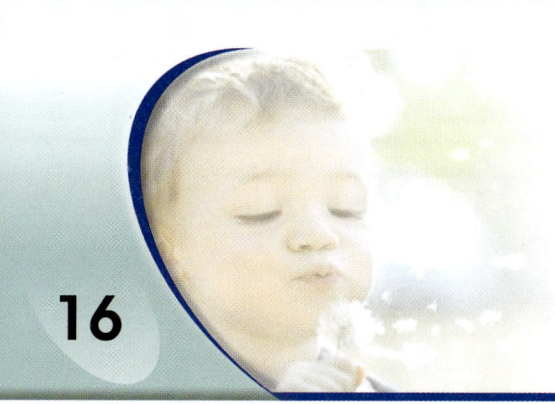

ANEMIA

Definition

Anemia is defined as when the hemoglobin level is more than two standard deviations below the mean for the child's age and sex.

Epidemiology

As per Third National Family Health Survey (NFHS 3): 79% of Indian children have anemia.

Based on Reticulocyte Count

Reticulocyte count reflects the number of immature RBCs in the circulation and, therefore, the activity of the bone marrow in producing RBCs. Normally, 1% of RBCs is reticulocyte (normal absolute count 40,000 cells/mm³).

In most anemias reticulocyte count should rise. Low reticulocyte count indicates bone marrow failure.

Hb as per Age

a. The Hb% is high at birth in most newborn. It declines physiologic low point between 2 and 3 months of age in the term infant and between 1 and 2 months of age in preterm infant (Tables 16.1 to 16.3).
b. Fetal hemoglobin (HbF) is major part of hemoglobin of early postnatal life. It declines gradually and disappears by 6–9 months of age.

Table 16.1: Hemoglobin value in infancy and childhood (g/dl)

Age	Mean	−2SD
Birth	16.5	13.5
1–3 days	18.5	14.5
1 week	17.5	13.5
2 weeks	16.5	12.5
1 month	14.0	10.0
2 months	11.5	9.5
3–6 months	11.5	9.5
0–5 years	12.0	10.5
2–6 years	12.5	11.5
6–12 years	13.5	11.5
Girls: 12–18 years	14.0	12.0
Boys: 12–18 years	14.5	13.0

Table 16.2: Hemoglobin level for diagnosis of anemia (WHO)

Age	Hb (g/dl)	Hematocrit
6 months to 5 years	<11.0	<33
5–11 years	<11.5	<34
12–13 years	<12.0	<36
Nonpregnant women	<12.0	<36
Men	<13.0	<39

Table 16.3: Hematocrit in infancy and childhood

Age	Mean	−2SD
Birth	51	42
1–3 days	56	45
1 week	54	42
2 weeks	51	39
1 month	43	31
2 months	35	28
3–6 months	35	29
0.5–2 years	36	33
2–6 years	37	34
6–12 years	40	35
Girls: 12–18 years	41	36
Boys: 12–18 years	43	37

Table 16.4: Classification of anemia

A. **Microcytic hypochromic anemia**
  1. Iron deficiency
  2. Thalassemia
  3. Sideroblastic anemia
  4. Lead toxicity
  5. Chronic disease
B. **Normocytic normochromic anemia**
  1. High reticulocyte count
    a. Hemangioma
    b. DIC
    c. Hemolytic anemia
      • *RBC intrinsic defect*
        – RBC membrane disorder
          Hereditary spherocytosis
          Hereditary elliptocytosis
        – RBC enzyme disorder
          G6PD deficiency
          Pyruvate kinase deficiency
      • *RBC extrinsic defect*
        – HUS
        – Autoimmune
        – Alloimmune
    d. Sickle cell anemia
    e. Blood loss
  2. Low reticulocyte count
    a. Red cell aplasia
      • TEC
      • Diamond-Blackfan syndrome
      • Parvovirus B19 infection
    b. Malignancy
    c. Fanconi anemia
C. **Macrocytic**
  1. Vit B_{12} deficiency
  2. Thiamine deficiency
  3. Folate deficiency

Classification

Depending on morphology and etiology
  i. Microcytic
  ii. Normocytic
  iii. Macrocytic

Based on morphology of RBC

a. *Normocytic:* Normal shape of RBC.
b. *Microcytic:* Small shape of RBC.
c. *Megaloblastic:* Large than normal shape of RBC (Table 16.4).

Based on Hb% in RBC

a. *Hypochromic:* Hb% is less than normal in RBC.
b. *Normochromic:* Hb% is normal in RBC.

Based on etiology

a. *Hemorrhagic:* Due to excessive bleeding.
b. *Dyshemopoietic:* Due to disorder of formation of RBC.
  i. *Due to deficiency of necessary factor*
    • Iron deficiency
    • Vit B_{12}, folic acid, vit C, vit B_6 deficiency
    • Malnutrition
    • Thyroxine deficiency
  ii. *Bone marrow depression*
    • Aplastic anemia
    • Others: Infections
        Drugs
        Renal disease

  iii. *Hemolytic anemia:* Due to excessive destruction of RBC.
    a. *Congenital disease:* Thalassemia, sickle cell anemia, hereditary spherocytosis.
    b. *Acquired:* Malaria, kala-azar, blood group incompatibility (RH, ABO), drug-induced, e.g. primaquine.

General features of anemia

Generalized pallor of the body, tachycardia, early fatigue on exertion, breathlessness, cardiomegaly. CCF in severe cases.

MICROCYTIC HYPOCROMIC ANEMIA

Causes

1. Iron deficiency
2. Thalassemia
3. Sideroblastic anemia
4. Lead toxicity
5. Chronic diseases
   - Malignancy
   - Infections
   - Kidney diseases

IRON DEFICIENCY ANEMIA

This is most frequent form of anemia, may be due to following causes in children.

Etiology

Causes of iron deficiency:

a. Deficiency of food: Normally iron store in body is sufficient for 6–9 months of age. Iron store is less in case of premature or excessive hemorrhage during delivery. If iron is not supplemented in food, child suffers from anemia.

b. Mother and cow milk do not contain sufficient amount of iron to fulfill the need. If baby's weaning is delayed and child is mainly on milk diet chances of iron deficiency anemia is more common in 9–24 months of age.

c. Due to excessive hemorrhage from GIT and hookworm infestation or other reasons.

d. Due to defective absorption of iron from GIT.

Histological abnormalities of the mucosa of gastrointestinal tract is present in severe cases. It leads to deficient absorption leading to diarrhea.

It is more common in two age groups:

1. 9–24 months of age.
2. Adolescent girls—because poor diet, rapid growth and loss of iron in menstrual blood.
3. Occult blood loss, e.g. hookworm infestation, other causes.

Clinical Features

Common features are generalized pallor of the body, irritability, loss of appetite, tachycardia, and splenomegaly is common; if hemoglobin is less than 5–9 gm%, on auscultation systolic murmur is present.

- Child suffers from loss of weight and malnutrition, in some children PICA is noticed due to iron deficiency.
- Lack of attention, alertness and learning ability are also noticed in infants and adolescents.

Laboratory Investigations

1. Blood smear: RBC, microcytic hypochromic, different shapes such as anisocytosis, polychromatophilias.
2. Hemoglobin is below normal: PCV, MCH, MCHC and MCV are reduced.
3. Serum iron level is reduced. Iron binding capacity of plasma is increased.
4. If facilities available, most characteristic investigation is erythrocyte protoporphyrin concentration which is reduced.
5. Iron store in bone marrow is absent or reduced.
6. Increased transferrin and decreased trasferrin saturation.
7. Normal or increased reticulocyte count.

Treatment

Specific treatment is administration of iron.

a. **Oral therapy:** Iron is given in the form of tabs or syrup. Iron sulfate is cheep and effective, recommended in dose of 6 mg per kg body weight three times in a day. Better given in between meals for best absorption. Iron is given up to hemoglobin reaches normal. It has to be given 1–3 months even after this.

b. **Parenteral therapy:** Given in following situation:
   - Intolerance due to oral administration or have diarrhea.
   - For rapid result.
   - If doubtful about patient self-administration.

Dose: Total iron required (mg) = Patient weight in lbs (pounds) × Hb deficit in % × 0.3 (Total iron in ml is calculated on the basis of 50 mg of iron in 1 ml).

How to give?

Parenteral intramuscular injection 1–2 ml every day (max 6 mg/kg) is given deep intramuscularly. It is painful, so given on separate sites. It is tested before administration by small amount for sensitivity.

Intravenous total dose calculated given in 5% dextrose or normal saline slowly. It is better to be avoided.

Other measures

1. Treatment of cause.
2. Blood transfusion: Slowly administered. It is better to give packed or sediment RBC. Plasma is avoided due to risk of CCF.
   Dose: 2–3 ml per kg of packed cells at any one time.
3. If patient is in CCF, packed red cells transfusion and frusemide are given. Digitalis is unnecessary.

MACROCYTIC (MEGALOBLASTIC) ANEMIA

Characterized by large RBCs with MCV more than 110 fl.

Causes

1. Folic acid deficiency
2. B_{12} deficiency

Folic acid deficiency: It may be due to:
a. Decreased folic acid intake
   - Diet lacking fresh fruits and vegetables.
   - Exclusive feeding with goat's milk.
b. Decreased intestinal absorption of folic acid
   - Diseases of small intestine
     – Coeliac disease
     – Chronic infectious enteritis
     – Crohn's disease
   - Medications
     – Anticonvulsants
     – Oral contraceptives

Clinical Features

1. Characteristic signs and symptoms of anemia.
2. Failure to thrive, chronic diarrhea and irritability.

Diagnosis

1. Blood examination—low serum folic acid
2. Blood film—large RBCs.

Management

1. Dietary folic acid, drug folic acid
2. Treatment of underlying cause.

Vitamin B_{12} Deficiency

Normal physiology—dietary vitamin B_{12} must first combines with intrinsic factor secreted by gastric cells then absorbed in the terminal ileum.

Etiology

Inadequate dietary intake

- Strict vegetarian
- Inherited inability to secrete intrinsic factor.
- Inability to absorb vitamin B_{12}.

Clinical Features

- General features of anemia
- Anorexia
- Smooth red tongue
- Neurological manifestations
- Ataxia, hyporeflexia, positive Babinski sign.

Diagnosis

- Peripheral blood smear—large RBC
- Blood PCV, serum B_{12} level low

Management

Monthly intramuscular B_{12} injections.

Normochromic Normocytic Anemias

In these type of anemias RBC size and shape is normal. It includes:
1. Hemolytic anemia
2. Red cell aplasia
3. Sickle cell anemia

Reticulocyte count: Reticulocyte count differentiate two types of anemia.

Reticulocyte count—low

Bone marrow suppression, failure
- Red cell aplasia
- TEC
- Diamond-Blackfan syndrome
- Parvovirus B19 infection
   Pancytopenia
   Malignancy

Reticulocyte count—high

- Hemolytic anemia
- Sickle cell anemia
   – Hemangioma
   – DIC
   – Blood loss

HEMOLYTIC ANEMIAS

A. Intrinsic RBC Defect

a. RBC Membrane Defect

- **Hereditary spherocytosis:** It is an autosomal dominant condition. There is a deficiency or abnormality of RBC cell membrane protein spectrin. RBC becomes spherical. So, there is increased destruction of RBC and diminished ability to pass into small vessels.
- Pallor, weakness, splenomegaly, formation of pigmentary gallstones or jaundice and anemia are clinical features.

Laboratory investigations

High reticulocyte counts, spherocytes on blood smear, hyperbilirubinemia, abnormal fragility.

Management

Blood transfusion, splenectomy cures the condition.
- **Hereditary elliptocytosis:** It is an autosomal dominant defect in spectrin of RBC cell membrane resulting elliptical RBC seen in blood smear.

Majority of patient have no symptom. Few has jaundice, splenomegaly and gallstones. If hemolysis is present splenectomy is advised.

b. RBC Enzyme Disorder (Glycolytic Enzymatic Defects of RBC)

A. *Pyruvate kinase deficiency:* Pallor, jaundice, splenomegaly, kernicterus, polychromatic RBC. Lab investigation shows low pyruvate kinase in the RBC. *Management* includes blood transfusion and splenectomy.

B. *Glucose-6-phosphate dehydrogenase deficiency* (G6PD deficiency): Symptoms appear after exposure to oxidant, hemolysis occurs resulting abdominal pain, fever, hemoglobinuria and jaundice. Smear shows 'bile cells', polychromasia, Heinz bodies.
Low level of G6PD in RBC is diagnostic. *Management:* Blood transfusion and splenectomy are needed.

B. Defect Extrinsic to RBC

1. Autoimmune hemolytic anemia—when antibodies are misdirected against RBC.
2. Alloimmune hemolytic anemia.
3. Sickle cell anemia

SICKLE CELL ANEMIA

Etiology and pathophysiology
1. Sickle cell disease is caused by single amino acid substitution of valine for glutamic acid on the number 6 position of the beta globin chain of hemoglobin (HbS).
2. When RBC is exposed to low oxygen or acidosis, the mutation results in polymerization of HbS within the RBC membrane. This results distorted RBC shape (sickled).
3. Sickled RBCs have decreased lifespan so more hemolysis and occlusion of small vessels resulting in ischemia, infarction and organ dysfunction.
   - *SS disease:* It is a result of two genes for HbS (homozygous).
   - *SS strain:* It is a result of only one gene for HbS (heterozygous).

Clinical features: Seen generally after 6 months of age.

1. Delayed growth.
2. Splenomegaly after 6 months of age.
3. *Leg ulcers:* Shallow ulcers near ankle due to vascular stasis and trauma.
4. *Hand–foot syndrome:* Painful swelling of hands and feet. It leads to destruction of metacarpals, metatarsals and phalanges.
5. *Occular:* Background and proliferative retinopathy, vitreous bleeding.
6. *CNS:* Stroke, dysarthria, hemiplegia.
7. *Heart:* Cardiomegaly.
8. *Priapism:* Painful, sustained erection.
9. Renal, enuresis, hematuria, chronic renal failure.
10. *Abdominal pain:* Due to infarction of abdominal viscera.
11. Acute chest syndrome.
12. Vertebral collapse, osteoporosis.
    Sickle chest syndrome: As a result of veno-oclusive crisis bone marrow infarction results in fat emboli to the lungs which causes sickling and infarction leading to ventilatory failure and death.
13. *Gall stones:* Pigmented gall stones.
14. *Cardiomegaly*—due to anemia.
15. *Infections:* Pneumonia, meningitis, osteomyelitis.

Diagnosis

Blood smear—sickled cells, target cells, Howell-Jolly bodies.

Sickling test—sickling test is induced by adding reducing agent like 2% sodium metabisulphite to blood HbA gives clear solution and HbS gives turbid solution. This is a basis of emergency screening test (Fig. 16.1).

Hb electrophoresis—hemoglobin in homozygous patient is chiefly (80–90%) hemoglobin SS (HbSS). Carrier will have 35–40% as HbSS. So, electrophoresis differentiates homozygous or heterozygous.

- *Reticulocyte count* is about 5–15%.
- *Bilirubin*—increased.
- *Bone marrow*—erythroid hyperplasia.

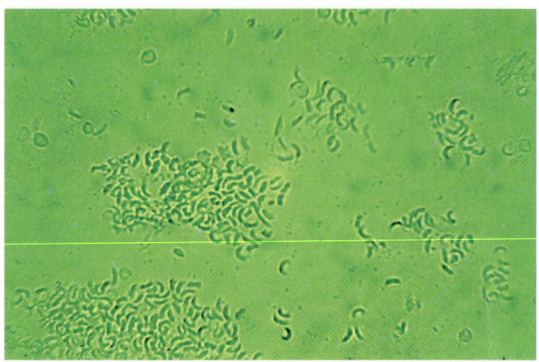

Fig. 16.1: Sickling test.

Both parents of the affected individual will have sickle trait.

Management

1. *Between crisis*
   a. Patient should be given folic acid regularly.
   b. Infections are treated early with antibiotics.
2. *During crisis:* Rest, analgesics, hydration and correction of acidosis, plasma volume expanders, oxygen.
3. *Exchanged blood transfusion:* To replace HbS with HbA if PCV falls dangerously.
   Regular blood transfusions to suppress HbS production and maintain HbS level below 30%.
4. *Bone marrow transplantation:* Potentially curative.

Preventive Care

1. Daily oral penicillin to reduce risk of *S. pneumoniae* infection.
2. Folic acid daily to reduce folic acid deficiency.
3. Routine immunization for influenza, pneumococcal, *Haemophilus influenzae* B and hepatitis B.

Prognosis

About 50% patients survive up to the age of 40 years.

THALASSEMIAS

This is quite common form of hemolytic anemia, reported from all over world. Depending upon defect in synthesis of chain of hemoglobin it is classified as follows:

1. *Beta thalassemia:* Due to suppression of synthesis of beta peptide chain.
2. *Alpha thalassemia:* Due to suppression of alpha peptide chain synthesis.
3. *Delta–beta thalassemia:* Due to suppression of both alpha and beta chain synthesis.
4. *Delta–gamma chain synthesis:* Suppression is rare.

Synonym

Colley's or Mediterranean anemia or beta thalassemia.

Pathogenesis

This is commonest form of thalassemia in which inherited genetic defect is in the synthesis of beta chain in hemoglobin, which is adult hemoglobin (HbA).

As a compensation increased production of fetal hemoglobin occurs. In blood normoblasts, target cells and microcytic hypochromic RBC are seen. Reticulocytes are increased.

Bone marrow hyperplasia is responsible for bone changes.

Clinical Features

The condition manifests insidiously from infancy at about 3 months of age. Early features are progressive pallor, diarrhea, fever, repeated respiratory tract infections and anemia. Spleen may be palpable with distension of abdomen.

The facial appearance is diagnostic with severe form. It is frontal bossing, prominent maxilla exposing the teeth, depressed nasal bridge and malocclusion of teeth, called *'thalassemic facies'*; this is due to expansion of marrow of face and skull bones (Fig. 16.2).

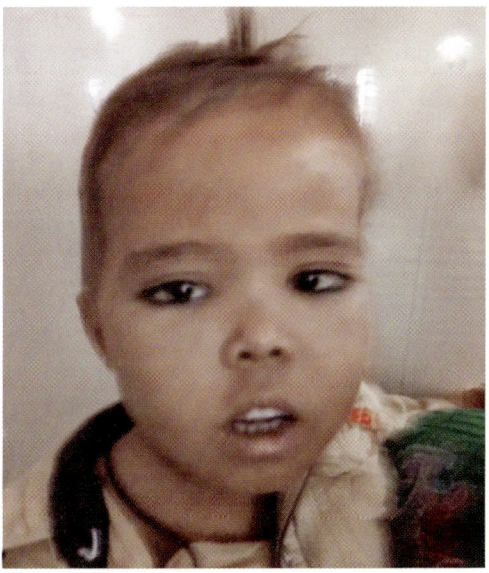

Fig. 16.2: Thalassemia.

Failure to thrive, underdevelopment, variable degree of hepatosplenomegaly and lymphadenopathy are associated features.

Increased pigmentation may occur skin due to high melanin in epithelium and hemosiderin in the dermis.

Cardiac complications such as pericarditis and congestive cardiac failure due to myocardial siderosis are common terminal events.

In blood dependent patient, death usually occurs in 2nd and 3rd decades of life.

Diagnosis

i. **Blood picture:** RBC microcytic hypochromic, anisocytosis, poikilocytosis, moderate basophilic stippling, nucleated RBC, target cells. Reticulocytes high (Fig. 16.3).

 Hb generally 4–9 gm% or below. Bone marrow—erythroid hyperplasia osmotic fragility reduced.

ii. Fetal Hb measured by electrophoresis is more than 40%. Skiagram skull shows 'hair on end' appearance due to prominent vertical trabeculae. Diploic space widened, overgrowth of maxilla, opacification of sinus are other features (Fig. 16.4).

Thinning of cortex, widening of medulla due to marrow hyperplasia, coarsening of trabeculations in bones (metacarpals and metatarsals).

Prominent vertical trabeculae (hair on end).

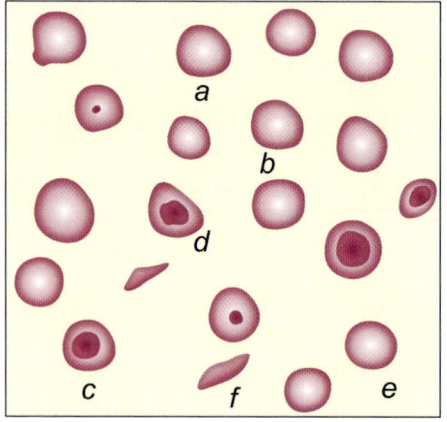

Fig. 16.3: Blood picture in thalassemia showing— (a) Microcytic hypochromic RBC; (b) Target cell; (c and d) Normoblast; (e) Basophilic stippling; and (f) Poikilocyte

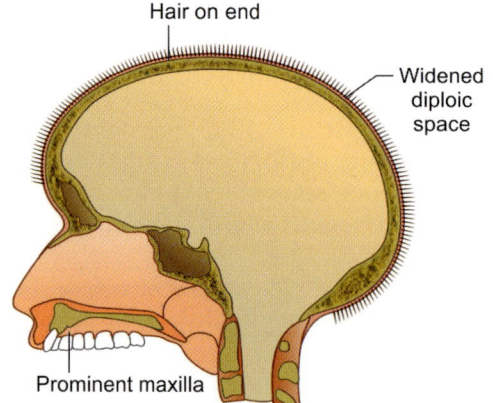

Fig. 16.4: Diagrammatic representation of skiagram of skull of thalassemia patient.

Treatment

No specific treatment is available.

1. Lifelong blood transfusion

   Repeated blood transfusion 'hypertransfusion is given 15 ml/kg (packed cells) every 4–5 weeks to keep hemoglobin level above 12 gm% and to completely suppress erythropoiesis. Hemosiderosis is inevitable due to prolonged transfusion because excess of iron produced by blood transfusion cannot be excreted by physiologic means and death occurs due to myocarditis due to hemosiderosis. Following measures are now enable to reduce hemosiderosis.

   a. Deferoxamine is an iron chelator given parenterally by subcutaneous injection 8–12 hourly daily. It is highly costly.

   b. Recently deferiprone (Kelfer-Cipla) is introduced as oral iron chelator, given in dose 7.5 mg/kg/day in 2–4 divided doses, cheep and orally administered. Dose may be increased 50–100 mg, if required.

2. Splenectomy

3. Bone marrow transplant is a potential option.

Prognosis

Prognosis is bad in spite of blood transfusions. Splenectomy is necessary, specially in children who require frequent transfusion or suffering from hypersplenism.

THALASSEMIA MINOR (HETEROZYGOUS, BETA THALASSEMIA, BETA THALASSEMIA TRAIT)

It causes mild asymptomatic anemia with HbE.

Lab blood: Hypochromia, microcytosis with target cells and anisocytosis on smear.

Treatment: No treatment is required. Many cases of thalassemia minor are misdiagnosed as iron deficiency anemia. However, iron level in beta thalassemia is normal or elevated.

Sideroblastic Anemia

In this group, ring sideroblasts are present in bone marrow. It may be inherited or acquired as a result of drugs or toxin (e.g. isoniazid, alcohol, lead poisoning, chloramphenicol).

Other causes: Lead poisoning
Malignancy
Infections
Kidney diseases

DISORDERS OF HEMOSTASIS

Hemostasis requires normal function of three important elements:
1. Blood vessels
2. Platelets
3. Soluble clotting factors

Bleeding may result from deficiency or dysfunction of any of these elements.

Causes of Disorders of Hemostasis

A. Disorder of clotting factors
- Congenital
  - Hemophilia A
  - von Willebrand's disease
  - Factor IX deficiency
- Acquired
  - Vitamin K deficiency
  - Liver disease
  - Disseminated intravascular coagulation

B. Disorders of platelets
1. Quantitative (low count)
   a. *Decreased production*
   - Congenital
     - Wiscott-Aldrich syndrome
     - Thrombocytopenia absent radius (TAR) syndrome
     - Fanconi anemia
   - Acquired
     - Drugs
     - Infections
     - Malignancy
     - Irradiation
   b. *Increased destruction*
   - Hemolytic uremic syndrome (HUS)
   - Disseminated intravascular coagulation (DIC)
   - Drugs
   - Immune mediated
     - Immune thrombocytopenic purpura (ITP)
     - Neonatal autoimmune
     - Neonatal isoimmune
   - Large hemangioma
   - Hypersplenism
2. Qualitative
   a. Congenital
   - Glanzmann thrombasthenia
   - Bernard-Soulier syndrome
   b. Acquired
   - Drugs
   - Uremia
   - Liver disorders
3. Blood vessel disorders
   a. HSP
   b. Hereditary hemorrhagic telangiectasia
   c. Scurvy
   d. Malnutrition

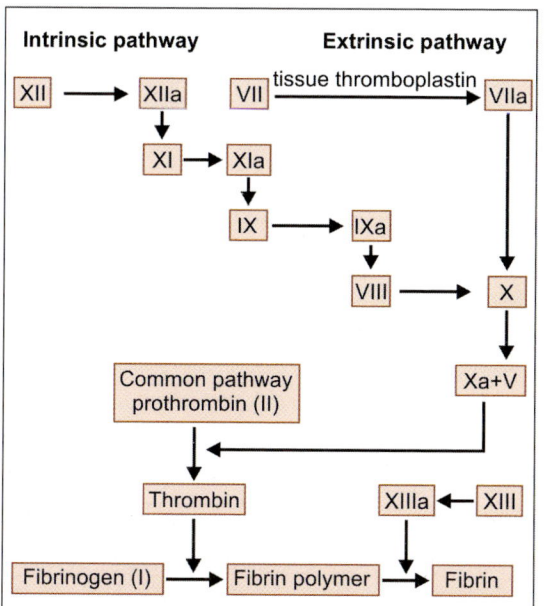

Fig. 16.5: Coagulation cascade.

e. Ehlers-Danlos syndrome

f. Corticosteroids

Clinical features of abnormal hemostasis

Child may suffer from cutaneous bleeding, e.g. ecchymosis, petechiae, epistaxis, prolonged bleeding during surgical procedure, hemarthrosis, deep venous thrombosis, pulmonary embolism or stroke.

Purpura is a group of diseases when small hemorrhages occur in the superficial layers of the skin give the area a purple discoloration, If it is shape of pinpoint (<1 mm)—petechiae, between 2 and 5 mm—purpuric spots, over 5 mm—ecchymosis (Fig. 16.6), finding in coagulation disorders (Tables 16.5 and 16.6).

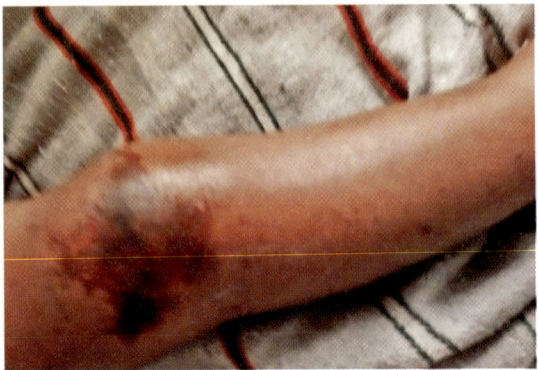

Fig. 16.6: Ecchymosis.

- Malaria
- Kala-azar
- Dengue
- Hepatitis B and C
- HIV
- Congenital (TORCH) infections
- Infection-associated with hemophagocytosis syndrome.

THROMBOCYTOPENIA

Causes

Idiopathic—thrombocytopenic purpura

Infections—disseminated intravascular coagulation.

Table 16.5: Differences in clinical and laboratory finding in coagulation disorders

Lab finding and clinical features	Factor VIII deficiency	Thrombocytopenia	von Willebrand disease	Platelet disorder function	Vit k deficiency	DIC
APTT	Prolonged	Normal	Prolonged	Normal	Prolonged	Prolonged
PT	Normal	Normal	Normal	Normal	Prolonged	Prolonged
Bleeding time	Normal	Prolonged	Prolonged	Prolonged	Normal	Prolonged
Platelet count	Normal	Low	Normal	Normal	Normal	Low
Patechiae	Absent	Present	Absent	Present	Present	Present
Hemarthrosis	Present	Absent	Rare	Absent	Present	Some time present

APTT—activated partial thromboplastin time; PT—prothrombin time; DIC—disseminated intravascular coagulation

Table 16.6: Differences between platelet disorders and coagulation disorders

	Platelet disorders	Coagulation disorder
Bleeding site	Skin mucus	Soft membrane, e.g. epistaxis joint, muscle
	GIT	
Pattern	Immediate after trauma	Delayed
	Mild	Severe
Petechiae	Present	Absent
Ecchymoses	Small, superficial	Large, deep

APTT—activated partial thromboplastin time; PT—prothrombin time; DIC—disseminated intravascular coagulation

Medication drugs
- Valproate
- Penicillin
- Heparin
- Quinine
- Digoxin

Thrombotic microangiopathy
- Thrombotic thrombocytopenic purpura
- Hemolytic uremic syndrome
- Malignancy
- Leukemia, lymphoma, neuroblastoma.

Immunodeficiency: Wiskott-Aldrich syndrome, HIV/AIDS
- Bone marrow failure
- Thrombocytopenia with absent radius
- Fanconi anemia
- Shwachman-Diamond syndrome
- Marrow replacement
- Osteopetrosis, Gaucher's disease

Others: Hypersplenism, Kasabach-Merritt syndrome.

Diagnostic Investigations

a. Complete blood count
b. Platelet count
c. Blood smear to identify platelet abnormality
d. Prothrombin time (PT)
e. Platelet function assay
   - Bleeding time—less accurate, not performed now.
f. Specific assay to identify factor.

PURPURAS

The purpuras are group of disease in which small hemorrhages occur into superficial layers of the skin, producing areas of purple discoloration.

Petechiae are minute extravasation. Ecchymosis is extensive hemorrhage.

Classification

1. *Thrombocytopenic purpuras:* Platelet count is reduced below 40,000/cu mm. Normal platelet count is 1,50,000–400,000/cu mm.
   a. Idiopathic thrombocytopenic purpura (ITP)
   b. Secondary purpuras
      i. Acute leukemia
      ii. Marrow aplasia
      iii. Secondary hypersplenism
      iv. Pernicious anemia
      v. Chemicals
      vi. Infectious disease, smallpox, measles, diphtheria.
2. Non-thrombocytopenic purpuras: Platelet count normal.
   a. Anaphylactoid purpura
   b. Thalassemia
   c. Congenital platelet function disorder
   d. Drug-induced.

IDIOPATHIC THROMBOCYTOPENIC PURPURA

This is most common form of purpura in childhood. The disease appears related to viral infections, e.g. rubella, rubeola, etc.

Clinical Features

Onset is acute with bruising and generalized patechial rash over any part of body, most prominent at legs (Fig. 16.7). Hemorrhages also occur in mucous membrane. Nasal bleeding and in few cases intracranial bleeding may occur. Acute phase lasts for

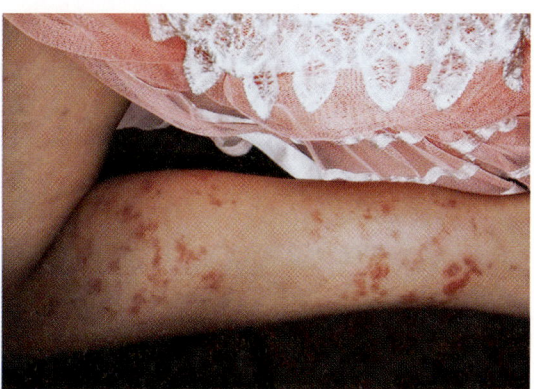

Fig. 16.7: Purpuric rash at legs.

1–2 weeks. Liver, spleen, lymph nodes are not enlarged.

Laboratory Investigations

i. Platelet count is low (below 20,000/cu mm).
ii. Torniquet test positive, prolonged bleeding time.
iii. Bone marrow—increased number of megakaryocytes.
iv. Myeloid and erythroid series of cells are normal. This differentiates it from purpura secondary to aplastic anemia and leukemia.

Management

This has excellent prognosis even when no specific therapy is given.

75% of patients recover completely within 3 months.

Relapses are unusual.

Management includes

i. Blood or platelet transfusion only temporary benefits due to short life of platelets, indicated in serious patient.
ii. Child should be protected from trauma.
iii. Infusion of plasma or gamma globulin causes sustained rise in platelet.

Steroids: Steroids reduce severity and shorten the duration of the illness.

Prednisolone given in dose 1–2 mg/kg/day for 3 weeks until the platelet count is normal, whichever comes first.

Second course is given, if thrombocytopenia persists.

Splenectomy: Splenectomy is indicated for chronic cases if thrombocytopenia persists for 1 year or resistant to steroid.

Immunosuppressive drugs are indicated for chronic and refractory cases.

HEMOPHILIA

Hemophilia is a constitutional anomaly of blood coagulation, characterized by lifelong tendency to excessive hemorrhage from trauma. This is most common hereditary bleeding disorder constituting 90–95% of such cases.

Classification

i. Hemophilia A (classical hemophilia, true hemophilia). This results due to qualitative or quantitative deficiency of a factor VIII, the antihemophilic factor (AHF).
   This is sex-linked recessive disorder occurring almost exclusively in males. Female acts as carrier and does not manifest disease. Incidence is 1 in 10,000. It accounts for 98% of all cases of hemophilias.
ii. Hemophilia B (Christmas disease): This results from deficiency of factor IX, the plasma thromboplastin components (PTC).
iii. Hemophilia C: This results due to deficiency of factor XII, the plasma thromboplastin antecedent (PTA).

Clinical Features

The tendency to bleed is not obvious at birth and excessive hemorrhage at umbilical cord is not seen because of AHG derived from mother. But, in many cases, due to slight trauma, excessive bleeding is noticed since early childhood.

Later, tendency to have excessive bleeding can be noticed following trauma, abrasion, contusion, during epistaxis and bleeding after tooth extraction.

Hemarthrosis especially at knees, ankles and elbows is a characteristic feature of the disease. Effected joint becomes swollen and painful. In earlier stages blood within joints absorbed but repeated attacks of hemorrhages cause inflammation and degenerative changes. The joint becomes immobile (fixed joints) (Fig. 16.8).

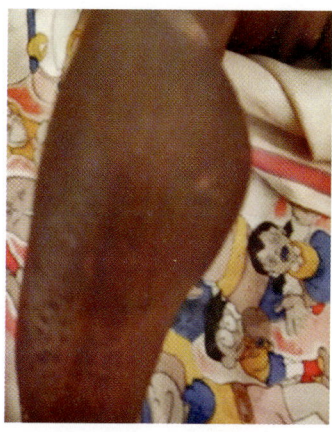

Fig. 16.8: Hemophilia—hemarthrosis.

Intramuscular hemorrhages and a large hematoma at sites of minor trauma may occur. Gastrointestinal hemorrhages (hematemesis or malena or both) may take place, often associated with pain. Bleeding may occur at CNS, genitourinary tract, liver, spleen, pleural or peritoneal cavity, in skin, unlike purpura, petechiae do not occur.

In mild hemophilia (subhemophilia) many of these features are absent.

Diagnosis

i. Clinical picture of disease and family history of disease on maternal side (especially maternal uncle).
ii. Blood examination
   a. Coagulation time is prolonged, while bleeding time is normal. Clot retraction normal, coagulation time may be normal when degree of deficit of factor VIII is not too pronounced.
   b. Prothrombin consumption is low and thromboplastin generation is high. These are more sensitive tests.
   c. Specific factor assay confirms the diagnosis.
iii. *Radiology:* X-ray joint of hemarthrosis. Initially, joint cavity is distended and synovitis. Later, synovial thickening, demineralization, erosion and contracture. Increased vascularization results acclerated bone growth. Premature appearance of ossification centers occur

at later stage. Articular surface is completely destroyed and juxta-articular cyst forms.

Prognosis and Course

Such patients are under constant threat to life from bleeding intracranially or into the tissues of the neck. Death may occur in infancy, childhood due to severe bleeding. If child survives, he should learn to adjust activities and avoid trauma lifelong. Timely medical helps also prolong life. Repeated hemorrhages in joints cripple him.

Treatment

i. Steps to prevent injury are taken.
ii. Local treatment of wound is aimed to create optimal conditions for the formation of clot, such as proper cleaning, application of cold compress, judicious local pressure, application of fresh plasma or thrombin powder or gel foam, adrenaline solution.
iii. Local treatment for hemorrhages into joints is done by application of ice bags just after injury and kept for 24–48 hours with involved joint wrapped in an elastic bandage.

After 48 hours, heat will aid in absorption of fluid from joints and should be applied cautiously. This is followed by gentle massage and passive exercise.

Specific Measures

Specific measures consist of giving replacement therapy for the missing clotting factor. In case there is severe bleeding, *fresh whole blood* is given to counteract shock and anemia.

In case of mild to moderate bleeding, *fresh plasma* is recommended, since factor VIII is labile.

Dose of fresh plasma—severe bleeding 2–3 ml/kg/hour for 6 to 12 hours, followed by 1 ml per kg per hour until a firm clot forms in 3–4 days.

If possible, concentrate of *antihemophilic factor* like *cryoprecipitate* of fresh plasma is given. It is useful, convenient and commercially available.

Normal AHF is achieved with transfusion of small volume of this preparation.

Genetics

In true classical hemophilia, only male will suffer. This is familiar, but due to mutation true classical hemophilia can occur without family history. Hemophilia B and C can occur in female also.

In classical hemophilia, if male (patient) marries healthy female, his son will not be sufferer but daughter will be 'carrier'. Son of these carrier daughter will suffer from disease.

For giving advise for marriage, detect female carrier only.

LEUKEMIAS

Definition

A condition of unknown etiology characterized by uncontrollable and abnormal proliferation of the leukocytes and precursors which infiltrate the body tissue. Leukemia is the commonest form of childhood malignancy. More than 95% cases of leukemia in childhood are of acute variety. 1–3% have chronic myeloid leukemia. Chronic lymphocytic leukemia is unknown in childhood.

Leukemias are most common cancer in children.

Subtypes

Main

1. Acute lymphocytic leukemia (ALL)
2. Acute myeloid leukemia (AML)

Others

1. Juvenile chronic myeloid leukemia (JCML)
2. Chronic myeloid leukemia (CML)

ACUTE LYMPHOCYTIC LEUKEMIA

Epidemiology

It is most common leukemia of children (75% of all acute leukemias).

Peak incidence is between 2 and 5 years, boy has higher incidence than girls.

High incidence is seen in children suffering from Down syndrome.

Etiology

Etiology in unknown various risk factors are as follows.

Genetic

- Down syndrome (most common)
- Fanconi syndrome
- Shwachman-Diamond syndrome
- Bloom syndrome
- Ataxia-telangiectasia
- Diamond-Blackfan anemia
- Kostmann syndrome
- Li-Fraumeni syndrome
- Severe combined immunodeficiency
- Paroxysmal nocturnal hemoglobinuria
- Neurofibromatosis type 1

Environmental

- Ionizing radiation
- Alkylating agents, e.g. cyclophosphamide, ifosfamide, epipodophyllotoxins—etoposide, tenoposide, nitrosourea (nitrogen mustard)
- Benzene

Immunophenotype

B cell derived	:	80–85%
T cell derived	:	95%
Mature B cell derived	:	1–2%

Cytogenetics

Hyperdiploidy	:	Good prognosis
Hypodiploidy	:	Poor prognosis

Incidence

Slightly more in boys than girls. Increase incidence is seen in immunodeficiency, chromosomal abnormalities and ataxia-telangiectasia.

Clinical Features

Onset is acute, early manifestations are anorexia, irritability and lethargy. Pallor, bleeding and fever are due to progressive failure of bone marrow.

On examination anemia, petechiae, lymphadenopathy and hepatosplenomegaly are seen. Bleeding from other orifices may occur.

Bone pain and arthralgia are common complaints. Infiltration in meninges results headache, vomiting and neck rigidity.

Laboratory Investigations

  i. Hemoglobin reduced
 ii. Leukocyte count in blood may be <500/cu mm or >50,000/cu mm or sometime normal.
     Peripheral smear shows blast cells which may be scanty or abundant.
iii. Bone marrow —leukemic lymphoblasts are seen in high number.
 iv. Skiagram bone—subperiosteal and sub-epiphyseal resorption of bone.
  v. Serum uric acid—high

Prognosis

Bad in children below 2 years and above 8 years of age.

Treatment

Treatment of ALL is divided in 4 steps.

1. Induction to Therapy

Aim: To eradicate leukemia from the bone marrow so that at the end of the therapy <5% leukemia blast cells remain in bone marrow.

Duration: 4–6 weeks.

Drugs: Induction 1
- Prednisolone—40 mg/m^2 orally on days 1–28.
- Vincristine—1.4 mg/m^2 intravenous (IV) on days 1, 8, 15, 22, 29.
- Daunorubicin—30 mg/m^2 IV on days 8, 15, 29.
- L-asparaginase—6000 U/m^2 (IM) alternate days 2–20 (10 doses).

Induction 2
- Methotrexate—intrathecal IT on days 1, 8, 15, 22.
- 6-mercaptopurine—75 mg/m^2 orally on days 1–7 and days 15–21.
- Cyclophosphamide—750 mg/m^2 IV on days 1 and 15.
- Methotrexate—intrathecal on days 1, 8, 15 and 22.
- Cranial irradiations—CGY for 9 days total (1800 CGY)
- Repeat induction—same as induction.

2. Consolidation (Intensification)

Aim: To reduce drug resistance
Drugs
- Cyclophosphamide—750 mg/m^2 IV on days 1 and 15.
  Vincristine—1.4 mg/m^2 IV on days 1 and 15
- Cytosine arabinoside—75 mg/m^2 subcutaneously every 12 hours (6 doses) day 1–3 and days 15–17.

3. Maintenance (Continuation) Therapy

Aim: To prevent relapse
Duration: 2–2.5 years
Drugs
- Prednisolone—40 mg/m^2 orally days 1–7
- Vincristine—1.4 mg/m^2 IV on day 1
- Daunorubicin—30 mg/m^2 IM on days 1, 3, 5 and 7.
- L-asparaginase—75 mg/m^2 orally daily for 3 of every 4 weeks for a period of total 12 weeks.
- Methotrexate—15 mg/m^2 orally once a week for 3 of every 4 weeks for a total 12 weeks.

4. CNS Protection (Prevention) Therapy

Aim: To eradicate leukemic cells which have passed blood–brain barrier because systemic therapy does not eradicate them. Many children with ALL have subclinical CNS involvement at early stage.

Management

1. Methotrexate is the drug used.
2. Cranial irradiation.

Treatment after relapse

If medical treatment fails, bone marrow transplantation has better prognosis than conventional treatment.

Prognosis

Poor prognosis is seen in:
1. Hypodiploidy
2. Philadelphia chromosome positivist
3. T cell ALL
4. IKZK1 gene detection
5. CNS disease
6. Age <1 year and >10 years
7. Leukocyte count >50,000/cu mm

ACUTE MYELOID LEUKEMIA (AML)

It results from clonal proliferation of hematopoietic precursors of myeloid, erythroid and megakaryocytic lineage (Fig. 16.9).

Epidemiology

Uncommon in children (about 2–3%).

More common in adolescence male affected as female. Congenital AML is mostly AML.

Etiology

Etiology is unknown. Most important predisposing factor is Down syndrome. Other factors are Fanconi syndrome, Kostmann syndrome, Bloom's syndrome, Diamand-Blackfan syndrome, anemia, medications—alkylating agents and epipodophyllotoxins.

Pathogenesis

Several genetic aberrations are identified which lead to changes in hematopoietic differentiation.

Classification

As per FAB classification several subgroups of AML are noticed $M_0, M_1, M_2, M_3, M_4, M_5, M_6, M_7,$ etc.

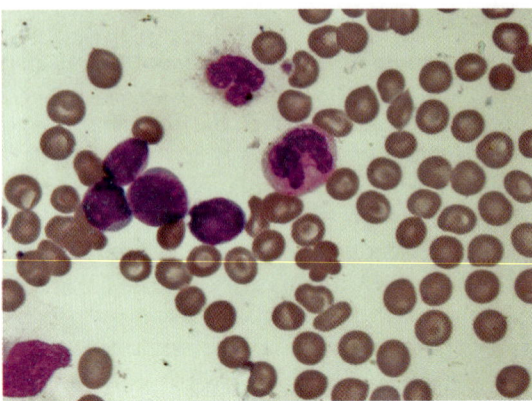

Fig. 16.9: Blood picture of acute myeloid leukemia.

Clinical Features

Clinically AML manifests as pallor, fatigue, bleeding and fever. Lymphadenopathy and massive hepatosplenomegaly are not common. Chloromas are localized collection of leukemic cells seen in AML at various sites—CNS, neck bones and skin. Pulmonary infiltration results respiratory distress.

Sometimes preleukemic phase is present characterized by refractory anemia, neutropenia, or thrombocytopenia.

Diagnosis

Diagnosis is confirmed by peripheral smear, bone marrow examination, cytochemical, immunophenotypic and genetic characteristic of blast cells.

Treatment

Drugs (induction therapy)

1. Cytosine arabinoside—100 mg/m^2/day given as continuous infusion for 7 days.
2. Anthracycline (daunorubicin)—42 mg/m^2/day for 3 days.

Other drugs: Etoposide, thioguanine may be given along with above drugs. Remission occurs in 70–80% of patients by this therapy.

Drugs (consolidation therapy)

1. Cytosine arabinoside
2. Etoposide

JUVENILE CHRONIC MYELOID LEUKEMIA

It is common below the age of 5 years characterized by acute course having anemia, lymphadenopathy, hepatosplenomegaly, skin involvement (eczema, xanthoma and *café au lait* spots), frequent infections and thrombocytopenia.

Leukocytosis usually less than 1 lac/mm². Peripheral smear—full of granulocytic precursors, increased normoblasts, monocytosis.

Management

Supportive care, packed cell and platelets transfusion, treatment of infections and stem cell transplantation. *Cis*-retinoic acid has some benefit. Survival rate is 30–50%.

Stem cell transplantation: Stem cell transplantation is indicated to patient with unfavorable genetic alterations.

Supportive care: It is indicated to all AML patients.

CHRONIC MYELOID LEUKEMIA (CML)

It is mainly disease of 2nd and 3rd decades of life but may occur at any age. It may be adult variety or juvenile variety.

Adult variety: Rare in children, manifests as pallor, fever, weight loss, headache, dizziness, visual disturbances. Splenomegaly, leukocytosis (<1 lac/mm³) mild anemia, thrombocytosis. Philadelphia chromosome is present in most of the cases.

Treatment is indicated to control increasing white blood cells by single chemotherapeutic agent either busulfan or hydroxyurea.

However, these agents are replaced by beta interferon, tyrosine kinase inhibitor, imatinib mesylate, stem cell transplantation is indicated in refractory cases.

Chronic myeloid leukemia is uncommon in children (about 3–5%). Common clinical features are as follows and differences between juvenile and adult types are given in Table 16.7.

Treatment

i. Remission is induced by busulfan in the dose of 4 mg/m²/day (0.06 mg/kg) daily till the count comes to 10,000 to 20,000/mm.
ii. If count is increasing, again treatment is started.
iii. Some cases may benefit by splenic irradiation.

Table 16.7: Differences between juvenile and adult types

Feature	Juvenile type	Adult type
i. Age of onset	Less than 2–4 years	10–14 years
ii. Skin rashes	Common	Uncommon
iii. Bleeding tendency	Common	Uncommon
iv Lymphadenopathy	Common	Uncommon
v. Splenomgaly	Mild	Marked
Laboratory investigations		
a. Total WBC count	Often below 1 lac/cumm	Often above 1 lac/cumm
b. Blast cells	Common	Less common
c. Monocytosis	Common	Rare
d. Platelet count	Often decreased	Not often decreased except in terminal stage
e. Nucleated RBC	Often increased	Normal
f. Fetal hemoglobin	30–60%	2–6%
g. Megakaryocytes	Deseased number	Increased number
h. Serum vit B$_{12}$ level	Increased	Increased
Response to treatment	Complete remission is rare	Complete remission (frequently)

PANCYTOPENIA (APLASTIC ANEMIA)

The term pancytopenia denotes bone marrow failure with decreased RBCs, leukocytes and platelets.

Types

1. Congenital
2. Acquired

CONGENITAL PANCYTOPENIA (FANCONI ANEMIA)

It is a autosomal recessive disease. Bone marrow failure occurs about at the age of 7 years.

Ecchymosis and petechiae are common presentations of the disease. Other features are skeletat deformities, short stature and absence or hypoplasia of thumb and radius. Skin is hyperpigmented. Renal abnormalities are also present.

Laboratory findings

Pancytopenia picture:
1. RBC macrocytosis
2. Raticulocyte low
3. Elevated HbF
4. Bone marrow hypocellularity

Management

1. Transfusion of RBCs and platelets.
2. Bone marrow transplant.
3. Immunosuppressive therapy (e.g. corticosteroids).

ACQUIRED

Etiology

Drugs: Sulfonamides, anticonvulsants, chloramphenicol.
Infections: HIV, Epstein-Barr virus (EBV) hepatitis C, cytomegalovirus (CMV)
Chemicals—arsenic
Radiations
Idiopathic
Clinical features: Pallor, bruising, petechiae or serious infections due to low WBC count.
Laboratory findings: RBC, WBC, platelets—low count.

Low reticulocytes, hypocellular bone marrow.
Treatment: Stop causative factor.

POLYCYTHEMIA

Polycythemia is defined as an increase in RBC relative to total blood volume.

Hematocrit (Hct) >60% or Hb% more than two standard deviations above normal values for age.

Causes

Primary —rare
Secondary—caused by increased erythropoietin production
1. *Appropriate*: Due to hypoxemia and cyanotic congenital heart disease
   - Pulmonary disease
   - Residence of high altitude
2. *Inappropriate:* Tumors of kidney, cerebellum ovary, liver, adrenal gland, kidney disease, e.g. hydronephrosis.

Relative—apparent increase in RBC mass due to decrease in plasma volume as seen in dehydration.

Clinical Features

Facial complexion is ruddy.

Management

Treat the cause, phlebotomy to keep Hct <60%. Dehydration management—treat dehydration.

NEUTROPENIA

It is defined as low absolute number of neutrophils.

It may be mild (1000–1500 cells/mm^3, moderate (500–1000 cells/mm^3 or severe <500 cells/mm^3.

Causes

Decreased Production

A. *Infections:* Viruses (HIV, EBV, CMV, hepatitis A and B, influenza, parvovirus)
   Bacteria: Typhus, Rocky Mountain spotted fever
   Protozoa (e.g. malaria)

B. Chronic benign neutropenia of childhood
C. Severe congenital agranulocytosis
D. Cyclic neutropenia
E. Genetic syndromes:
    a. Chédiak-Higashi syndrome
    b. Cartilage hair hypoplasia syndrome
F. Shwachman-Diamond syndrome
G. Drugs (antibiotic, anticonvulsant, aspirin)
H. Metabolic diseases

Hyperglycemia, methylmalonic acidemia, Gaucher's disease.

Increased Destruction

A. Infections (mostly viral)
B. Drugs
C. Hypersplenism
D. Autoimmune neutropenia
E. Alloimmune neutropenia.

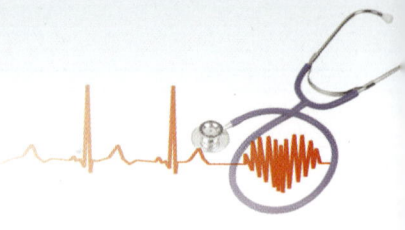

Behavioral Disorders
(Psychosomatic Disorders)

17

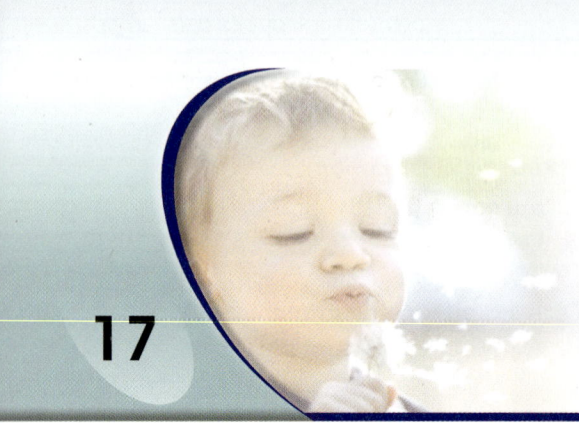

Body consists of soma and psychi. A child develops some abnormalities in behavior due to emotional abnormalities, which are out of control of his will. They are called behavioral or psychosomatic disorders.

Etiology

Causes of abnormalities may be:

i. **Personal factors**
   a. Genetically determined, e.g. in Klinefelter's syndrome in the form of aggressive behavior.
   b. Acquired—as during steroid therapy psychosis is more common in adolescents than adults.

ii. **Environmental factors:** Environment affects the child behavior in which he lives. Father, mother, other siblings, school and other classmates behavior affects the child. Excessive overprotection, guilt, over anxiety, under affection, rejection or disturbances, overcriticism, parenteral incompatibility, sibling rivalry, psychosis, adoption; all affects child personality.

Classification

1. Problems related to intellectual functioning
   a. Truancy—remaining away from school without leave.

   b. School phobia—child recent going school because dread of school situation.
2. Developmental disorders
   a. Disorders of motility
      i. *Delayed motor development:* Some children sit and walk much later than expected and do not show any mental subnormality.
      ii. *Hyperactivity:* Children are constantly in motion which is accompanied by distractibility, short attention span and visual motor defects.
      iii. *Clumpsiness:* Difficulty in performing everyday task, e.g. dressing or undressing.
   b. Right and left indiscrimination. These are mentally dull.
   c. Disorders of speech
      i. *Cluttering:* Rapid, confused, jobed speech and associated with changes in behavior personality.
      ii. *Dyslaxia:* Abnormal substitution, insertion or omission of speech sounds.
      iii. *Lipsing:* Inability to pronounce correctly one of the sibilant sounds like S, She, Z, Ch, J.
      iv. *Aphonia:* Voice is lost suddenly but articulation is present.

v. *Falsetto voice:* High-pitched voice.

vi. Incessant talking: To get attention from parents.

vii. Tachylalia (rapid speech).

viii. Slow speech.

ix. *Idioglossia:* Speech that is barely comprehensible. Children may develop a language of their own.

d. Reading disorders: Dyslaxia—difficulty to read in spite of normal intelligence.

e. Hearing defects

i. Auditory verbal imperception: Difficulty in understanding spoken words.

ii. Auditory verbal indiscrimination—difficulty in discriminating individual sounds especially words which sound alike, e.g. beek or seek.

iii. Defective auditory memory span: Difficulty in retaining information in the proper sequence.

f. Enuresis

g. *Motion sickness:* Symptoms result from repeated oscillatory movements of the body.

3. Problem related to emotional development.

a. Anxiety

b. *Phobias:* Unwarranted fears which continually impose themselves on consciousness.

c. Obsession and compulsions: Ideas which persistently obtrude themselves into the reground of consciousness against the will and better judgment of the individual. Compulsions which result from obsessions.

d. *Impulsions:* Children who are preoccupied to an unusual degree with various interests, ideas and actions.

e. *Circumscribed interest patterns:* Children in whom the main characteristic is a concentration of interest in a specialized field of thought or endeavor.

f. *Hypochondriasis:* Anxiety concerning health or exaggeration of somatic symptoms for the purpose of getting attention.

g. *Temper tantrum:* Outbursts of anger.

h. *Breath holding:* Breath holding during the course of violent crying, cyanosis, unconsciousness and convulsive twitching are rare.

i. *Excessive aggression:* Child who attempts to dominate every situation.

j. *Hostility:* Those feelings and impulses which contain an element and ill will towards others.

k. Shyness

l. *Cruelty:* The child hurts for the pleasure of hurting and for the satisfaction of seeing others suffers.

m. *Depression:* Child feels unloved, rejected and a failure.

n. *Emotional deprivation:* Emotionally deprived children show listless, relative immobility, unresponsiveness to stimuli, indifferent appetite, failure to gain weight in spite of proper diet.

o. *Sensory deprivation:* Performance of the individual is markedly impaired if all the sensations are blocked.

p. *Sex problems:* Masturbation, petting, homosexuality.

q. *Problems of everyday habit:* Thumb sucking and finger sucking, nail biting, lip sucking and lip biting. Nose picking, hair pulling, teeth grinding, psychogenic cough, day-dreaming, imaginary playmates, ties.

r. *Disturbance of eating:* Anorexia, pica, rumination (ingested food is regurgitated), aerophagia colic (no cause apparent).

s. Obesity

t. Constipation

u. *Disorders of sleep*
- Nightmares—terror from a disease.
- Night terror—not associated with dreaming but hallucination.
- Somniloquy—talking during sleep.
- Somnambulism—sleep walking.
- Narcolepsy—paroxysmal and diurnal attacks of irreversible sleep.

Organic disturbance having large psychic component, e.g. asthma, ulcerative colitis.

Antisocial Behavior

Juvenile delinquency: Violation of law and antisocial act such as lying, stealing, running away, fire setting, homicide.

General Management

General management is directed towards correction of causative situation and make psychologic environment.

PICA (GEOPHAGIA)

Eating of substances other than food, e.g. earth, flakes of paint, plaster from wall. This may be:
1. *Pshychosomatic disorders:* Due to abnormal atmosphere creating emotion abnormality.
2. Due to deficiency of iron, vitamins and minerals.
3. Due to worm infestations.

Treatment

Treat the reason. Psychotherapy is essential.

ENEURESIS

Bed wetting after 3 years of age.

Causes

a. Psychosomatic disorders, over strictness of parents.
b. Threadworm infestation, especially in girls.
c. Genitourinary tract infection.
d. Congenital anatomic defect in spine.
e. If child is not trained properly.

Treatment

Child is treated psychologically:
1. Give less fluids in night. Empty bladder before sleep and in-between in night. Do not punish or say anything if he fails, it will create tension and increase illness. If he succeeds, encourage him.
2. *Imipramine:* Dose 25–75 mg before going to bed.
3. If pinworm infestation is associated, it is treated.

BREATH-HOLDING SPELLS

In breath-holding spells, child cries vigorously, takes long breath and followed by holding of breath. Face becomes cyanosed or pale. Sometimes convulsions occur. Child recovers soon without any treatment. This is common in 6–8 months age. This is attraction seeking phenomenon. Cause of this is tense atmosphere in the child environment.

Treatment

Child and parents should be dealt psychologically to reduce tension in them. No treatment is necessary. Parents should be assured about benign nature of problem and that it is not going to harm the baby.

BRUXISM

Grinding of teeth at sleep. This is due to mental tension. This also occurs due to mental retardation and in unconscious patient.

No treatment is necessary. Psychologically treated to reduce tense atmosphere.

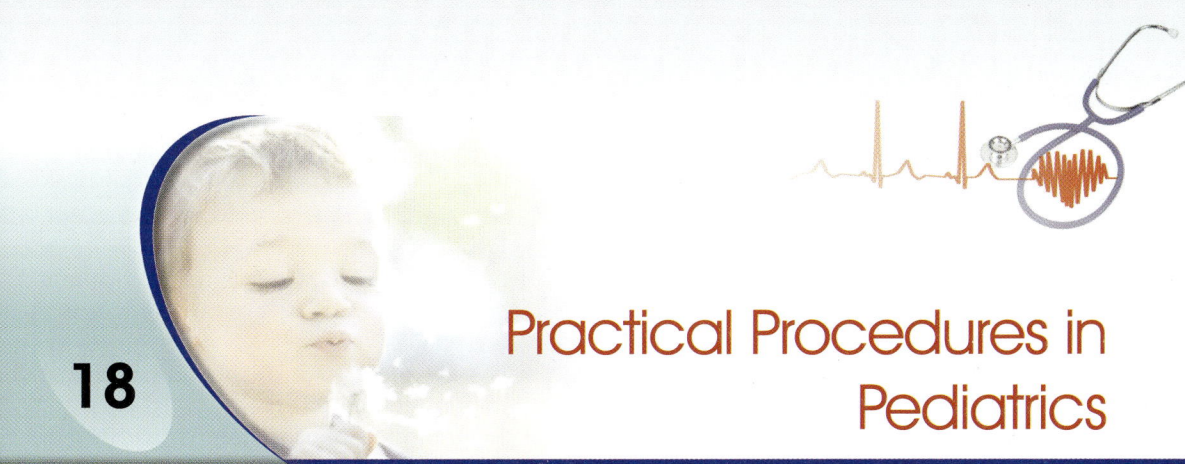

18

Practical Procedures in Pediatrics

Collection of Urine Sample

Method

1. Midstream sample is collected. The patient passes a small amount of urine and stops. Then next part of urine is collected in clean container.
2. Wash the genitalia before collecting urine. Avoid collecting urine during menstrual period in females.
3. Collection of urine in infant:
   a. In boys test tube strapped to penis
   b. In baby girls plastic bags can be strapped around vulva. The bag is fixed around the baby's genitalia and left in place for 1–3 hours.
   c. Catheterization for collection of urine should be avoided because of danger of starting an infection.
   d. Occasionally suprapubic puncture may be required in sick neonates or small infants.

Collection of Blood Sample

Blood is collected for small amount for Hb examination, smear, RBC, WBC count from finger or heel prick method. When large quantity is required, peripheral vein is selected for collection. Femoral vein is avoided as far as possible due to risk of hazards.

UMBILICAL VEIN CATHETERIZATION

Indicated for exchange transfusion and blood sample collection.

Anatomy

Umbilical vein is situated at about 12 o'clock position in umbilical cord. Lumen gaps: It is single, while two umbilical arteries are situated laterally. Their lumen is obliterated, thin walled, color is whitish.

Method

i. Before procedure, catheter is marked for distance to be inserted. Umbilical vein is identified, stump is held with forceps, clot or debris is removed from vein and artery is dilated with artery forceps (Table 18.1).
ii. Catheter is pushed into vein forward. Free flow of blood is obtained. Ideally catheter should reach up to lower part of inferior vena cava or right atrium. X-ray chest (lateral and PA view) may identify position.
iii. Catheter is filled with heparinized saline (1000 units of heparin to 100 ml of normal saline) stopped and labelled as venous.

VENESECTION OR 'CUT DOWN'

It is an emergency procedure when every attempt to intravenous administration in vein fails. Vein is dissected out.

Table 18.1: Approximate length of catheter to be passed for umbilical vein catheterization

Length of baby (crown heel length)	Venous catheter (IVC)
36 cm	6.0 cm
40 cm	7.0 cm
44 cm	8.0 cm
50 cm	9.0 cm

Removal: Catheter is removed. Purse string suture is tied. Bleeding controlled.

Site

Most common site is great saphenous vein situated just anterior to and above the medial malleolus of foot. Next common site is vein above cubital fossa.

Steps (Fig. 18.1)

1. Secure the foot firmly with splint or any attendant in position of external rotation.
2. Clean the area with antiseptic lotion.
3. Test the Xylocaine sensitivity then infiltrate the site with 2% Xylocaine.
4. A small incision over skin is made transverse to direction of vein.
5. Dissect underlying fat and fascia and tissue with dissecting forceps and vein is exposed.
6. The vein having been cleared, an aneurysm needle or artery forceps is passed under it threaded with catgut or silk suture and drawn back loop is cut. Forms two ligatures.
7. Distal (lower ligature) is tied to occlude venous return. Ends are caught in artery forceps.
8. Dissect the sheath of the vein with the help of needle.
9. A small incision is made over surface of the skin sufficiently to allow insertion of a cannula or polythene tube. It is inserted about 2 cm within vein.
10. Blood begins to flow in polythene tube. Now vein is tied by proximal ligature.
11. Polythene tube attached with needle is connected with drip set.
12. Wound is closed with fine stitches, polythene tube is fixed with help of adhesive and sterile gauze.

Abdominal Paracentesis

In newborn procedure is same except that the tap should be done in left iliac fossa to avoid puncturing of liver, if it is grossly enlarged.

Bone Marrow Aspiration

Usual site is iliac crest. In children less than 2 years anteriomedial aspect of tibia.

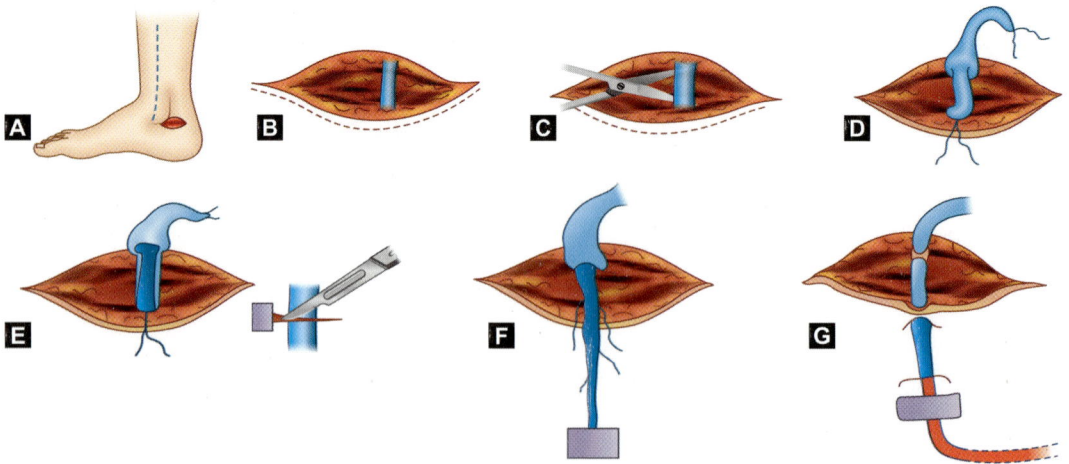

Fig. 18.1A to G: Steps of venesection.

ENDOTRACHEAL INTUBATION

Anatomy

Epiglottis is a lid-like structure overhanging the entrance to the trachea.

Vallecula: A pouch formed by the base of tongue and the epiglottis.

Esophagus, cricoids, glottis, vocal cords, trachea, bronchi.

Position of newborn: On the flat surface with head in a midline position, neck slightly extended with the help of roll placed under baby 'shoulder'. Do not hyperextend or flex the neck.

How to hold laryngoscope: Hold the laryngoscope in your left hand between your thumb and first two or three fingers with the blade pointing away from you.

Visualize the glottis and insert the tube

1. Stabilize the baby's head with over right hand and by helping person.
2. Slide the laryngoscope blade over the side of tongue pushing the tongue to the left side of the mouth.

Advance blade until the tip lies in the vallecula; just beyond the base of the tongue. Your right index finger may be open to open the baby's mouth to easier the insertion.

Lift the blade of laryngoscope slightly, thus lifting the tongue out of the way to expose the pharyngeal area (Fig. 18.2).

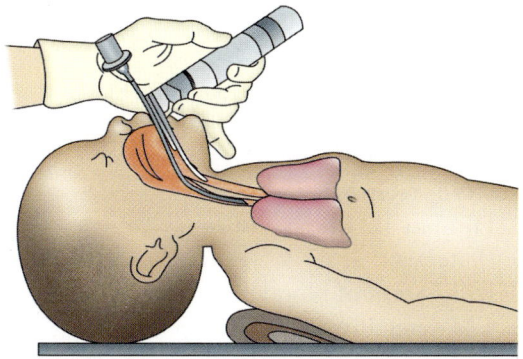

Fig. 18.2: Endotracheal intubation.

During lifting the blade, raise the entire blade by pulling up in the direction the handle is pointing. Take care do not elevate the tip of the blade by using a rocking motion and pulling the handle towards you.

See the epiglottis, vocal cords as stipes on each side of the glottis or as an inverted letter V. Adjust the blade until structures come into view.

Insert the tube holding the tube in your right hand, introduce it into right side of the baby's mouth with the curve of the tube lying in the horizontal plane.

Keep the glottis in view, when the vocal cords are apart, insert the tube until the vocal cord guide is at the level of the cords.

If the cords are together, wait for them to open. Do not touch the closed cords with the tip of the tube because it may cause spasm.

1. Position of the tube in the trachea—about half way between the vocal cords and carina.
2. Stabilize the tube with one hand and remove the laryngoscope by other hand. Do not press the tube firmly.

To ventilate the baby—attach the tube with ventilation bag. Resume positive pressure ventilation.

For meconium suction—connect the tube to a meconium aspirator which has been connected to suction force. Occlude the suction control part of the aspirator.

Gradually withdraw the tube suctioning any meconium that may be in trachea.

Repeat intubation and suction as necessary a little or no meconium is recovered.

NASOGASTRIC TUBE

A nasogastric tube is a narrow bore tube passed into stomach via the nose. These are used for short term feeding and also for aspiration of stomach contents.

Wide bore tube is used for drainage and fine born tube (gauze less than 9) for feeding because it reduces risk of rhinitis, pharyngitis or esophageal erosions.

Inserting a Nasogastric Tube

- Measure the tube from bridge of nose to the earlobe, than to the point midway between the lower end of sternum (xiphisternum) and the navel.
- Mark the measured length with marker.
- Explain the procedure and obtain consent of patient.
- Sit the patient in a semi-upright position with head supported with pillow and not tilted forward or backward.
- Examine the nostril for any deformity obstruction.
- Lubricate the tubing (2–4 inch) of stomach and with lubricant (2% Xylocaine).
- Pass the tubing with either nostrils gently.
- Insert gently past the pharynx, esophagus, and then into the stomach.
- Ask the patient to swallow
- If resistance is felt do not force but rotate it gently and advance.
- Stop the advancing if patient starts coughing, cyanosed, distressed or coil of tube returns in mouth or buccal cavity.
- Advance up to mark
- Check the tube for its position:
  a. Test the pH of aspirate (less than 4) by blue litmus.
  b. X-ray will confirm.

Old test of introducing of air into stomach and checking the bubbling sound in epigastrium with the help of stethoscope not very much reliable.

- Secure the tube with adhesive tape.
- Tube should be flushed with water regularly to prevent occlusion due to feeding or medication.

Contraindications

- High risk of aspiration
- Gastric stasis
- Gastroesophageal reflux
- Upper GIT stricture

- Nasal injuries
- Basal skull fracture

Removal—pinch the tube and remove the tube.

Feeding with Tube

Various types of feeding tubes (small, large size) are available. Approximate distance of tube to reach at stomach is measured from nose to ear and then tip of xiphisternum. Nostrils are cleaned and tip of tube lubricated and passed through nose backwards up to stomach which is confirmed by pushing air by syringe into tube and listening the voice with stethoscope at left upper part of stomach. Sometimes, fluid is seen in tube. It also confirms.

Feeding with tube is done with the syringe, piston is withdrawn. Child is lying and feeding material (milk, etc.) is filled in barrel. Hold the tube up so feeding material goes by gravity. After feeding push some water and close it.

Gastric wash may be done with the help of syringe. Contents in the stomach are sucked and thrown. Then push some normal saline, again contents are withdrawn. It is repeated until returning fluid is same (normal saline). Tube is removed being firmly caught between thumb and finger so to prevent food escaping from tube at the end when it is withdrawn.

BLOOD TRANSFUSION

It is a common medical procedure in which blood is given through an intravenous (IV) in one of the blood vessels.

Types

1. Red blood cells transfusion
2. Frozen plasma transfusion
3. Prothrombin complex concentrate (PCC)
4. Cryoprecipitate
5. Human albumin solution
6. Platelets
7. Irradiation of blood components
8. CMV negative blood components
9. Use of anti-D immunoglobulin (Anti-D Ig).

Blood transfusion is indicated if patient has lost blood or not producing blood this can be in illness, surgery, cancer, infection, burns, injury or other medical conditions.

RBC TRANSFUSION

ABO and RH (D) groups of patient and blood (donor) should be matched where possible. For all patients should be confirmed by two samples taken at different time.

Indications
* Anemia
* Hemorrhage

Process: The sample of blood is sent to laboratory for typing and crossmatching. Typing means when the lab determines blood type (group), crossmatching means to determine if patient's blood is compatible with donor's blood.

Blood types (group)	Rh group may be (+) or (−)
A positive	A negative
B positive	B negative
O positive	O negative
AB positive	AB negative

Blood group detection is important because RBC contain antigen or protein markers corresponding to these blood groups.

If wrong blood is given to patient, his immune system will detect and react to it and make attempt to destroy it.

Transfusion Reactions
* Back pain
* Blood in urine
* Chills
* Fainting
* Dizzinss
* Fever, flank pain
* Skin flushing

Cause of reaction: Antibodies in the recipient blood attack the donor's blood if both are not compatible. If antibodies attack on red blood cells of donor's blood, it causes hemotype reaction. If antibodies attack on WBC of donor blood then it causes febrile reaction.
* Allergic reaction—itching and hives
* Acute lung injury (TRALI).

It is due to donor plasma antibody damage cells of lungs. It reduces oxygen supply to body. It occurs after six hours of receiving blood.
* Infection, shock death—may occur if bacteria are present in donor's blood.
* CCF—if blood amount given is too much.

Serious Complications
* Acute renal failure
* Anemia
* Pulmonary edema
* Shock
* Allergic anaphylaxis.

PHLEBOTOMY

Drawing blood by venepuncture.

Steps
1. Select suitable site for venepuncture
   * Veins above cubital fossa
   * Veins at dorsum of hand and foot
   * Veins at scalp in infant
2. Use of the following articles keep ready
   * Gloves
   * Torniquet
   * Alcohal swab/disinfectant
   * Gauze pads, cotton balls
   * Blood collection table
   * Marking pens, sharp container, label
3. Watch hands in warm, running water with chlorhexidine gluconate (hand washing product)
4. Wear globes
5. Apply tourniquet 3–4 inches above the puncture site. It should be so much tight so as to stop the blood flow in veins and not in arteries. Duration should not be more than 1 minute. Release the tourniquet as soon as the blood starts coming in tube.

6. Clean the site of venepuncture with 70% isopropyl alcohol. Allow to dry for 30–60 seconds. Do not touch site after cleaning.

Venepuncture using butterfly wing set and syringes:

1. Use 25- or 23-gauge needle with bevel up with attach syringe. 21-22-gauge should be preferred as it ensures rapid blood flow.
2. Clean the site, apply tourniquet.
3. Perform venepuncture, keep needle's bevel up.
4. Grasp the syringe barrel firmly and pull the plunger until required quantity of blood drawn (if venepuncture is done for IV fluid, fit the IV set end). If venepuncture is done to give medication, keep ready medicine in syringe before venepuncture. Push gently medicine slowly.
5. If venepuncture is done for collection of blood sample. Pour blood in evacuated tube.

Mixing

Tubes should be gently inverted to ensure thorough mixing of the blood with additive.

Tubes with anticoagulant such as EDTA, heparin, etc. must be mixed to ensure that the specimen does not clot.

VENEPUNCTURE USING SYRINGE

- Pull the skin light with your thumb or index finger just below the puncture site (fix the vein).
- Holding the needle in line with vein use a quick, small thrust to puncture the skin and vein.
- Draw the blood by pulling back slowly on the syringe if venepuncture is done for collecting blood.
- If venepuncture is done to give IV fluid medication. Fit the IV tube. Give medicine, if venepuncture is done for giving medicine.
- After removal of syringe with needle place a gauze pad over the puncture site, quickly remove the needle. Apply pressure for about 2 minutes. When bleeding stops apply fresh gauze or tape.

IV CANNULATION

Intravenous catheterization is most common procedures performed in hospitals, clinics for various purposes such as fluid and electrolyte replacement, drug administration blood products and to draw blood for investigation.

Selecting the Vein

In adult—site selection should be initiated from distal to proximal.

In children—in infants and children
1. Anticubital fossa
2. Dorsum of hand or foot
3. Saphenous veins in lower leg
4. Scalp veins

Cannula Selection

Three types of IV cannula are present
1. *Over:* The needle plastic cannula—a plastic cannula mounted over a needle. After the venepuncture is made, the cannula is guided off the needle and into the vein. This is most common device.
2. *Through:* The needle cannula after venepuncture, a cannula is threaded through the needle into vein.
3. *In lying cannula:* It is softer and causes less intimal damage; and is kink resistance which reduces the incidence of cannula failure.

Most cannulas contain a flashback chamber. This provides visual indication that the cannula entered the vein (Figs 18.3 and 18.4).

Size of Cannula

- Most of the cannulas range from 0.5 to 2 inches in length
- Diameter of cannulas range from 14 to 26 gauge.

For pediatric usage

Infant	0.56–0.75 inch length
	24–26 gauge size
Adult	0.5–2 inch length

Use the cannula depending size of vein

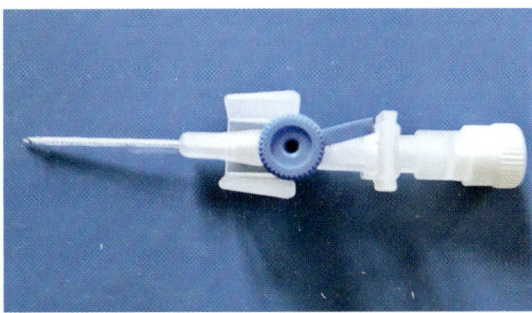

Fig. 18.3: IV cannula.

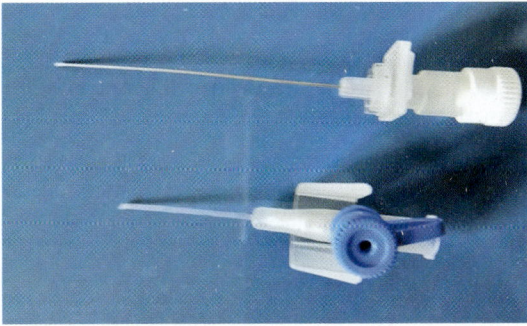

Fig. 18.4: Parts of cannula.

General Guideline

- Infant and children : 26–24 gauze
- Children and elder : 24–22 gauze
- Medical elder and post- : 24–20 gauze
  operative surgical patient
- For rapid blood transfusion : 18 gauze
- Trauma patients and those : 16 gauze
  require large volumes of
  fluid (fast)

Before inserting cannula see it carefully as problems with catheter tip.

Site Preparation

- Clean the site—visible dirty skin should be cleaned with soap and water, hairy sites should be clipped. The antimicrobials solution (e.g. 10% povidone iodine, 70% isopropyl alcohol, chlorhexidine)
- Aqueous benzalkonium like compounds should not be used.

Note
- Cannula should be inspected for integrity before use discard if not.
- Only one cannula should be used for each cannulation.

Cannula Placement

Equipment required

1. Antiseptic
2. Swab
3. Gauze square
4. Adhesive tape
5. Clear dressing
6. Torniquet
7. Gloves
8. IV cannula (Figs 18.3 and 18.4)
9. IV bottle, drip set, medicine, syringe.

Steps

1. Apply tourniquet 2–3 inch above the intended venepuncture site. Patient should be asked to open and close his fist several times. This will make venous distension.
2. Identify desirable vein, palpate the vein seen. It is soft and bouncy.
3. Some clinicians prefer BP cuff instead of tourniquet. In such cases cuff is inflated than deflated to just below the patient diastolic pressure to make vein visible without engorging.
4. Vein stabilization
   a. Use thumb the skin down over the knuckles to stabilize the vein.
   b. To stabilize vein on the forearm with the left hand or assisting person used to encircle the patient arm and thumb. Used to pull downward on the skin below the venepuncture site.
5. Approaching the vein
   a. IV cannula is inserted at 5 to 15° angle depending upon vein location and its depth, e.g. in superficial hand vein.
   b. From sides—approach the vein from side. It reduces risk of piercing vein's back wall.

c. If vein is situated at deeper tissues where it cannot be seen or felt. The cannula is inserted about 1 to 2 cm below the vein's visible segment and then cannula is turned through the tissue to enter the vein.

d. Avoid insertion of cannula where two veins bifurcate.

Inserting the Cannula

- Right hand should be used to grasp the cannula or its wings (in butterfly needle, scalp vein set).
- Proceed with venepuncture insert cannula at a 10 to 30° angle depending upon depth of vein. Cannula's bevel should be up to reduce the risk of piercing vein's puncture wall.
- Look at flash chamber for blood.
- If blood flow is seen then cannula is in correct position.
- Keep the vein immobilized and the cannula advanced through the skin with gentle and quick motion.
- Back flow of blood in cannula tubing or hub should be observed (Fig. 18.5).
- If backflow of blood occurs briefly it means stylet passed the lumen out of vein lumen.
- Cannula is pushed off the stylet and look at transparent tubing of cannula for presence of blood. Now push the cannula without stylet in the vein.

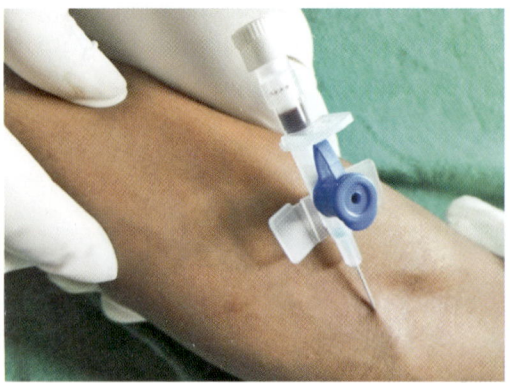

Fig. 18.5: Insertion of cannula.

- It is not successful then repositioning of the cannula tried as long as stylet has not pulled back compeletly.
- If it is unsuccessful, remove the cannula. If any swelling or blood is seen at puncture site, press the site with swab.
- Again try with new venula.
- If it is successful—cannula is advanced into vein. Tourniquet released.

Apply digital pressure beyond the tip and thumb stabilized.

Securing and Dressing

- 1–2 inch wide strip of tape is placed across the cannula hub keep in mind that it should not cover puncture site.
- 2 inch strip of adhesive tape is placed under the cannula bulb in a way that adhesive side facing up.
- The tops strip is folded around the cannula hub.
- Cover the venepuncture site and catheter hub with the dressing. The hub tubing function is not covered.
- A 2 × 2 gauze pad is folded in halt and covered with inch wide tape strip, it is placed under cannula hub tubing function. Tubing is curled to the side.
- A inch wide tape strip is placed over the tubing directly on the top of the tape under the hub.

Flushing IV cannula—2 ml of normal saline and 3 ml after administration of drug.

Flushing should be done every 6 hourly to maintain patency.

Remove the cannula—if signs of phlebitis (pain, tenderness around insertion site, swelling, tissue damage).

LUMBAR PUNCTURE

Indication: Lumbar puncture is indicated to obtain cerebrospinal fluid for the diagnosis of meningitis, encephalitis, intracranial bleeding, metastatic leukemia or benign intracranial hypertension.

Procedure

Spinal needle—choose appropriate size of the needle as per age of the baby.

Position of Baby

1. Make the baby sit up with dorsal and lumbar spine flexed, or
2. Baby may be made to lie on his side with spine flexed as much as possible. Small and sick babies may not withstand the too much flexon.

Steps

1. Position the baby with the help of assistant.
2. Clean the site with antiseptic povidone iodine and then with alcohol.

Site

Sites for lumbar puncture are:
1. Interspace between L3 and L4, or
2. Interspace between L4 and L5

In newborn baby spinal cord down to L3 level, therefore, higher taps are fraught with dangers to injury to the spinal cord.

1. Spine of 4th lumbar vertebra is located by drawing a line joining the two iliac crests.
2. The spinal needle is grasped firmly making facing upward towards calling and inserted in selected interspace in the midline sagittal plane slowly slightly oblique in towards head of the baby.
3. When the ligamentum flavum and then dura are punctured a decreased resistance (Pop) are felt.
4. Remove the stylet and cheek flow of CSF. Collect CSF in sterile tube (about 1 ml).
5. Stylet is reinserted to remove the spinal needle.
6. Puncture site is cleaned and cover.

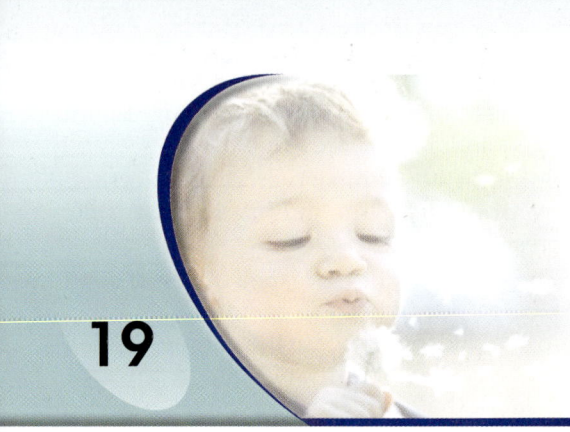

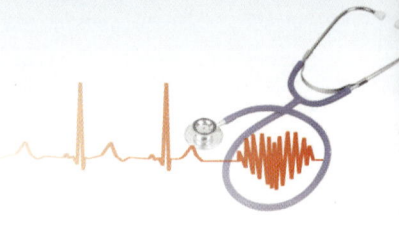

19

Miscellaneous

SCABIES

Scabies is caused by *Sarcoptes scabiei,* an insect mite. This is most common skin disease in children.

Clinical Features

Contrary to adult, it may occur in skin of any part of the body. Generally, this occurs in spaces between fingers in hands or toes, wrist, elbow or axilla. This also occurs in skin of palm and soles. In infants, this may occur in head also. Papule, burrow formation and vesicles are characteristic lesions. Infections at itching point causes pyoderma or causes eczema like symptoms. Oozing or hardening of skin at itching point is other features.

Treatment

If infection due to bacteria is superimposed in scabies, antibiotics are prescribed to control it. Nails should be cut, clothes should be changed and boiled. If other persons also suffering in the family; everybody is treated simultaneously.

Specific Treatment

Specific treatment is as follows:
  i. *Benzyl benzoate:* 25% solution of drug is applied all over body after bath except head. Bath is taken for 2nd day. Permethrin 5% cream—apply locally.
  ii. Gamma benzene hexachloride (ointment or lotion). Drug is applied all over body. Drug should be avoided in infants and young children due to its harmful effects.

MONILIASIS

Oral Thrush

This is caused by *Candida albicans* (fungus). White brown layer is deposited over tongue, palate, mucosa, gums of the patient, which can be removed easily. Red colored raw spots are seen at the point of removal of layer.

Difficulty in feeding, weakness and deficiency of nutrients occur due to lack of feeding.

Infections on other parts of the body

  i. In girls, it causes vulvovaginitis. White layer is deposited over mucous membrane of genitalia and white frothy discharge comes out from genitalia.
  ii. Infections are also common at diaper area because it is good source due to wetting by urine. Itching and erythma is found between thighs.

Treatment

i. Nystatin (one lac unit per ml) 3–4 times should be applied locally.
ii. Gentian violet is another drug. 1% of aqueous solution should be applied. It causes blue discoloration. Blue color can be removed by paste of soda.

PHENOTHIAZINE TOXICITY

Signs of toxicity are seen after giving anti-emetic drugs such as triflupromazine (Siquil) or prochlorperazine, etc. Toxicity is more common after parenteral administration and in high doses.

Clinical Features

Features are of acute onset and signs and symptoms are of extrapyramidal involvement. The features are torticolitis muscular rigidity, ophisthotonus, marked deviation of eyes, oculogyric crises.

Other features are tremors, ataxia, swallowing difficulty, drooling, consciousness is not altered. Convulsions are rare.

Treatment

Diphenhydramine hydrochloride (Benadryl) is an excellent antidote and gives dramatic response.

Dose is 2 mg/kg, maximum 50 mg, given intravenously or orally.

ORGANOPHOSPHORUS
(POISONING)

It is very common poisoning because pesticides and insecticides are used for various purposes, associated with high mortality.

Clinical Features

Clinical features of organophosphorus poisoning are due to increased sympathetic activity. Symptoms are blurred vision, headache, giddiness, nausea, chest pain, profuse salivation and sweating.

Pupils are constricted, papilledema may occur. Muscarinic symptoms are common.

Nicotinic and central muscarinic symptoms predominate in same intoxication such as tachycardia and hypertension.

Death is due to respiratory failure.

Treatment

1. Gastric decontamination.
2. **Atropine:** 0.05 mg/kg IV is given, dose is repeated after every 15 minutes till signs of atropinization appear, maximum 1 mg/kg/24-hour intravenous infusion of atropine in better than bolus dose.
3. **Pralidoxime aldoxime methiodide (PAM):** It is used for reversing nicotinic effects, weakness, respiratory failure.

DHATURA (BELLADONNA) POISONING

Accidental ingestion of dhatura seeds is common in children.

Clinical Features

Dhatura poisoning manifests as delirium confusion, visual disturbances, photophobia. Pupils are dilated, sluggishly reacting, dryness of mouth and skin, tachycardia and urinary retention are common.

Treatment

1. Gastric levage.
2. Physostigmine: Dose 0.1 mg/kg (max 2 mg) intravenous slowly.

SNAKE BITE

Snake bite is common in tropical countries, many snakes are nonpoisonous. Poisonous snakes may cause various symptoms and signs.

Nonspecific symptoms are abdominal pain, nausea and vomiting.

1. Neurotoxiciy—ptosis, diplopia, bulbar palsy, generalized weakness.
2. Coagulopathy—bleeding from various sites—gum bleeding, epistaxis, intracranial bleeding.
3. Rhabdomyolysis—muscle pain, tenderness, dark urine due to acute tubular necrosis.

4. Hypotension, shock
5. Tissue necrosis—pain, tenderness, blisters at the site of bite.

Treatment

- Local—at the site of bite, cleaning with antiseptic.
- Pressure immobilization is not advised because it may worsen local necrosis.
- Envenomation—administration of anti-snake venom is advocated in patient having symptoms of poisoning. Doses are same as adult.

HYDROCARBON POISONING

Karosene, turpentine, lubricating oil and tar are accidental poisoning commonly seen in children.

Poisoning results pulmonary symptoms as aspiration pneumonia, restlessness, fever, abdominal distension and signs of pneumonitis are major clinical manifestations. Skiagram chest shows infiltration, pleural effusion, emphysema and pneumatocele.

Convulsions or coma may occur.

Management

1. Gastric lavage is contraindicated but if large quantity of turpentine is ingested, then it can be done.
2. Symptomatic treatment.
3. Steroids have no beneficial effect.
4. Phenobarbitone is given for the control of convulsions.

SCORPION ENVENOMING

Mesobuthus tamulus, an Indian red scorpion is a lethal species.

Etiology and Pathogenesis

After envenoming serum venom concentration peaks at about 2 hours and its level in directly related to clinical manifestations. Children are more likely to develop rapid deterioration because of their lesser body weight.

Venom is a potent sodium channel activator which results in autonomic storm followed by sustained adrenergic activity.

Severity of envenomation and mortality are related to cardiorespiratory dysfunction, cardiac failure and pulmonary edema.

Myocarditis due to direct effect of venom on myocardium, hypoxia in the presence of increased catecholamines and altered permeability of myocardial cell membrane affecting electrical propulsion and abnormalities in electrolytes fluxes.

Coronary microvascular spasm due to catecholamine overstimulation may be triggering the myocardial perfusion derangement.

Pulmonary edema may be due to direct effect of toxin on the myocardium and impairment in the clearance of alveolar fluid mediated by epithelial sodium channel and sodium potassium pump.

Toxin causes massive release of vasoactive peptide hormone including endothelin 1 which impairs the clearance of alveolar fluid.

High morbidity and fatality due to scorpion envenomation is associated with features of severe vasoconstriction, hypertension, tachycardia, cool extremities, increased myocardial injury, cadiogenic shock due to long lasting sympathetic excitation.

Clinical Features

Parasympathetic effects like vomiting, profuse sweating, salivation, priapism in males, bradycardia, hypotension, premature ventricular ectopics and coronary sinus rhythm disturbances.

Excessive respiratory secretion may cause early respiratory failure. These effects are short lasting and less severe.

In severe cases, clinical features of pulmonary edema develop. Cardiogenic shock, local pain, convulsion also may be present.

Myocardial dysfunction is diagnosed if

a. Congestive cardiac failure or cardiomegaly.

b. Hemodynamics compromise that requires vasopressor (dobutamine or dopamine).

c. Echocardiography shows left ventricular dysfunction.

Investigations

1. Elevated CPK—MB levels in the blood
2. Echocardiography—to evaluate cardiac function.
3. ECG—abnormal
4. Cardiac troponin—important diagnostic and prognostic tools to assess myocarditis. Normal value suggests non-involvement of myocardium.

Management

Effects of SAV and oral prazosin combined are better than only oral prazosin.

1. *Scorpion antivenom (SAV):* It is administered within four hours of the sting, it neutralizes circulating scorpion venom.

   Dose: 30 ml of monovalent antivenom add into 100 ml of normal saline and infuse intravenously over 30 minutes, look for anaphylaxis or allergic reaction.

2. *Prazosin (oral):* Prazosin is called physiological and pharmacological antidote to scorpion venom action. It antagonizes the after effects of venom liberated catecholamines and has no action on the venom *per se*. It neutralizes overstimulated autonomic nervous system.

   The venom deposited at the sting site acts like a depot and gradually releases into the circulation.

   With oral prazosin patient take 12–48 hours to recover.

   Its phosphodiesterase inhibitory action results in cellular accumulation of cyclic GMP an endothelin inhibitor and insulin release from beta cells of pancreas rectifying the metabolic effects caused by excessive alpha receptor stimulation and circulatory catecholamines.

   Dose: 30 µg/kg every 3 hourly

3. *Dobutamine:* 10% of the pediatric patient develop tachycardia, hypotension, pulmonary edema and shock with warm extremities.

   In such cases intravenous dobutamine, nitroglycerine and ventilator support are required for 24–96 hours.

   Dose: 6–20 µg/kg/min

Avoid

1. *Steroids* enhance the necrotizing effect of circulating catecholamine which further damages myocardium and worsen the clinical manifestations.
2. *Antihistamines* by inhibiting the potassium channels, prolong the QT interval which may result in sudden unexpected death in recovering patient.
3. *Calcium channel blockers* can depress the myocardium and precipitate pulmonary edema.
4. Diuretics enhance the development of pulmonary edema and shock.

   Pulmonary edema: Managed by:
   a. Oxygen
   b. Mechanical ventilation.
   c. Sodium nitroprusside.
   Intravenons infusion (0.3–5 µg/kg/min)

   Encephalopathy: Managed by:
   a. O_2
   b. Mechanical ventilation
   Midazolam or phenytoin for control of convulsion.

ACCIDENTAL PROBLEMS

Swallowed Object

Sometimes child engulfs small objects such as stones, coins, pins, button. If object is smooth, it passes through the body via anus. Banana or smooth foods are given. But laxatives are not given, it may cause harmful effects.

If objects are sharp or rough and child suffers from pain in abdomen; surgery may be indicated.

ATOPIC DERMATITIS
(INFANTILE OR ATOPIC ECZEMA)

Atopic dermatitis is achronic, recurrent, inflammatory skin disease, characterized by differing manifestations are erythema, edema, intense pruritus, exudation, crusting and scaling.

The 'atopy' signifies the hereditary to develop allergies to food and inhalant substances as manifested by eczema, asthma and hay fever. Atopic dermatitis can be divided into three stages:

i. Infantile AD (from 2 months to 2 years of age
ii. Childhood AD (from 2 to 10 years) and
iii. Adolescent and adult stage of AD.

Infantile AD

This is seen mainly after introduction of artificial milk, cow milk, eggs, cereals in infant's diet and symptoms are manifested with it.

This usually begins as an itchy erythema of cheeks. In the erythematous patches, minute epidermal vesicles develop, vesicle rupture and produce moist crusted areas, the eruption may rapidly extends other parts of the body mainly the scalp, the neck, the forehead, the wrists and the extremities. The buttocks and diaper area are often involved.

Lesions which are infiltrated exudative areas, take a characteristic lichenified appearance. Itching is intense and is the chief symptom.

In some cases, especially in older children, drier lesions are found where there is excessive dryness, which due to pruritus predisposes to eczematization.

In majority of the infants, the skin symptoms disappear to the end of second year. Flare up lesions are often seen following immunization, during teething, during attack of common cold and in winter (especially seen in cases aggravated by wool irritation and low humidity). Food allergy may play a significant role in few selected cases of young atopic dermatitis.

Childhood Atopic Dermatitis

In childhood, atopic dermatitis is less acute, less exudative, drier and more papular. The classical locations are antecubital and popliteal spaces, the wrists, eyelids, face and neck.

Pruritus is constant feature. Other cutaneous changes are secondary to it. Scratching induces lichenification and secondary infection.

During childhood, there is tendency of a decrease in the frequency of sensitization to egg, wheat and milk and an increase in sensitization to non-ingested substances particularly wool, cat hairs, dog hairs and pollens. Sensitivity to neomycin and nickel is more frequent than normal persons. This is an exception to rule that atopies have diminished ability to acquire delayed hypersensitivity.

Susceptibility to Infections

This increases susceptibility to superimposed infection. Staphylococcus flare the lesion. There is increased susceptibility to respiratory infections, herpesvirus or vaccinia virus infection.

Immunology

Frequent immunologic peculiarities in AD are elevated serum IgE, decreased ability to be sensitized to dinitrochlorobenzene or bacterial or fungal antigens. Other peculiarities are decreased antibody dependent cellular cytotoxicity, decreased T cytotoxic cells, decreased chemotaxis and activation of polymorphonuclear leukocytes and decreased cytotoxicity and chemotaxis of monocytes.

Diagnosis

Diagnosis is made on the basis of history, the morphology and distribution of the lesions and the presence of associated features. A family history of atopy may also be present.

Differential diagnosis: Dermatoses resembling atopic dermatitis may be seborrheic dermatitis, irritant or allergic eczematous contact dermatitis, nummular dermatitis, scabies and psoriasis.

Treatment

a. Avoid nutrients in food which increase it.
b. Avoid excessive cold and hot atmosphere, woolen clothes; sunlight is helpful.
c. Local: In severe cases 1:5000 solution of potassium permanganate wet compresses is effective for oozing, eczematous lesion. The primary and important therapeutic tool in the treatment of eczematous lesions is use of *topical corticosteroids*. These suppress inflammation and stop pruritus. Start with high potency to quickly quell inflammation and pruritus, later on for maintenance therapy low potency steroids are more appropriate.
Lubricants applied alternated or applied at same time with topical steroids lessen the risk of prolonged corticosteroid therapy.

Internal Treatment

Antihistamines are useful to suppress pruritus, allay anxiety and allow sleep. Acute flare ups of AD can be suppressed by a short-term course of steroids (oral or parenteral).

Photochemotherapy (PUVA) is useful in selected patients with recalcitrant chronic AD.

Secondary *Staphylococcus aureus* should be treated with appropriate oral antibiotics which often may be useful even without clinical evidence of infection.

FAILURE TO THRIVE

In this category those children under 5 years of age come, whose physical growth is significantly less than that of other children of similar age and sex.

Causes

1. Causes resulting lack of sufficient food.
2. Food is sufficient but child suffers from emotional deprivation due to lack of love and affection.
3. Environment is changed all of a sudden.

Physical

1. CNS disease
2. Heart disease
3. Endocrine disease
4. Lack of absorption of food in the intestine
5. Worm infestations
6. Disease like cancer
7. Long duration illness like tuberculosis.

COMMON SIGNS AND SYMPTOMS

Cough

Common conditions which cause acute cough are:
A. Acute respiratory conditions
   1. Nasopharyngeal: Viral infections (common rhinovirus)
   2. Laryngeal: Viral and bacterial infections
   3. Tracheobronchial
     a. Viral and bacterial infections
     b. Allergic causes (asthma and asthmatic bronchitis)
     c. Foreign body
     d. Aspirants (milk, fluid)
   4. Pulmonary:
     a. Viral and bacterial infections including measles, whooping cough.
     b. Parasitic infestations
     c. Hypersensitivity reactions (asthma and asthmatic bronchitis)
     d. Aspirants (fluid, milk)
     e. Inhalants—dust, smoke, gases
     f. Irritants—chemicals, thermal
   5. Pleural—irritants
B. Recurrent and persistent cough in children
   Recurrent cough
   1. Recurrent tonsillitis or adenoiditis
   2. Dripping from upper airways
   3. Recurrent respiratory infections, tracheitis, bronchitis
   4. Increased bronchial reactivity (asthma)
   5. Occasional aspiration (as in pharyngeal incoordination)
   6. Idiopathic pulmonary hemosiderosis

Persistent cough

1. Postinfectious hypersensitivity of cough receptors (asthma, asthmatic bronchitis)
2. Chronic bronchitis and tracheitis
3. Bronchiectasis
4. Immotile cilia syndrome
5. Foreign body aspiration
6. Aspiration (due to pharyngeal incompetence, tracheoesophageal cleft, fistula, gastroesophageal reflux)
7. Pertussis syndrome
8. Compression of trachea, bronchi (vascular ring, neoplasm, lymph nodes, lung cyst)
9. Endobronchial or endotracheal tumors and tuberculosis
10. Habit cough
11. Hypersensitivity pneumonitis
12. Fungal infections

C. Cough due to involvement of other systems are:
1. Congenital heart disease
2. Immunodeficiency of alpha antitrypsin deficiency or cystic fibrosis.
3. Chalasia of esophagus.

Cyanosis

In newborn: Pulmonary—pneumonia, hyaline membrane disease, airway obstruction, congenital pulmonary anomalies, diaphragmatic hernia. Non-pulmonary—congenital heart disease, congestive heart failure, effects of maternal anesthesia and drugs, CNS disease, shock, sepsis, acidosis, polycythemia; metabolic—hypoglycemia, hypocalcemia.

In infancy and childhood

a. Respiratory system
   i. Respiratory distress syndrome
   ii. Congenital lung anomalies
   iii. Diaphragmatic hernia
   iv. Pleural effusion
   v. Pneumothorax
   vi. AV fistula

b. Cardiovascular system
   i. Right to left shunts (congenital heart disease)
   ii. Congestive heart failure
c. Shock: Due to blood loss, metabolic acidosis
d. Miscellaneous: Polycythemia, methemoglobinemia.

BOSSING OF SKULL

Causes

Rickets, thalassemia major, congenital syphilis, achondroplasia, Hurler's syndrome, cleidocranial dysostosis, ectodermal dysplasia, Ehlers-Danlos syndrome, Mallermann-Streiff syndrome.

MACROCEPHALY

Causes

Hydrocephalus, subdural hematoma, hydranencephaly, porencephaly, achondroplasia, osteopetrosis, pycnodysostosis, rickets, cerebral gigantism, cerebral lipoidosis, metachromatic leukodystrophy.

MICROCEPHALY

Causes

Craniosynostosis, familial microcephaly, intrauterine infections (CMV, rubella, toxoplasmosis), Cockayne's syndrome. Smith-Lemli-Optiz syndrome, cri du chat syndrome, trisomy 13 and 21, fetal alcohol or hydantoin syndrome, Rothmund-Thomson syndrome, Wolf-Hirschhorn syndrome.

SPARSE LIGHT BROWN AND BRITTLE HAIR

Causes

Protein energy malnutrition (kwashiorkor), cretinism, chronic systemic debilitating diseases, progeria, ectodermal dysplasia, hypervitaminosis A, zinc and copper deficiency, congenital syphilis, acrodynia, idiopathic hypoparathyroidism.

LYMPHADENOPATHY (GENERALIZED)

Causes

1. Inflammatory or infective group—rubella, rubeola, typhoid, tularemia, infectious mononucleosis tuberculosis.
2. Malignancy—leukemia, lymphoma, reticuloendotheliosis, malignant tumors such as neuroblastoma sometimes metastasize to lymph nodes, Gaucher's disease, lipoidosis.
   Causes (solitary)—involvement of single node is due to infections in area that it drains.

CERVICAL LYMPHADENOPATHY

Causes

Tuberculosis, acute lymphadenitis due to infection in throat, from lesion on scalp, Hodgkin's disease, leukemia, brachial cyst.

PUFFINESS OF EYELIDS/FACE

Familial, conjunctivitis, hypoproteinemia (nephritis, nephrotic syndrome, anemia, kwashiorkor), excessive crying, angioneurotic edema, congestive cardiac failure, constrictive pericarditis, mediastinal obstruction, myxoedema, spasmodic cough (e.g. whooping cough), chronic sinusitis, cavernous sinus thrombosis, chronic cor pulmonale, dermatomyosis.

Abdominal Pain

See Chapter 8: Diseases of 'Gastrointestinal System'.

Ascites and Anasarca

See Chapter 8: Diseases of 'Gastrointestinal System'.

Hepatomegaly

See Chapter 8. Page 160.

Splenomegaly

1. Physiological
   a. In neonatal period spleen is frequently palpable.
   b. In young children spleen is often palpable.

2. Infections
   a. Bacterial—septicemia, bacterial endocarditis, syphilis, typhoid, tuberculosis
   b. Protozoal—malaria, kala-azar
3. Congestive: Portal hypertension, congestive splenomegaly (band)
4. Cirrhosis: Indian childhood cirrhosis, other types of cirrhosis
5. Neoplasm: Leukemia, Hodgkin's disease.
6. Metabolic: Gaucher's disease, amyloidosis, Niemann-Pick disease, Hand-Schüller-Christian disease.
7. Blood disease: Hemolytic anemias—thalassemia, sickle cell anemia, hypersplenism (primary and secondary), infectious mononucleosis.

Arthritis

i. Rheumatic fever
ii. Rheumatoid arthritis
iii. Arthritis associated with infections: Gonococcal, tuberculosis, syphilitic, brucellosis, mumps, rubella, pyogenic
iv. Traumatic
v. Neuropathic
vi. With connective tissue disorders—SLE, polyarteritis nodosa
vii. Arthritis with blood disorders
viii. Allergy and drug reactions
ix. Degenerative osteoarthritis

HEMOPTYSIS

Causes

Bronchiectasis, lung abscess, resolving lobar pneumonia, pulmonary hemosiderosis, pulmonary edema, mitral stenosis, tubercular cavity and bleeding disorders. Acute infectious fevers of hemorrhagic variety—smallpox, measles, diphtheria, trauma to chest.

Hematemesis/Malena

i. Swallowed blood following epistaxis, dental extraction, swallowed maternal blood (in newborn).
ii. Esophagitis
iii. Tumors, e.g. hemangioma

iv. Peptic ulcer
v. Poisoning—certain poison
vi. Portal hypertension
vii. Blood diseases—hemophilia, leukemia, purpura, polycythemia. Malena is altered blood in stool.

HEMATOCHEZIA

In stool, red blood is known as hematochezia.

Causes

i. Necrotizing enterocolitis
ii. Hemorrhagic disease
iii. Anal fissure or excoriated buttocks
iv. Colonic polyp
v. Intussusception
vi. Infectious colitis (dysentery)
vii. Meckel's diverticulum
viii. Crohn's disease and ulcerative colitis
ix. Fissures and hemorrhoids
x. Intestinal neoplasms.

TRISMUS (LOCK JAW)

i. Tetanus
ii. Temporomandibular joint arthritis
iii. Encephalitis
iv. Brain tumors
v. Phenothiazine toxicity, strychnine poisoning
vi. Infantile Gaucher's disease
vii. Tumors of jaw
viii. Primary hypoparathyroidism

ACRODYNIA (PINK DISEASE)

This is caused by chronic mercury poisoning in infants and young children. Which may be due to repeated contact with mercury product such as hour paints, wall papers, teething powder.

Clinical manifestations include listlessnees. restless, irritability and characteristic rashes at tip of fingers, toes and nose which is pinkish in color. Later hands and feet become dusky pink.

Profuse perspiration at skin, extreme pruritus, nail becomes dark, photophobia and extreme hypotonia are also distinctive features, later on neurological symptoms appear.

Treatment is specific, BAL is affective antidote. L-penicillamine is also better and successful antidote.

DUCHENNE'S MUSCULAR DYSTROPHY
(PSEUDOHYPERTROPHIC MUSCULAR DYSTROPHY)

The muscular dystrophies are group of disorders of which the essential feature is a progressive degeneration of certain group of muscles of the body. Duchenne muscular dystrophy (DMD) is the most common of muscular dystrophies.

This is an X-linked recessive disorder due to deletion of genetic material at Xp 21 site (Xp = short arm of X chromosome, 21 = number of color band from centromere when X chromosome is stained with vital dyes). Males are sufferer (like hemophilia) and females are carrier; in about one-third cases fresh mutation can lead to DMD.

Etiopathogenesis

'Dystrophin' is a protein which gives stability to the muscle plasma membrane (sarcolemma). It is synthesized by above gene thus it is grossly deficient in DMD cases. This defect in sarcolemma leads to entrance of large amount of calcium inside the muscle fiber. This activates calcium dependent proteolytic enzymes and produces poisoning to mitochondria. Enzymes produce necrosis of muscle fibers and release of enzymes in blood. The degenerated muscle fibers are replaced by fibrofatty tissue. So, muscles look grossly enlarged (pseudohypertrophy) but weak in power.

Incidence

One in 3000 to one in 5000 male births.

Clinical Features

As stated earlier disease primarily affects males. Most of the cases, child is normal at birth. Onset is usually between 3 and 5 years of age. Disease is characterized by clinical triad of peculiar waddling gait, large calves the 'climbing the legs' phenomenon (Gower's sign) in early childhood.

The pelvic girdle muscles are affected first and weakness slowly spreads to the shoulder girdle. Some muscles (gastrocnemii, glutei, quadriceps, infraspinatus and deltoid) show pseudohypertrophy. The term 'pseudo-hypertrophy' is used because early in disease, hypertrophied muscles have considerable strength, but later on enlarged muscles are often weak, since most of the increased bulk is due to fatty infiltration. The hypertrophic muscles of leg (calf) are stronger than anterior leg muscles resulting toe walking are contracture of heal cords.

Weakness of muscles of knees and spine leads to characteristic method of rising detected by Gower's sign: In getting up from floor the first rolls to prone position, kneels and then raises himself to standing by pushing with his hands against shins, knees and thighs. (*refer to* Fig. 1.41, Chapter 1).

Some muscles show wasting (latissimus dorsi, sternal head of pectoralis major) weakness of shoulder muscles are detected by lifting the child with hands under the axillae, he will slip through the examiner's hands rather than adducting the arms. At later stage, child becomes unable to lift the arms above the head.

Dystrophy of thoracic muscles and diaphragm and kyphoscoliosis comprises breathing and coughing resulting respiratory tract infection.

Mental retardation is associated in two-thirds of cases and is not progressive.

The proximal muscles of the limbs are more liable to waste than distal ones. Muscles of hands and face escape.

Later on lumbar lordosis, scoliosis and increased tendency to fractures are common skeletal changes.

Death occurs due to respiratory tract infection, malnutrition, respiratory failure or cardiac failure.

Investigations

1. *ECG:* Sinus tachycardia and abnormal ECG in cardiac involvement.
2. *Muscle biopsy:* It shows necrosis, degeneration and 'supercontracted' or hyaline muscle fibers. Fibrosis and replacement of degenerated fibers by fatty tissue.
3. *Electron microspcopy:* Dystrophic changes in posterobasal and prelateral walls of left ventricle. Septum and atrial myocardium are relatively not affected.
4. *PET scan* (positron emission tomography scan): It shows metabolic abnormality in plasma membrane of cardiac muscles, skeletal muscles, RBC and fibroblast.
5. *EEG:* Diffuse non-specific changes.
6. *Serum enzymes:* Serum enzymes like aldose, CPK, MB, SGPT, SCOT and LDH-S are elevated. CPK is elevated 10–20 thousands units in early stages and failing with progress of the disease.
7. *EMG* (electromyography): It shows short duration, low amplitude, polyphasic, MUAPs and mean normal interference pattern.
8. *Cinematography:* SA node artery occlusion.
9. *Genetic studies:* Deletion of Xp 21 site. Prenatal diagnosis is possible by using DNA probe.
10. Serum creatine kinase elevated <10 times upper limit of normal.
11. *Muscle biopsy:* Absence of (dystrophin 1, 2, 3) staining in immunohistochemical analysis.

Management

Aim of management is to maintain strength and joint movements by exercise, physiotherapy and avoid prolonged immobility.

1. *Corticosteroids:* Improves strength and ambulation.

   Prednisolone (0.3–0.75 mg/kg/day) or Deflazacort 0.9 mg/kg/day is given if excessive weight gain or behavior change.

2. Surgery for fixed contractures and spinal deformity.
3. Supportive care for respiratory and cardiac gastrointestinal problems.

Newer Therapy

Exon skipping, gene therapy, all therapy, pharmacological approaches.

Carrier Female Identification

Carrier female may be identified by high CPK level, ECG, EMG and muscle biopsy. It is done by chronic biopsy at 8–10 weeks of pregnancy with 70% accuracy. So, non-effected fetuses can be saved and effected fetuses can be aborted.

Course and prognosis: The disease progresses slowly to involve all muscles of the body and death occurs in 10–12 years of the onset of clinical manifestations.

Prevention and Genetic Counseling

Early prenatal diagnosis and carrier detection is possible. Male siblings of an affected child have 50% chances of being affected; sisters have 50% chances of being carrier.

INBORN ERRORS OF METABOLISM

These are rare genetic (hereditary) conditions in which body cannot properly turn food into energy. The disorders are usually caused by defects in specific enzymes that help to metabolize parts of food. These disorders are suspected in newborn or in children when all well baby have sudden seizures, altered sensorium, sepsis, hypoglycemia, acidosis without cause. Consanguineous marriages may be risk factor.

Classification

1. Disorders due to carbohydrate metabolism
2. Disorders due to amino acid metabolism
3. Urea cycle disorder or urea cycle defects
4. Disorders of organic acid metabolism
5. Disorders of fatty acid metabolism
6. Disorders of porphyrin metabolism
7. Disorders of purine and pyrimidine metabolism
8. Disorders of mitochondrial metabolism
9. Disorders of perioxysomal function
10. Lysosomal storage disease

DISORDERS OF CARBOHYDRATE METABOLISM

1. Glycogen storage disease
2. Galactosemia
3. Hereditary fructose intolerance

Glycogen Storage Disease

It is an autosomal recessive disorder of glycogen.

Two Types

1. **Type 1:** Glerke disease (most common). It is due to deficiency of glucose-6-phosphatase enzyme.
2. **Type 2:** Translocase enzyme deficiency.
   Gierke disease is most common. Glucose-6-phosphatase is not converted into glucose due to deficiency of glucose-6-phosphatase enzyme.

Clinical Features

Fasting hypoglycemia—in early morning child is lethargy, have seizures because in night baby may not be fed well.
- Hepatosplenomegaly, doll-like facies seen.
- Investigations—done to detect.
- Hypoglycemia, hyperlipidemia, lactic acidosis, elevated uric acid.

Important Glycogen Storage Diseases

Liver Glycogenesis (Liver is Effected)

Type 1: Von Gierke disease—due to deficiency of glucose-6-phosphatase enzyme.

Type 3: Kori disease—due to glycogen debranching enzyme deficiency.

Type 4: Anderson disease—glycogen branching enzyme deficiency.

Type 6: Hers disease—liver phosphorylase deficiency.

Muscle Glycogenesis *(Muscles are Effected)*

- **Type 2:** Pompe disease—due to lysosomal acid α-glucosidase enzyme deficiency. Skeletal muscles, hypotonia, heart muscles weak.
- **Type 5:** McArdle disease
- **Type 7:** Tarul's disease

Differential Features Between Type 1 GSD and Type 2 GSD

	Type 1 GSD	Type 2 GSD
Kidney	Enlarged	Normal
Muscle	Not involved	May be involved
CK level	Normal	May be elevated
LFT	Normal	Altered
Effect of glucagon	No	Blood glucose elevated

Galactosemia

It is a autosomal rescessive disorder of galactose metabolism. It may be due to deficiency of following 3 enzymes.

1. GALT (galactose-1-phosphate uridylyltransferase—mostly
2. Galactokinase
3. Epimerase

Breast milk contains lactose. During digestion it breaks into glucose and galactose. Galactose cannot be digested due to deficiency of enzyme.

Sepsis with *E. coli* is most common.

Clinical Features

Diarrhea, vomiting, failure to thrive, hepatomegaly, jaundice are its clinical manifestations.

Treatment

Avoid milk and milk product. Breast milk is contraindicated.

Hereditary Fructose Intolerance

It is due to aldolase B enzyme deficiency.

Sucrose is break down to glucose and fructose during digestion. Fructose is not digested due to deficiency of above enzyme. So, aversion to sweet is noticed. If sweet is given vomiting, hepatomegaly, jaundice, hypoglycemia are presenting feature.

Reducing substance detected in stool by Benedict reagent.

Treatment

Avoid fructose in diet. Avoid sugar-based suspension of drug. Give drug in form of crushed tablets.

Some Common Diseases of Inborn Error of Metabolism

Gaucher's Disease

It is an autosomal recessive genetic disorder. It is result of build up of fatty acids in certain organs particularly in liver and spleen and bones and brain.

Common is type 1 have clinical features as hepatosplenomegaly, fractures of bones, easy bruising, anemia, severe fatigue, muscle rigidity, seizures. Diagnosis is done checking of enzyme level in blood and genetic analysis. Dual energy X-ray absorptiometry and MRI are investigations to be done. Treatment—no cure. Drugs are given to control symptoms. These are enzyme replacement therapy (imiglucerase, taliglucerase, velaglucerase) and substrate reduction therapy (miglustat, eliglustat). Bone marrow transplant and removal of spleen are surgical treatment.

Phenylketonuria

It is an inherited condition caused by a defect in PAH gene. The PAH gene is responsible to create phenylalanine enzyme which is responsible for breaking down phenylalanine amino acid of protein.

Clinical features are seizures, eczema, tremors, stunted growth, hyperacidity and must odour to their breath, skin or urine. Diagnosis is done by detecting enzyme in the blood. Diagnosis can be done during antenatal period.

Treatment

Low protein diet, low phenylalanine diet, PKU diet having no phenylalanine. Prevent PKU by diet plan.

Alkaptonuria

It is a rare inherited disorder. It is due to deficiency of homogentisic dioxygenase (HGD) enzyme. This enzyme is responsible of break down a toxic substance called homogentisic acid. This acid is build up in body which causes bones and cartilase become brittle.

Clinical Features

Dark spots on sclera, thickened and dark cartilase in ears, blue discoloration in skin around sweat glands, dark-colored sweat, black ear wax, kidney stones, arthritis. Dark spots at diaper arouse suspicion about it.

Diagnosis

It is done by gas chromatography to detect homogentisic acid in urine. Urine becomes dark or black on standing.

Treatment

No specific treatment. Low protein diet is given.

Some Important Clinical Findings of Disorders

Clinical finding	Disorder
Coarse facies	Lysosomal disorders
Cataract	Galactosemia, Wilson disease, DM
Retinitis pigmentosa	Mitochondrial disorders
Cherry red spots	GM1, NDP, Tay-Sachs disease
Eczema, alopecia	Biotinidase disease
Abnormal kinky hairs	Menkes disease
Decreased pigmentation	Phenylketonuria, albinism

Chromosomal Disorders

A chromosomal disorder occurs from a change in number or structure of chromosome. Each chromosome has characteristic banding pattern stained by stain. A set of chromosome as seen under microscope is known as karyotype. Any deviation from normal karyotype is known as chromosomal abnormality.

Some chromosomal abnormalities are harmless, some are associated with clinical disorders. Abnormalities may be in number or structure of chromosomes.

Numerical Abnormalities

There is change in number of chromosomes. They are most severe form of disorders, are usually fatal. Few survive to term. Most common is Down syndrome.

Syndrome	Abnormality
Down syndrome	Trisomy 21
Edward syndrome	Trisomy 18
Patau	Trisomy 13
Turner	Monosomy (X)
Klinefelter	XXY
XXX	XXX
XYY	XYY

Turner Syndrome (TS, 45X, Or 45 X0)

It is a chromosomal abnormality results when one of X chromosome (sex chromosome) is missing. This condition affects only female. It is not inherited. Gene defect occurs during formation of reproductive cells.

Clinical Features

Short stature, lymphedema (swelling) of hands and feet of newborn. Webbed neck, broad chest and widely spaced nipple, lower posterior hairline, low set ears, micrognathia.

Congenital heart diseases associated are bicuspid aortic valve (most common), aortic stenosis, coarctation of aorta.

Child may have hypothyroidism, cubitus valgus, high arched palate. At later age amenorrhea, sterility.

Prenatal Diagnosis

- Detected by amniocentesis, chorionic villi sampling.
- Diagnosis is made by karyotyping

Treatment

No cure. Symptoms can be minimized by drug therapy. Growth hormone alone or with low dose of androgen, estrogen replacement, moderate reproductive technologies.

Klinefelter Syndrome

It is a genetic disorder characterized by extra copy of X chromosome (XXY). Boys suffer from this disorder.

Clinical Features

In early childhood—weak muscles, slow motor development, delay in speaking, undescended testes.

Afterward

Tall stature, tall legs shorter torso and broad hips as compared to normal child. Absent or delayed puberty, small firm testes, gynecomastia, behavioral disorders.

Adult

Low or no sperm count, small genitalia, low sex drive, gynecomastia, less body and facial hairs.

Diagnosis

As per clinical features especially genitals, hormone test, karyotyping.

Treatment

No cure, symptoms can be minimized by testosterone replacement therapy, breast tissue removal, speech and physical therapy, fertility treatment such as removal of sperm from testes and injecting into ovum.

Structural Abnormalities

This occurs when large sections of DNA are missing or are added to a chromosome. It occurs by deletion, duplication, translocation, inversion and ring. Balance abnormality involves rearrangement of genetic material so overall no loss or gain. Unbalanced structural abnormality occurs when genetic material is gained or lost.

Unbalanced Structural Abnormalities

Syndrome	Abnormality
Hirschhorn	Chromosome 4
Cri du chat	Chromosome 5
WAGR	Chromosome 11
Angelman/Prader-Willi	Chromosome 15
DiGeorge	Chromosome 22
Fragile X	X Chromosome

Fragile X syndrome is second most common chromosomal abnormality characterized by elongated face, prominent jaw, large ears, learning disabilities.

SINGLE LINE ANSWER OF MCQs

Based on Memory

- Most common congenital acyanotic heart disease is VSD.
- Most common congenital cyanotic heart disease is TOF.
- Rate of increase of weight and height is best indicator of growth of child.
- MAUC is age-dependent indicator of growth (between 6 to 60 months of age)
- Protective effect of breast milk is due to IgA antibody.
- Para-aminobenzoic acid in breast milk protects newborn against malaria. Lipase in breast milk protects baby against Giardia and *E. histolytica*.
- Persistence of Moro's reflex in baby after 6 months is abnormal.
- Newborn baby if suffers from frothing after feed, esophageal atresia is suspected. Diagnosis is confirmed by passing the tube and take X-ray chest and abdomen. Recoil of tube is seen.
- Mouthing appears 5–6 months of age. Stranger anxiety appears at 7 months.
- Most common sequel of bacterial meningitis is hearing loss due to vestibular infection.
- Most common bacteria causing bacterial meningitis are *Streptococcus pneumoniae*.
- In infantile spasm drug of choice is ACTH, then vigabatrin.

- Coarctation of aorta is associates with turner syndrome.
- Apnea in newborn is cessation of respiration for 20 seconds.
- For diagnosis of vesicoureteric reflux, best investigation is micturating cystourethrogram.
- Most common cause of nephrotic syndrome is MSD (minimal change) which is steroid responsive good prognosis.
- Pyuria is diagnosed more than 10 WBC/HPF in urine.
- UTI diagnosis investigation is done:
  <1 year—USG, DMSA, MCU
  1–5 years USG, DMSA. If these are abnormal then MCU.
  >5 years USG, if abnormal, then DMSA, MCU.
- Eisenmenger syndrome is reversal of shunt. Blood flows right to left.
- PICA is consumption of non-nutritious substances like clay, MUD, chalk, etc.
- Unidextrous ulnar grasp by baby is attained at 6–7 months of age, and radial grasp at 6–7 months of age.
- Rh incompatibility is type 2 hypersensitivity reaction.
- Temper tantrum is childhood disorder which increases as per advancing age.
- If temporary teeth are not erupted up to 13 months of age, it is called delayed dentition.
- Most common ASD is osteum secundum.
- Cystic fibrosis is diagnosed by sweat chloride test.
- Transient tachypnea of newborn baby (TTNB) disappears after 24 hours of age.
- Celiac disease—most common clinical manifestation is iron deficiency. BROW (barley, ray, oat, wheat) diet should be avoided.
- Congenital varicella syndrome and clinical features are—deafness, cataract, PDA.
- Omphalocele is midline defect.
- Umbilical hernia is benign self-limiting disease.
- Umbilical granuloma is due to hypertrophy of granulation tissue.

- Maximum concentration of dextrose given from peripheral line to newborn is 12.5%.
- Bradicardia in newborn is due to hypoxia, hypothermia, head injury, apnea.
- In ASD—left atrium does not enlarge.
- TOF—X-ray chest shows boot-shaped heart due to upturned apex of heart, cardiomegaly not seen.
- In pulmonary stenosis—right ventricular hypertrophy seen.
- Ebstein anomaly—atrialization of right ventricle seen, shape of heart becomes box-shaped.
- Down syndrome—common associated congenital heart disease is ASD.
- Coarctation of aorta—femoral pulse is not palpable, common site of coarctation is juxtaductal.
- Croup (laryngotracheal bronchitis)—most common causative organism is parainfluenza B virus.
- Stridor—most common congenital anomaly causing it is laryngomalacia.
- Pneumonia in measles is also known as 'HECHT' pneumonia.
- Most common complication of measles is otitis media.
- Most severe complication of measles is pneumonia.
- Most rare and delayed complication of measles is SSPE, which is treated by recent drug isoprinosine.
- In baby less than 1 year common causative organism of pneumonia is *Staphylococcus aureus*.
- Apgar score is taken in newborn after 1 minute and after 5 minutes of birth.
- In a case of first episode of febrile seizures lumbar puncture is indicated in:
  1. All baby <6 months of age because clinical signs of meningeal irritation are not well developed and difficult to elicit so meningitis cannot be diagnosed on clinical basis alone.
  2. All babies 6–12 months of age who are unimmunized against pneumococcus (Hib vaccine) or immunization status is unknown.

- Breast milk can safely stored at room temperature up to 4 hours; in refrigerator up to 24 hours; in freezer up to 1 month, in deep freezer up to 6 to 12 weeks.
- Erythema toxicum is most common skin lesion in newborn appears 2–3 days of life, require no treatment.
- IUGR baby not occurs in diabetic mother. Diabetes of mother results large-for-date baby.
- Tachypnea is diagnosed if RR is >60/min in 0–2 months baby, >50/min in 2–12 months, >40/min in 12 months to 5 years baby.
- Pathological jaundice is diagnosed if serum bilirubin exceeds 5 mg/dl on day 1, 10 mg/dl on day 2, 15 mg/dl on day 3.
- Baby born with PDA—prostaglandin E_1 drug is given to survive the baby till surgical intervention is done.
- Red urine without RBC in urine seen in hemoglobinuria. Which may be due to intravascular hemolysis.
- Causes of red urine are due to drugs taken—sulphonamide, rifampicin, pyrazinamide, phenytoin.
- Most common refractory rickets is hypophosphatemic rickets.
- Most common cause of congenital hydrocephalus is congenital aqueductal stenosis.
- Most common form of acquired hydrocephalus is post-infectious.
- 'Shakir' tape is used to measure mid-upper arm circumference.
- Growth rate of length in adolescence is 9–10 cm/years.
- first sign of puberty in girls is thelarche; testicular enlargement in boys.
- First sign of success of iron therapy in anemia is seen in 12–24 hours of beginning of therapy. It is decrease irritability, increase alertness, rise in Hb seen in 1 month, iron store repletion in 3 months.
- Neonatal conjunctivitis—cause in day 1—chemical, up to day 5—*N. gonorrhoea*, day 5 to 2 weeks—Chlamydia.
- DPT vaccination is contraindicated in progressive neurological illness. Absolute contraindication is hypersensitivity reaction to previous dose or development of encephalopathy within 7 days of administration of DPT.
- DPT vaccination is safe in child of cerebral palsy because it is a stable neurological disease.
- Reaction due to DPT vaccine is due to pertussis component.
- Death in thiamine deficiency is due to cardiac involvement.
- Cephalhematoma is not present at birth.
- For Kangaroo mother care—baby should be stable.
- Craniopharyngioma is most common supratentorial tumor.
- Intussusception is most common cause of acute abdomen in 6 months to 2 years of age.
- Supraventricular tachycardia is most common tachyarrhythmia in children. Drug of choice for treatment is adenosine.
- Casein/whey ratio in human milk is 40:60 while in cow milk is 80:20. It causes easy digestibility of human milk.
- Croup (acute laryngotracheal bronchitis LTB). X-ray of front of neck shows steeple sign due to subglottic narrowing of trachea.
- Hydrops fetalis is due to Rh isoimmunization.
- Dose of adrenaline in neonatal resuscitation is 0.1–0.3 ml in 1:10000 dilution.
- Acute bronchiolitis cause—most common organism is RSV virus, X-ray chest is not needed to diagnose, treatment is oxygen, nebulization by hypertonic saline. Ribavirin is drug of choice.
- Pneumonia classification
  Pneumonia (0–2 mo)
  1. No pneumonia
     - Cough, cold present
     - No tachypnea
     - No retraction of chest
  2. Pneumonia
     - Cough, cold, and
     - Tachypnea present
     - Retraction of chest present

3. Severe pneumonia

All features of pneumonia as above and inability in feeding, lethargy, unconsciousness, hypo- or hyperthermia. Treatment (0–2 months) give first dose of antibiotic, urgent referral.

Pneumonia (2 months to 5 years)

1. No pneumonia
   – Cough and cold
   – Tachypnea, retraction of chest wall absent.
   – Treatment.Give first dose of antibiotic then refer.
2. Pneumonia
   – Above plus
   – Tachypnea, retraction of chest wall present.
   – Treatment—give antibiotic, urgent referral.
3. Severe pneumonia
   – As above of pneumonia
   – Plus
   – Lethargy, poor feeding, convulsions.
   – Treatment—give first dose of antibiotic then urgent refer.

- Subtle seizures are most common seizures of newborn.
- Myoclonic seizures have worst prognosis in newborn.
- Hypoxic ischemic encephalopathy (HIF) is most common cause of newborn seizures.
- Neurofibromatosis—chromosome 17 is affected.
- Acute flaccid paralysis (AFP): Cerebral palsy is not AFP because its onset is not acute.
- Acute watery diarrhea without abdominal pain suggest *Vibrio cholerae* infection.
- Anemia due to iron deficiency occurs due to chronic blood loss in hookworm infestation.
- Evening colic in infant more common in cow milk fed babies.
- Hemolytic disease of newborn is due to vit K deficiency. So, vit K is given to every newborn, 1 mg IM to term baby and 0.5 mg IM to preterm baby.

- Meconium is first stool pass by newborn baby. Greenish black in color. It is generally passed up to 3 days. At 7th days stool becomes golden yellow.
- Umbilical cord usually seperates at about 7th day due to dry gangrene.
- Incidence of UTI is more in male during infancy and more in female after infancy.
- UTI is diagnosed by urine examination—routine and microscopic, nitrite test, leucocyte esterase test, micturating cystogram, USG, DMSA scan to evaluate kidney function.
- Mission Indradhanush covers all the vaccination of child included in National Immunization Program. Vaccination against mumps is not included.
- Umbilical cord contains two artery and one vein (left)
- Dexamethasone or betamethasone is given to preterm to prevent RDS.
- Intrahepatic cholestasis occurs in neonatal hepatitis, extrahepatic cholestasis occurs in biliary atresia.
- Nephrotic syndrome (minimal change)—features are selective proteinuria, light microscopy normal, electron microscopy shows fusion of podocytes.
- Nephrotic range of proteinura is >40 mg/m^2/day, >3.5 gm/day, >7.1 gm/m^2/day.
- Last fontanelle to close—anterior fontanelle.
- Two live vaccines should not be administered on same day, e.g. BCG and measles vaccine. Keep 4 weeks interval.
- Hydroamnios in mother—chances of baby to suffer esophageal atresia is more.
- Erythema toxicum in newborn never seen on day 1.
- Infective endocarditis least occur in ASD.
- HRCT is investigation of choice for diagnosis of bronchiectasis.
- Vitamin C deficiency may occur in child on breastfeed.
- Congestive heart failure is not occur in TOF.
- Varicella vaccine is live attenuated vaccine.

- Most common systemic presentation of tuberculosis in children is tuberculous lymphadenitis.
- Diagnosis of metabolic alkalosis—high bicarbonate in blood, in metabolic acidosis—low bicarbonate in blood.
- Antibodies in neonates acquired during intrauterine life is IgM.
- Congenital rubella syndrome—infection occurs before 26 weeks of intrauterine life.
- Neural tube defect occurs due to nonclosure of neural tube at 3–4 weeks of gestation.
- Specific marker of neural tube defect is acetylcholinesterase.
- Most common neural tube defect is meningomyelocele.
- Phenytoin is not used to treat absent seizures.
- Infantile spasm is treated by ACTH.
- Temporal lobe epilepsy is treated by carbamazepine.
- Child presented with mental retardation, infantile spasm, hypopigmented patch on back—most likely diagnosis is tuberous sclerosis.
- Neurofibromatosis is generally associated with defect in chromosome 22.
- Brain tumor in children is usually infratentorial.
- Most common infratentorial tumor is glioma.
- Most common posterior fossa tumor is astrocytoma.
- Urine color is green in phenylketonuria, dark in alkaptonuria.
- Earlier cardiac lesion in rheumatic carditis is MR.
- Most common cause of secondary hypertension in children is renal disease.
- Bat wing appearance in X-ray chest is seen in cardiogenic pulmonary edema.
- Hypoplastic left ventricle causes death within 1st week of life.
- Measles virus is also known as paramyxovirus.
- Rubella never cause conduction defect.
- Chickenpox never cause enteritis.
- Klinefelter syndrome is diagnosed by karyotyping.
- Phacomelia is congenital absence of long bones. It is side-effect of drug thalidomide taken by mother in antenatal period.
- Barr body is absent in female in turner syndrome.
- SRY gene differentiate gonad—ovary or testes.
- Pseudohermaphrodite in children is mainly due to 21α-hydroxylase deficiency.
- HbA$_2$ is hepful in diagnosing β-thalassemia.
- Highest cure rate is seen in retinoblastoma
- Commonest site of recurrence of acute lymphatic leukemia is CNS.
- Most common presentation of Wilms' tumor is asymptomatic abdominal mass.
- Height of child at birh doubles at the age of 4 years.
- Molar is first permanent tooth to appear.
- Nails formed at 10–12 intrauterine life.
- Short stature secondary to growth hormone deficiency have normal body proportion.
- Marasmus—hepatomegaly never seen.
- Flaky paint dermatosis is seen in kwashiorkor.
- Wing sweft deformity seen in rickets.
- In asymmetric IUGR brain is not effected.
- Hyline membrane in lung mainly composed of fibrin.
- Fetal lung maturity is assessed by L/S ratio.
- Hyperglycemia in newborn if blood glucose >125 mg/dl.
- Heart lesion usually associated in congenital rubella syndrome is ASD.
- CCF in infant mainly diagnosed by liver enlargement.
- Bronchiolitis treatment—drug of choice is ribavirin.
- Symptoms improve with crying—choanal atresia.
- Common cause of portal hypertension in children is extrahepatic obstruction.

- Profuse watery diarrhea in children is caused by Giardia.
- Unilateral renal agenesis is associated with single umbilical artery.
- Most common cause of hemolytic uremic syndrome is *E. coli.*
- Most common brain tumor is glioma.
- Figure of 3 sign is seen in X-ray chest of coarctation of aorta.
- Primary site of Ghon's focus in congenital tuberculosis is liver.
- Erythromycin should be given to contact of diphtheria for 7 days irrespective of previous immunization against diphtheria.
- Gluten-free diet is given in celiac disease. So, avoid wheat.
- HMD (hyaline membrane disease RDS) treatment—surfactant (lecithin) is given.
- 15 years boy suffering from fever, enlarged cervical lymph nodes. Biopsy of lymph node shows Langerhans' cell. Diagnosis is TB.
- Child with chest indrawing and RR 38/min. Diagnosis is severe pneumonia, give antibiotic and refer.
- Hymen in children does not rupture easily because it is deeply situated in children.
- Child with protuberant abdomen, edema, hypoproteinemia but no proteinuria. Diagnosis—kwashiorkor.
- Low osmolarity ORS does not contain lactate. Na and glucose concentration is same.
- Resomal (rehydration solution for malnourished) is prepared by dissolving 1 pkt of ORS in 2 litres of water.
- Dyslexia is most common learning disability.
- In central hypotonia reflexes are normal.
- In peripheral hypotonia reflexes are poor or absent.
- UTI common organism—*E. coli.*
- Zinc deficiency causes growth retardation, dementia, poor immunity, delayed wound healing, hypogonadism.
- Hypoglycemia in neonates—blood glucose <45 mg/dl
- Cerebral palsy—legs are affected more than upper limb.
- Congenital umbilical hernia may be associated with congenital hypothyroidism.
- Bed wetting is normal up to 4 years in boys and up to 5 years in girls.
- Neuroblastoma cross midline, while Wilms' tumor does not cross midline.
- Flag sign in hairs is seen in kwashiorkor.
- Rotavirus infection is most common cause of early childhood diarrhea.
- Most severe complication of mumps—meningoencephalitis, aseptic meningitis.
- Breast milk—fore milk is rich in water so satisfy thirst while hind milk is rich in fat so provide nutrition.
- Rise in heart rate is good indicator of success of positive pressure ventilation during neonatal resuscitation.
- Most common calcification seen infant abdomen is due to meconium peritonitis.
- Prenatal teeth appear in lower jaw—not effect normal dentition.
- Triceps skin fold thickness represents total subcutaneous fat up to 60 months age.
- Mitochondrial inheritance is transmitted from mother to daughter. Male does not transmit.
- PIGN (post-infectious glomerulonephritis) is diagnosed by streptozyme test.
- Calcifications are best seen in CT scan.
- For diagnosis of posterior urethral valve best investigation is MCU.
- Renal stone not diagnosed by MRI.
- Ureteric stones are diagnosed by CT scan.
- Rapid sequence excretory urography used for detection of renovascular hypertension.
- Intraperitoneal air is best detected by CT scan.
- Gold standard investigation for diagnosis of rickets is PET.
- Best investigation to diagnose GERD is intragastric pH monitoring.

- Cork screw sign is seen in diffuse esophageal spasm.
- Tertiary contraction seen in barium examination of diffuse esophageal spasm.
- Spring water cyst is also called pleuro-pericardial cyst.
- Water lily sign seen in X-ray chest of Echinococcus.
- Karley B lines seen X-ray of mitral stenosis.
- Handedness develop at 3 years of age.
- Maximum growth spurt in girls occur at menarche.
- Infantile colic occurs at age of 0–3 months mostly.
- Typhoid polysaccharide vaccine is administered at the age of 2 years.
- Oral typhoid vaccine 21 is given alternate days 1, 3, 5.
- Vaccine derived paralytic poliomyelitis is due to poliovaccine serotype 2.
- Zebra bodies are feature of Niemann-Pick disease.
- Flask-shaped deformity in femur seen Gaucher's disease.
- Cerebroside accumulation in cells seen in Gaucher's disease.
- A child with phenylketonuria may develop microcephaly, mental retardation and congenital heart disease.
- Hydronephrosis may not be seen if kidney obstruction is due to staghorn calculi.
- Best method to detect minimal ascites is USG.
- Most important investigation to diagnose Hirschsprung disease is rectal biopsy.
- Double bubble sign is seen in esophageal atresia.
- Inferior rib notching is seen in X-ray chest of coarctation of aorta.
- Congenital adrenal hyperplasia (CAH)

  11β-hydroxylase deficiency
  - Female virilization (ambiguous genitalia in female)
  - Hypertension

  21β-hydroxylase deficiency
  - Ambiguous genitalia in female
  - Salt wasting

  17β-hydroxylase deficiency
  - Male ambiguous genitalia
  - Hypertension

  3β-hydroxysteroid deficiency
  - Male ambiguous genitalia
  - Salt wasting

Tetralogy of Fallot

- Heart failure is not feature of TOF until unless complicated by anemia, myocarditis, systemic hypertension, endocarditis.
- On auscultation no murmur of VSD is heard, if VSD is so large and unrestricted that both ventricular chambers work as single chamber so there is hardly any pressure gradient between two chambers and no turbulence in blood flow so no murmur.
- Ejection systolic murmur on pulmonary area is due to pulmonary stenosis.
- 2nd heart sound is single and is due to only aortic component. Pulmonary component is not heard because it is soft and behind aorta.
- Hypoxia causes cyanosis and clubbing of fingers.
- Cyanotic spells are seen when right to left shunt increases. Sqatting position helps in aborting cyanotic spells because there is kinking of lower limb vessels so less blood goes to right side of heart from systemic circulation. Less blood results less right to left shunt and help in relief from cyanotic spell.
- X-ray chest is better investigation for diagnosis. Cardiomegaly is not seen, boot-shaped heart seen due upturning of apex due to right ventricular hypertrophy.
- ASD is not a part of TOF but is part of Fallot's tetralogy and pentalogy.
- Pink tetralogy of Fallot means no cyanosis or less seen, if pulmonary stenosis is very mild.

Height/Length

- Length is up to 2 years of age—taken by infantometer in lying down.
- Height is after 2 years of age—taken by stadiometer during standing. Normal height/length is as:
  - At birth—50 cm, 3 months—60 cm, 9 months—70 cm, 1 year—75 cm, so length increases 50% from birth to 1 year
  - At 2 years, 90 cm, 4 and half years—100 cm. So, height is double of birth at 4 years (100% increase), so maximum growth rate in length is at first year and at puberty.
  - Expected height = 6 X + 77 cm (X is age in years)

Upper and lower segment ratio

- Upper segment (US) is length of body above symphysis pubis. While lower segment (LS) is length of below symphysis pubis.
- US/LS ratio (US:LS) at different ages:
  - At birth 1.7–1.9:1
  - 3 years 1.3:1
  - 7–10 years 1:1

Growth

- Growth is measured by anthropometric measurement—weight, height, head circumference, skin fold thickness, MAUC, chest circumference.
- At birth, head circumference is more than chest circumference. At 9 months to 1 year both are equal. Beyond 1 year chest circumference becomes more than head circumference.
- Skinfold thickness is measured by Harpenden calipers at suprascapular, subscapular, biceps, triceps area.
- MAUC is measured by Shakir's tape.
- Growth chart is graphical representation of anthropometric parameters.
  - NCHC charts came in years 1977
  - CDC charts came in years 2000
  - WHO charts are used most commonly Came in years 2006 .
  - WHO charts for under 5 years children used now all over the world prepared

after survey from 6 countries including India. These are based on multicentre growth reference study (MGRS)
  - In survey those babies are enrolled who were on exclusive breastfeed for few month of life.
  - These growth charts are: Weight for age, weight for height, height for age, head circumference for age, mid-upper arm circumference for age, BMI for age, major motor mile stones.
  - Charts are separate for boys and girls. Two types of charts: Percentile and SD (Z score) charts are available.
  - Who charts are used up to 5 years of age in India. Beyond this they are not preferred. For them Indian growth charts are:
    - IAP growth charts
    - KN Agrawal growth charts
    - Khadilkar growth charts

Short Stature

- Length/height of baby is <3 percentile or below –2 SD is called short stature.
- Classification: Proportionate and disproportionate.
- If US:LS ratio is normal—proportionate; if change disproportionate short stature.

Proportionate Short Stature

Causes are:
1. Normal variant
2. Intrauterine causes
3. Postnatal causes
1. **Normal variant may be**
   a. Familial short stature
   b. CDGP (constitutional delay in growth and puberty)
a. *Familial short stature*
   - Both parents are of short statures. But child height is < –3 SD or <3 SD percentile. But his height is normal as per target height.
   - Target height is height which is aspected for that age and sex as per mid-

parental height. (FH = Fater's height; MH = Mother's height)

Mid-parental height for boys

$$= \frac{FH + MH + 13\ cm}{2}$$

$$Girls = \frac{FH + MH - 13\ cm}{2}$$

– Child has normal puberty, have family history of short stature. Bone age is equal to chronological age.

b. *CDGP:* It is most common cause of short stature in children:

– Here there is delay in achieving height for his age. For, example, 6 years child have height of 4 years age. So, height is less than aspected of during childhood but final adult height attained is normal.

– Bone age is less than chronological age. Delay in ossification also.

– Delayed puberty is present. There is also history of delayed puberty in parents.

2. **Intrauterine causes:** IUGR, intrauterine infection, e.g. TORCH, genetic syndromes (Turner syndrome, Down syndrome, Seckel syndrome)

3. **Postnatal or acquired causes**

– Severe long-standing malnutrition, chronic systemic disease such as chronic renal disease, celiac disease, endocrine causes (growth hormone deficiency, hypothyroidism, Cushing syndrome), psychosocial deprivation.

– Single test of growth hormone is not correct but tests should be dynamic. Growth hormone stimulation tests should be performed.

– Most common cause of Cushing syndrome is iatrogenic.

Disproportionate Short Stature

It is of two types:

1. **Short trunk dwarfism:** US/LS ratio decreases than normal. Causes are spondyloepiphyseal dysplasia (vertebral column is effected), metabolic diseases (mucopolysaccharidosis, mucolipidosis), carries (Pott's spine) hemivertebra, congenital butterfly vertebra.

2. **Short limb dwarfism:** US/LS ratio increased than normal. Causes are rickets, achondroplasia, osteogenetic imperfecta, congenital, chondroectodermal dysplasia.

Achondroplasia

It is autosomal dominant disorder shows clinical manifestations as champagne glass pelvis, hand abnormality, obesity, neurological problems, bowing of legs, shortening of legs (proximal part shortening), large head, interpedicular distance of vertebra decreases.

Clinical features may be seen even at birth. Gene FGFR 3 is effected.

Osteogenesis Imperfecta

It is defect due to collagen type 1 diagnosed by triad of symptoms:

1. Recurrent fractures so also known as brittle bone disease, bone deformity

2. Blue sclera

3. Deafness.

• **Bone age:** Bone age is the skeletal maturity determined by looking ossification of different bones. For determination X-rays are taken and see the ossification developed. X-rays are taken as follows:

– Newborn (term)—X-ray knee

– Infant (3–9 m)—X-ray shoulder

– 1–13 years—hand and wrist (left)

• **Weight:** Weight of child at birth is 2.8–2.9 kg.

Rules: At birth—W (birth weight)

5 months—2 months W (double)

1 years— 3 W (triple)

2 years—4 W

3 years—5 W

5 years—6 W

7 years—7 W

10 years—10 W

Expected weight of baby less than 1 year of age

$$\frac{X+9}{2} \quad X \text{ is age in months}$$

Expected weight of baby less than 1–6 years of age

$$2X + 8 \quad X \text{ is age in years}$$

Expected weight of baby less than 7–12 years of age

$$\frac{7X-5}{2} \quad X \text{ is weight in years}$$

- Intrauterine growth restriction (IUGR). Two types of IUGR are given in Table 19.1.

Rh Isoimmunization

- Rh positive person is said when D antigen is present at short arm of chromosome 1 of the person.
- Rh negative pregnancy—when mother is Rh negative and fetus is Rh positive. Fetus Rh blood group may be known by detection of husband blood group. If father is Rh positive chances of fetus to become positive are 50% or 25%.

- If mother is Rh negative and fetus is Rh positive, Rh antigen present in RBC of fetus but not present in mother's RBC. Due to any reason fetal blood enters into mother's blood so immune system of mother take antigen as foreign substance and form antibodies (Rh D). Initially antibody formed are IgM antibodies which cannot cross placental barrier. Then after 5–6 months IgM antibody convert into IgG antibodies which can cross placental barrier. By this time patient is delivered. So, first pregnancy is spared.
- In subsequent pregnancy if mother is Rh negative and fetus is Rh positive, due to some reason if fetal blood enters mother's blood again mother immune system is stimulated. Mother's immune system is now already prepared so it forms IgM antibodies very quickly and IgM antibodies change to IgG antibodies occurs quickly. This is called amnestic response.
- IgG antibodies enter fetal circulation because they can cross placental barrier. So,

Table 19.1: Difference between IUGR type 1 and IUGR type 2

IUGR type 1	IUGR type 2
1. Defect is at the time of early pregnancy At the time of zygote formation, embryo formation due to effect on mitosis so number of cells are less	1. Defect is at the time of late pregnancy at about 32–34 weeks of pregnancy Cells are normal because mitosis is complete up till now. Size of cell is less
2. Number of cells cannot be regained, so prognosis is bad	2. Cell size can be increased, so prognosis is good
3. All parameters seen in USG such as abdominal circumference, head circumference, biparietal diameter, femur length are effected they are less	3. Less amount of blood is coming to fetus, so blood collected from peripheral organs is sent to brain (brain sparing effect). So, last organ effected is brain. Head circumference is normal. Liver is first organ effected Abdominal circumference is decreased, weight is decreased. Rest all parameters are normal
4. Ponderal index is normal	4. Ponderal index is decreased
5. Causes are—chromosomal abnormality, TORCH infections, genetic disease	5. Causes are—placental insufficiency, PIH, chronic renal disease
6. More complicated.	6. Less complicated
7. Also called symmetrical IUGR. Because all parameters are decreased	7. Also called asymmetrical IUGR. Because abdominal circumference is decreased, rest are normal

$$\text{Ponderal index} = \frac{\text{Estimated fetal weight (g)}}{(fl)^3 (cm)} \times 100 \quad fl \text{ is femur length}$$

antigen–antibody reaction takes place at fetal RBC level resulting hemolysis of fetal RBC.

- Antibodies are formed in mother but problem occurs in fetus, this phenomenon is known as isoimmunization.

Hydrops Fetalis

Causes

Immune causes

1. Antibody to Rh antigen (Rh isoimmunization) most common
2. Antibodies to Kele antigen
3. Antibody to ABO antigen

Nonimmune causes

1. Cardiovascular abnormalities ASD.
2. Hematological—anemia, homozygous α-thalassemia.
3. Parvovirus 19 infection

Diagnosis: It is diagnosed radiologically. Look for pleural effusion, pericardial effusion, ascites, subcutaneous edema. Effusion in two or more cavities is diagnostic.

Celiac Disease

It is a disease in which immune reaction occurs to eating gluten, a protein found in wheat, barley and rye.

Reaction to eating gluten creates inflammation and damages to small intestine villi so prevents absorption of some nutrients (malabsorption).

Symptoms are diarrhea, stomachache, flatulence, indigestion, constipation. General symptoms are fatigue, failure to thrive, iron deficiency anemia, vit B_{12} deficiency. This condition is associated with Down syndrome, Turner syndrome.

Treatment—gluten-free diet is given.

Tropical Sprue

It is a rare digestive disease in which small intestine's ability to absorb nutrient is impaired resulting nutritional deficiency (malabsorption).

Exact cause is not known but environmental and nutritional condition in tropics is supposed to be responsible.

Symptoms are abdominal cramps, diarrhea, indigestion, muscle cramps, failure to thrive, iron, folic acid, vit B_{12} deficiency symptoms. Diagnosed by intestinal biopsy.

Treatment—antibiotics are given to kill overgrowth of bacteria for 2 weeks to one year. Antibiotics are tetracycline (not in children), sulphamethoxazole and trimethoprim, ampicillin. Supportive treatment gives iron, folic acid, vit B_{12}.

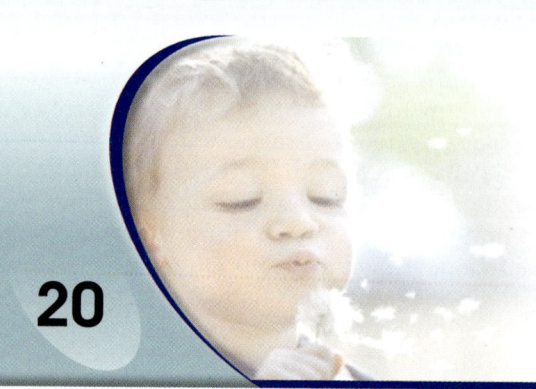
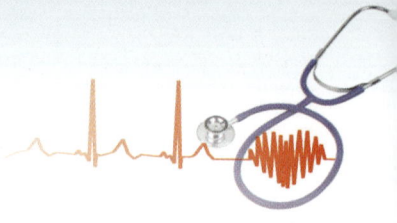

20

Endocrinology

THYROID DISORDERS

General Considerations

1. Thyroid hormones are involved in the regulation of physical and intellectual growth, intermediary metabolism and thermoregulation.
2. Hypothalamic-pituitary—thyroid axis is regulated by feedback mechanism between thyroxine, triiodothyronine (T_3), thyrotropin-releasing hormone (TRH) and thyroid-stimulating hormone (TSH).
3. Most of the triiodothyronine (T_3) is produced by conversion of thyroxine (T_4) to T_3.

$$T_4 \xrightarrow[\text{Enzyme}]{\text{Monodeiodinase}} T_3$$

If T_3 level falls. Blood protective mechanism involves to produce T_3 from T_4 in hypothyroid state. So, T_3 level is last to fall in hypothyroidism.
4. If T_3 and T_4 levels fall. TSH level increases to produce more T_3 and T_4.
5. Thyroid function is assessed by estimation of TSH, and free and/or total T_3–T_4 in blood.
6. TSH estimation in serum is most sensitive indicator of primary hypothyroidism.
   - T_4 estimation is best indicator in assessment of thyroid depleted state.

- Both free T_3 and T_4 (unbound FT_3, FT_4) are the biological active forms of each hormone, so its level estimation indicates hypothyroidism.
- Elevated FT_3 and undetectable TSH level are indicative of hyperthyroid state.
- Low FT_4 and high TSH is indicative of hypothyroid state.

HYPOTHYROIDISM

Causes of Hypothyroidism

Primary

a. Hashimoto's thyroiditis
b. Iodine deficiency (endemic goiter): Trapping, organification, thyroglobulin synthesis, deiodination.
c. Dysgenesis: Aplasia, dysplasia, ectopic
d. Thyroid injury: Surgery irradiation, ectopic
e. Goitrogens in foodstuffs, pollutants
f. Transient causes: Maternal TSH receptor blocking antibody, iodine excess, maternal antithyroid drugs.

Secondary or Tertiary

a. Malformations: Septo-optic dysplasia, holoprosencephaly
b. Genetic defects

c. CNS insults: Trauma, surgery, radiation, infection

d. CNS: Tumours

Peripheral

Resistance to thyroxine, TSH.

CONGENITAL HYPOTHYROIDISM

Epidemiology: This is a most common congenital metabolic disorder. About 1 in 40,000 newborns have congenital hypothyroidism.

Etiology

Primary

1. Autoimmune thyroiditis
2. Iodine deficiency: In some area of India, it is most common cause.
3. Thyroid dysgenesis: Common cause. Thyroid aplasia (absent thyroid gland), hypoplasia or ectopic thyroid gland (found at base of the long to midchest).
4. Thyroid dyshormonogenesis: It is an inborn error of thyroid hormone synthesis, autosomal recessive and associated with goiter.

Pendred syndrome is a common disorder of pendrin gene, defect is decreased intracellular transport of iodine. It is associated with sensorineural hearing loss.

1. Propylthiouracil (PTU) use during pregnancy for maternal Graves' disease may result transient hypothyroidism in newborn.
2. Maternal autoimmune thyroid disease also results transient hypothyroidism because maternal thyroid blocking antibodies may cross placenta and black TSH receptors on the newborn thyroid gland.
3. *Thyroid injury:* Surgery, radiation, infections.
4. Enzyme defects.

Secondary or Tertiary *(Hypothalamus or Pituitary)*

- Malformations: Septo-optic dysplasia, holoprosencephaly genetic defect.
- CNS injury: Trauma, surgery, radiation, infection
- CNS tumors: Craniopharyngioma, germinoma
- Peripheral (rare): Resistance to thyroxine.

Clinical Features

Most of the newborns with hypothyroidism are asymptomatic and do not show any sign. Because T_4 is not essential for fetal growth.

Thyroid hormone is essential for normal brain growth during first 2 years of life in hypothyroid state, following features become apparent:

1. Prolonged jaundice, poorfeeding
2. Lethargy and constipation
3. Large anterior and posterior fontannele protruding tongue, umbilical hernia, myxedema, mottled skin, hypothermia, delayed neuromotor development and poor growth (hypotonia) (Fig. 20.1).
4. Hoarse cry, thyroid goiter at neck.

Diagnosis

1. High TSH
2. Radionuclide uptake and thyroid ultrasound—to confirm presence of thyroid gland.
3. Radiotracer uptake study with radioactive iodine or technetium.
4. Low TSH level—hypopituitarism.

Management

1. Thyroid hormone replacement (thyroxine T_4) should begin immediately at dose of 10–12 µg/kg/day.
2. Thyroxine level (T_4) becomes normal at 1 week of treatment and TSH level normalizes at 1 month of treatment. Monitoring is done. Level of T_4 is adjusted at upper limit.
3. In suspected transient hypothyroidism—thyroid replacement is stopped for 1 month at the age of 3 years. If no abnormality in T_4 and TSH levels occur, discontinue treatment.

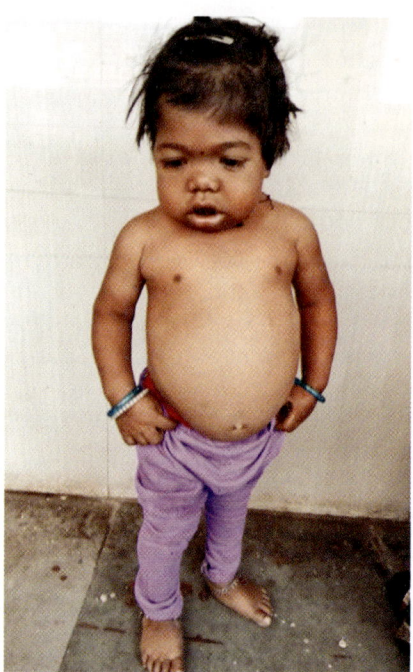

Fig. 20.1: Hypothyroidism—12-year-old girl (dwarf).

Prognosis

Early diagnosis and continuous treatment following neonatal screening results a normal intellectual outcome.

Sequelae

If treatment is delayed, mental retardation and short stature are common sequelae.

ACQUIRED HYPOTHYROIDISM

Etiology

Autoimmune thyroiditis, most common cause—thyroid peroxidase antibody is usually present. It may be associated with other autoimmune endocrinopathies such as diabetes mellitus, adrenal insufficiency and hypoparathyroidism.

Iodine deficiency and goitrogens are other causes of acquired hypothyroidism.

Secondary hypothyroidism is due to hypothalamopituitary defects such as CNS injury tumors.

Clinical Features

Common clinical manifestations are short stature and mental retardation. Cold intolerance, lethargy, constipation, delay in dentition are other features. Goiter is common in iodine deficiency. Goiter is firm in consistency. It may be associated with Down syndrome, celiac disease and diabetes mellitus type 1.

Evaluation

- Short stature and mental retardation.
- Pituitary function test
- T3, T4, TSH estimation
- Antibodies to thyroid peroxidase enzyme (anti-TPC).

Treatment

Thyroxine is given as follows:

Age	Dose (µg/kg/day)
1–6 mo	10–15
1–5 yr	6–10
5–12 yr	3–5
12–18 yr	2–3
>18 yr	1–2

Initial treatment is started with 25–50% of the dose then gradually increased every 3–4 weeks, follow-up every 3 months up to 2 years, then 6 monthly interval. Mild elevation of TSH <8 U/L in the selling of normal FT4 (subclinical hypothyroidism) is self-resolving and does not require any treatment.

IODINE DEFICIENCY DISORDERS

This is an endemic disease caused by iodine deficiency in food. Clinical manifestations include goiter, delayed growth and development. Depending on size of goiter, it is classified in 4 stages.

- 24-hour urine excretion or urinary iodine concentration is done for evaluation.

Prevention and control: Iodinated salt or oil intake is best prevention method used to prevent the disease.

HASHIMOTO'S DISEASE

Chronic Lymphocytic Thyroiditis (CLT)

This is an autoimmune disorder characterized by lymphocytic infiltration of thyroid gland, resulting in varying degrees of follicular hyperplasia, fibrosis and atrophy.

Epidemiology

More common in girls. It is most common cause of acquired hyperthyroidism, hypo-thyroidism may be associated with Down syndrome, Turner syndrome, celiac disease and DM type 1.

Etiology

Thyroid antibodies develop because of imba-lance in immunoregulation. It causes thyroid cell cytotoxicity or stimulation. There is also genetic predisposition. Thyroid peroxidase antibodies are usually present.

Clinical Features

Child may be asymptomatic. Goiter at front of neck characteristic firm in nature. Short stature and mental retardation (unexplained), poor school performance are clinical mani-festations. Cold intolerance, lethargy, constipation are other associated symptoms.

Management

Thyroid hormone replacement.

HYPERTHYROIDISM

Etiology

Infancy: Transplacental passage of thyroid antibodies. TSH receptor activating mutation.

After infancy

- Graves' disease (TSH receptor stimulating antibody)
- Subacute thyroiditis
- Toxic thyroid nodule
- Toxic multinodular goiter
- Iatrogenic
- Pituitary resistance to T_3

Epidemiology

Hyperthyroidism is relatively uncommon in children. Most commonly seen in girls, caused by Graves' disease.

Clinical Features

Hyperthyroidism manifests clinically in children as weight loss with increased appetite, tremors, diarrhea, warm extremities, increased sweating and anxiety.

Eyes examination may demonstrates lid lag exophthalmos, ophthalmoplegia, absence of wrinkling. Thyroid gland is enlarged and usually smooth in texture (Fig. 20.2).

Cardiac examination demonstrates tachy-cardia, cardiac arrhythmia, high output cardiac failure.

Pubertal evaluation may be notable for delayed menarche and gynecomastia in boys.

Graves' disease diffuse toxic goiter is an autoimmune disorder characterized by excessive thyroid hormone by the thyroid gland mediated by TSH look alike antibody. It is a short genetic factor.

Laboratory Findings

1. T_3 and T_4 levels increased TSH levels sup-pressed or undetectable.
2. Ultrasonography and nuclear scan for radioactive iodine uptake (RAIU) differen-tiate toxic nodule or diffuse goiter.

Management

Antithyroid Medications

- PTU and methimazole are two most commonly used antithyroid medications. Both inhibit thyroid synthesis.

Beta blocker (propranolol 2 mg/kg/day) is effective to treat sympathetic symptoms.

Iodinated contrast
- Idopate 0.001 µg/kg/day
- Lugol's iodine: 5% iodine and 10% potassium iodide

Prednisolone (1–2 mg/kg/day)

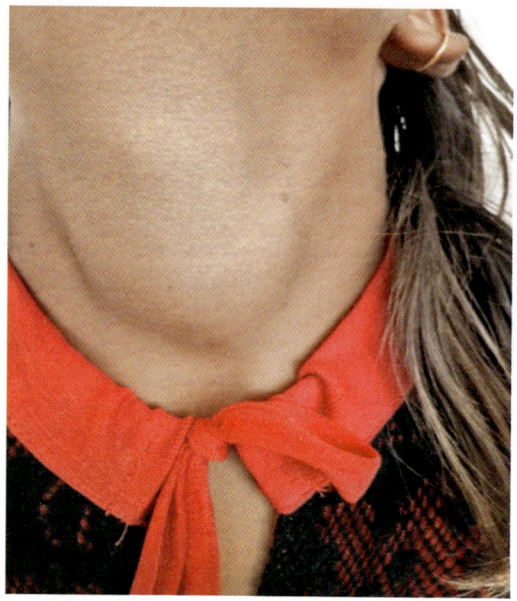

Fig. 20.2: Thyroid goiter.

Inhibits conversion of T_4 to T_3 and useful in treatment of hyperthyroid storm.

If cardiac failure: Digitalis.

Surgery: Subtotal thyroidectomy may be considered, if antithyroid medication fails.

DIABETES MELLITUS

This is a metabolic disorder that is characterized by hyperglycemia and glycosuria.

Epidemiology

Incidence of diabetes is increased due to obesity. Peak is about 5–12 years of age. Seasonal variation has been identified maximum cases occurs in spring and fall. It is second most common chronic disease of childhood. Incidence is 1 of 500 children.

Types of Diabetes

1. Type 1: Insulin deficiency (insulin dependent)
2. Type 2: Insulin resistant (noninsulin dependent)

TYPE 1 DIABETES MELLITUS (TYPE 1 DM)

Etiology

It is multifactorial. Following factors are identified:

1. *Genetic factor:* Genetic influences involve multiple genes. About 95% patients with type 1 DM have haplotype DR3 or DR4. Inheritance has not seen found to fit into autosomal or X-linked as seen in Mendelian pattern.

   Type I DM incidence in monozygotic twin is 30–70%.

2. *Environmental factors*

   Triggering factors are:
   - Viruses
   - Cow milk protein—it is controversial
   - Nitrosourea compounds

Autoimmune factors and autoimmunity

Autoimmune distraction affects only B cells of the islets.

Islet cell antibodies (ICA) are present in 85% of patients. They are detected in asymptomatic children.

Other immunologic markers antibodies against insulin and against glutamic acid decarboxylase (GAD) may be detected.

About 10% of general population may have ICA, therefore, to develop type 1 DM children must have ICA, environmental factors and genetic predisposition.

Clinical Features

Symptoms of type 1 diabetes mellitus include polyuria, polydipsia, nocturia, polyphagia, fatigue, and weight loss.

As symptoms progress weight loss, vomiting and dehydration occur.

Diabetes ketoacidosis occurs in 50% of patient.

Recent acute infection may be only presentation. Such as monilial vulvovaginitis in girls.

Diagnosis

1. Clinical features—polyuria, polyphagia, polydipsia, weight loss.
2. Random blood sugar more than 200 mg/dl.
3. Elevaled glycated hemoglobin (HbA1c).

Management

Most children respond to insulin therapy.

Insulin

- Insulin analog Lispro [Lys (B28), pro (B29)] human insulin has a better control of blood sugar as its action is faster than regular insulin and duration of action is shorter.
- Insulin aspart has longer duration of action than Lispro (Table 20.1).

  Short acting preparations have faster onset and shorter duration while long acting have slower onset and longer duration.
- Insulin requirement 0.5–14 unit/kg/day—initiated with 4 doses to achieve normal blood glucose level.
- Insulin pumps are now being used in children to achieve better glucose control.

  Administration of insulin is newly diagnosed patients may involve combination of short acting, intermediate acting, long acting or very long acting insulin.

  Two main types of regimen are used.
  1. NPH with short acting insulin analogues.

Table 20.1: Different types of insulin preparations

Preparation	Effective duration
Short acting	
1. Lispro	3–4 hr
2. Insulin aspart	3–6 hr
3. Regular	
Intermediate	
NPH insulin	10–16 hr
Lente	12–18 hr
Long acting	
Ultralente	18–20 hr
Glargine (lantus)	24 hr

2. Long acting insulin, typically insulin Glargine (lantus) with short acting insulin.
   - NPH + short acting—before breakfast
     Short acting—at dinner or bedtime
     As NPH—2/3 Total in morning
     1/3 Total—at evening
     Pre dinner—1/2–2/3 of evening insulin as NPH
     1/3–1/2 insulin given as short acting prior to dinner

Monitoring

- Blood sugar level is monitored at least four times a day (prior to meals and at bedtime).
- Variation in meal, any physical activity may result fluctuation in blood sugar level.
- Watch for hypoglycemia—all patient should have parenteral glucagon available. In case of seizure or coma secondary to low blood sugar.
- Watch for honeymoon period—within a few weeks after the initial treatment 75% patients exhibit progressive reduction in daily insulin requirement or insulin-free period. It lasts few days to month. It is due to transient recovery of residual islet cell function insulin-free period rarely 1 year.
- Watch for Somogyi phenomenon
  When evening dose of insulin is too high causing hypoglycemia in the early morning. This results in the release of counter-regulatory hormones (epinephrine and glucagon) to counteract this insulin-induced hypoglycemia.
  Patient has high blood glucose level in the morning. Treatment of this is to lower bedtime insulin dose, not to raise it.

Diet

1. Avoid simple sugars. Sweeteners, aspartate, are allowed under limit.
2. Food with low glycemic index and fibers are advised.
3. Intake of saturated fats should be limited and minimum intake of *trans* fat is advised.
4. Insulin intake and caloric intake are adjusted.

Exercise: Simple activity walking, jogging and swimming are recommended.

Complications (long-term complications)
1. Diabetic retinopathy
2. Diabetes nephropathy
3. Diabetic neuropathy
4. Atherosclerotic disease
5. Hypertension
6. Heart disease, strokes
7. Diabetic ketoacidosis (DKA)

DIABETIC KETOACIDOSIS

Diabetic ketoacidosis is termed when hyperglycemia is greater than 300 mg/dl with ketonuria and serum bicarbonate level less than 15 mmol/L or serum pH more than 7.30.

Clinical Features

Vomiting, polyuria, polydipsia and mild to moderate dehydration and presenting features. In severe cases, abdominal pain rapid and deep (Kussmaul) breathing and coma are noted. Fruity breath in DKA patient is due to ketones.

Laboratory Diagnosis

1. Blood—elevated glucose level
2. Urine—sugar present, ketones body present
3. Hyperkalemia—due to metabolic acidosis.

Management

1. Fluid and electrolyte therapy.
2. Potassium—if urine output is established potassium acetate or potassium phosphate administered.
3. Regular insulin infusion 0.1 U/kg/hr.
4. Cerebral edema is treated with IV mannitol or hypertonic saline.

TYPE 2 DIABETES MELLITUS

Epidemiology

Occurs in 2–3% of all children with diabetes.

Etiology

1. Hereditary component type 2 is more stronger than type 1.

2. Progressing decline in insulin secretion and peripheral tissue resistance to insulin are both etiological factors responsible for type 2 DM.

Clinical Features

About half of the type 2 patients is asymptomatic. Diabetic ketoacidosis is uncommon. Obesity is important feature. Acanthosis nigricans (velvety and hyperpigmented skin of the neck and axillary folds) is common.

Treatment

1. Oral hypoglycemia drugs.
2. If ketosis is present—insulin is drug of choice.

DISORDERS OF ADRENAL GLAND

Adrenal gland composed of two parts:
a. Adrenal cortex which synthesizes:
   1. Adrenal corticoids
   2. Gucocorticoids (cortisol)
   3. Androgens (DHEA)
b. Adrenal medulla: Mineralocorticoids synthesis is controlled by the renin angiotensin system and glucocorticoids androgen synthesis is regulated by a negative feedback by hypothalamic-pituitary-adrenal axis via ACTH.

   Children may suffer from adrenal insufficiency or adrenocortical excess.

Adrenocortical Insufficiency

Classification: Primary or secondary
1. *Primary* (problem at the level of adrenal gland): Destruction of adrenal cortex or from enzyme deficiency.

   Examples are Addison's disease, CAH and adrenoleukodystrophy.
2. *Secondary:* It is due to interference with the release of cortisol releasing hormone (CRH) from hypothalmus or ACTH from pituitary examples are—pituitary tumors, craniopharyngioma, Langerhans' cell histiocytosis. Iatrogenic due to long-term exposure of dosages of glucocorticoids (>2 weeks), hypothalmic pituitary axis is suppressed.

Congenital or Acquired

a. Acquired adrenal insufficiency
   - Addison's disease
   - Long-term steroid taking
b. Congenital adrenal hyperplasia (CAH)

Acquired Adrenal Insufficiency

Etiology

Causes are:

1. Chronic supraphysiological steroids use usually more than 2 weeks.
2. Addison's disease: It is an adrenal insufficiency resulting from autoimmune destruction of the adrenal cortex. Antibodies to the adrenal gland may be detected on examination.
3. Acute adrenal hemorrhage in neonates and septicemia (especially associated with meningococcemia, known as Waterhouse-Friderichsen syndrome.

Clinical Features

Anorexia, weakness, hyponatremia, hypotension and morning hypothermia and episodes of shock during severe illness. Failure to thrive, hyponatremia and hyperkalemia.

Primary adrenal insufficiency is characterized by hyperpigmentation seen in exposed areas such as elbows and palmar creases, areola, genitalia, and hyperpigmentation is not present in secondary adrenal insufficiency.

Evaluation

1. Serum electrolytes and sugar—low, cortisol level—low or normal.
2. ACTH stimulation test—0.25 mg of ACTH intramuscular or intravenous given and serum cortisol level estimated after 60 minutes. Less than 18 µg/dl are suggestive of adrenal insufficiency.
3. ACTH level elevated—suggestive of primary adrenal insufficiency, low level suggests pituitary defect.
4. Abdominal CT scan and work-up for tuberculosis.

Management

a. Crisis management: Correction of shock by intravenous fluids boluses. Hydrocortisone at a dose of 50 mg/m^2 followed by 100/m^2/day in four divided doses.

   Cortisone is tapered gradually if child is stable. Hydrocortisone is reduced to 10 mg/m^2/day. Fludrocortisone acetate (0.1 mg/day) should be added once the hydrocortisone is less than 50 mg/m^2/day.

b. Long-term treatment requires lifelong replacement of glucocorticoids and mineralocorticoids.

   Doses should be increased 2–3 times in conditions of minor stress, e.g. fever and 4–5 times in severe infections and surgery.

Secondary adrenal insufficiency—only glucocorticoids synthesis (6–10 mg/m^2/day) is required. Mineralocorticoids replacement is not suggested.

Congenital Adrenal Hyperplasia

Congenital adrenal hyperplasia (CAH) is autosomal recessive congenital enzyme deficiency in the adrenal cortex. It is a primary adrenal insufficiency of childhood.

CAH is most common cause of ambiguous genitalia when no gonads are palpable. It is a most common adrenal disorder.

Enzyme Deficiency

a. **21-hydoxylase deficiency**
   Classic salt wasting form
   Both mineralocorticoids and glucocorticoids pathways are affected, resulting in both cortical and aldosterone deficiency.

   Girls present with ambiguous genitalia. After 1–2 weeks of life both boys and girls present with failure to thrive vomiting and electrolyte misbalance.
   Simple virilizing form
   Only glucocorticoids pathway is affected, resulting only in cortisol deficiency.

   Girls present as ambiguous genitalia at birth (Fig. 20.3) and boys present after

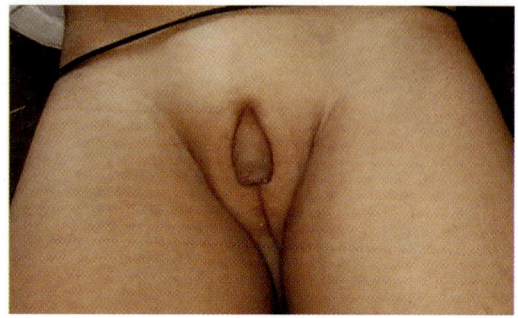

Fig. 20.3: Ambiguous genitalia.

1–4 years of age with tall stature, advance bone age, pubic hair, penile enlargement (sign of precocious puberty).

Nonclassic form

In this form onset is late, cortisol deficiency is mild and no mineralocorticoids invovement.

It presents 4–5 years of age. Girls present with premature adrenarche, clitoromegaly, acne, hirsutism, infertility and rapid growth. Boys present with premature adrenarche, rapid growth and premature acne.

b. **11β-hydroxylase deficiency** (5% cases): Clinical presentation is similar to 21-hydroxylase deficiency except that they suffer from hypertension and hypokalemia.

c. **3β-hydroxysteroid dehydrogenase deficiency:** They suffer from salt wasting crisis, glucocorticoids deficiency and ambiguous genitalia.

Diagnosis

a. 21-hydroxylase deficiency has increased 17-hydroxyprogesterone deficiency.

b. 11β-hydroxylase has increased level of 11-deoxycortisol.

c. 3β-hydroxysteroid dehydrogenase deficiency has increased level of DHEA and 17-hydroxypregnenolone.

Management

The patient requires lifelong treatment. Salt wasting and virilizing forms are treated with hydrocortisone (10–15 mg/m²/day and fludrocortisone (0.1 mg/day).

Cortisone suppresses ACTH production so that androgen production decreases but is not excessive enough to interfere with proper growth. Mineralocorticoid (fludrocortisone) is given to normalize the plasma renin activity (PRA) because patient also has aldosterone deficiency.

Monitoring: Monitor growth velocity, physical examination, bone age, laboratory test (17-OHP, PRA), parents should be educated about importance of compliance and medicines at the time of fever, vomiting, surgery which requires additional dose of drug to prevent adrenal shock.

Glucocorticoid Excess

Causes

a. Iatrogenic: When corticosteroids are given for long period in chronic disease.

b. Cushing syndrome is most common cause. There is excessive glucocorticoids production due to adrenal tumors.

c. Cushing disease: There is excessive glucocorticoids production caused by excessive ACTH production by pituitary tumor such as microadenoma.

Clinical Features

Excess of glucocorticoids manifests as poor growth, delayed bone age, moon facies, nuchal pad, easy bruisability, obesity, delayed puberty, behavioral problems, bone pain and muscle weakness (Fig. 20.4).

Laboratory Investigations

a. Elevated free cortisol in 24-hour urine collection.

b. Absence of expected cortisol suppression seen in overnight dexamethasone suppression test (dexamethasone is given in the evening normally suppress the morning physiological rise in cortisol).

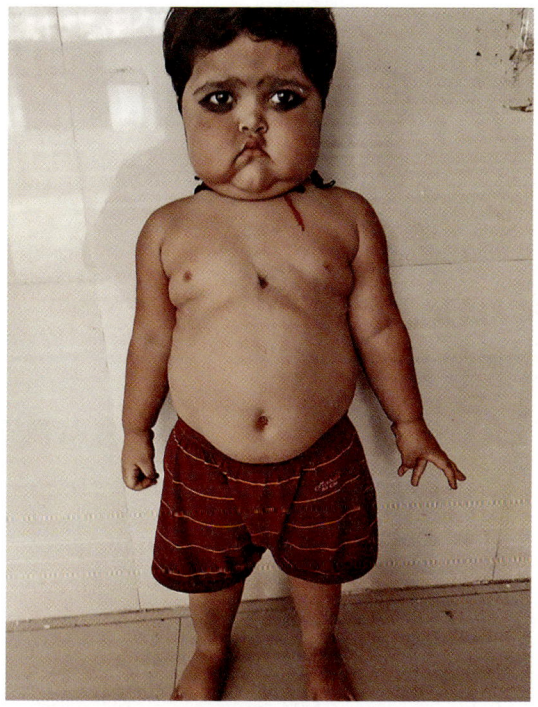

Fig. 20.4: Iatrogenic glucocorticoid excess.

c. Adrenal tumors are detected on ultrasound.
d. MRI of hypothalamic pituitary regions.
e. Inferior petrosal sinus sampling is done to detect ACTH production.

Management

1. Resection of adrenal adenoma and carcinoma.
2. Medical management is done by inhibitors of steroidogenesis, e.g.
   - Ketoconazole, aminoglutamide
   - Cyproheptadine, metyrapone, mitotane
   - Results are variable.

Aldosterone excess: Excess of aldosterone causes fluid, sodium retention and increased urinary loss of potassium. It may be primary or secondary.

a. Primary hyperaldosteronism caused by hyperplasia or adenoma.
b. Secondary hyperaldosteronism
   - Renal failure
   - Congestive cardiac failure
   - Liver disease
   - Nephrotic syndrome
   - Other state of mineralocorticoids excess.

Clinical features of primary hyperaldosteronism are hypertension and hyperkalemic alkalosis.

Management

Management includes salt restriction and by aldosterone antagonist such as spironolactone or eplerenone. Surgery is indicated for adrenal adenoma.

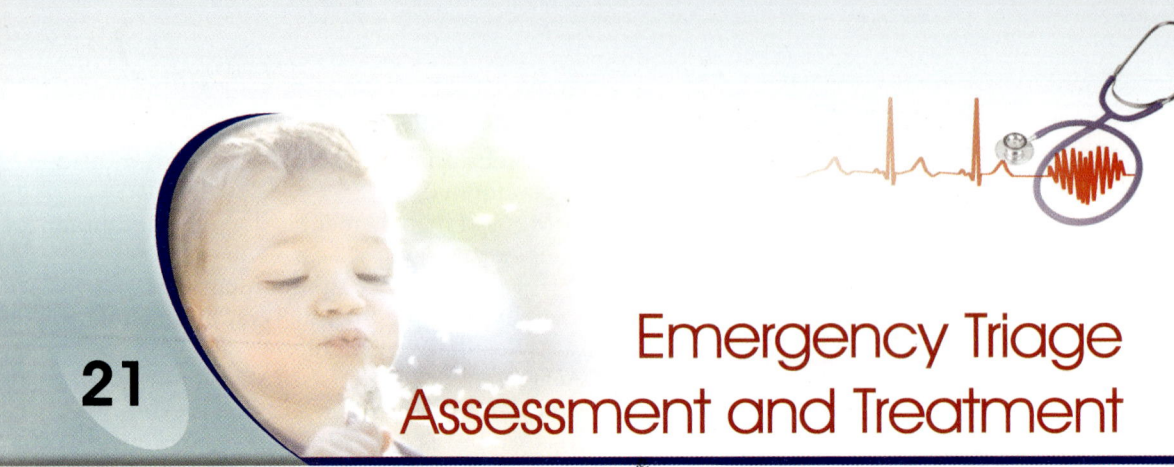

21

Emergency Triage Assessment and Treatment

CHILD MORTALITY

Causes of death of child 0–5 years of age are:
1. Neonatal death : 57.9%
2. Pneumonia : 11.9%
3. Diarrhea : 9.4%
4. Meningitis : 1.8%
5. Malaria : 0.6%
6. Measles : 1.8%
7. Others : 16.5%

TRIAGE

Triage is the process of rapidly screening all sick children on their arrival in hospital.

All sick children can be placed in following categories.

E—emergency
P—priority
Q—queue (nonurgent)

All children with emergency signs require immediate emergency treatment.

The triaging process

Assess several emergency signs quickly (average in 20 seconds).

Assessing emergency signs (E)

Quickly assess the patient for serious illness. You can easily remember them as ABCD.

A—Airway
B—Breathing
C—Circulation/convulsion/consciousness/ coma
D—Dehydration

Steps to check for emergency signs

Step 1: Assess for airway or breathing problem.

Step 2: Assess for circulation (shock, impaired circulation and convulsion, unconsciousness or not.

Step 3: Assess for severe dehydration.

Assessing priority signs

Priority signs may be sick child below 2 months age, high temperature (fever), trauma, severe pallor, poisoning, pain, respiratory distress, restless or lethargic, severe acute malnutrition, edema, burn.

Airway and breathing A and B

Assess the child look—active, talking or crying as follows:
a. Not breathing or gasping—assess for neck trauma
b. Obstructed breathing—in foreign body aspiration
c. Central cyanosis—bluish purple discoloration of tongue and inside mouth.
d. Severe respiratory distress. Assess:
   • For labored breathing
   • Needing much more effort to breathe than normal.

- Difficulty in breathing while talking, eating or breastfeeding.
- Fast breathing chest indrawing, using auxiliary muscles for breathing, breathing which causes head to nod or bob.
- Oxygen saturation less than 90% (SpO_2).

Abnormal Respiratory Noises

- *Stridor*—a harsh noises on breathing in inspiration
- *Grunting*—short noise when breathing out.

How to check pulse: Palpate carotid or femoral pulse within 10 seconds.

Carotid pulse: Locate the trachea using 2 or 3 fingers, slide finger into the groove between the trachea and muscles at the side on neck, feel carotid.

Femoral pulse: Femoral pulse is palpated midway between hip bone and pubic symphysis, view at the junction of thigh and abdomen.

Respiratory arrest: Respiratory arrest is the absence of respiration (e.g. apnea) during early phase of respiratory arrest, heart rate may be slow, cardiac arrest may develop if rescue breathing is not provided.

Cardiac arrest: In children, cardiac arrest does not usually from cardiac arrest but it is terminal result of respiratory failure or shock.

Positioning of child to improve the airway

To open the airway lift the chin.

Neck is slightly extended and head is tilted by placing one hand onto the child's forehead. Lift the mandible up and outward by placing the fingertips of other hand under the chin.

- Neutral position—nose up
- Sniffing position—chin up

If child has neck trauma: Above method is not used it may aggravate cervical injury jaw thrust is used by placing two or three fingers under the angle of the jaw on both sides and lifting the jaw upwards and outwards.

It is also used in bag and mask ventilation.

Ventilate with bag and mask: See Chapter 2: Neonatology for detail.

Management of the airway in chocking child

If child is brought with a history of aspiration of a foreign body resulting respiratory distress.

When sudden respiratory distress is associated with coughing, gagging, stridor, cyanosis or wheezing.

Foreign body may be coin peanuts, etc.

Management

Conscious Child

- Lay the infant on your arm or thigh in a head down position. Hold the jaw to support the head, give five blows to the infant's back with the hand between the both scapular regions.

  If not improved turn the infant and give two thrusts at midline of the chest with two fingers, one finger below nipple level.
- Abdominal thrusts (Heimlich maneuver): Position of child may be sitting or standing encircle him by putting both arms under the axilla.

  Place the thumb size of one fist on abdomen of child between xiphoid process and navel.

  Place the other hand over the fist and pull upwards in abdomen repeat 5 times check inside mouth if foreign body found, remove.

Unresponsive child with palpable pulse

Do CPR along with chest compression.

Chest compression

Indication pulse is not detectable, heart rate 60/min, child shows poor sign of circulation after adequate oxygenation.

1. Child should be supine on hard flat surface.
2. Two techniques.

Thumb technique encircles the infant's chest and supports the infant's back with the fingers of both hands use both thumbs of hand be depress the sternum.

Two-finger technique: The tips of middle finger and either index finger or ring finger of one hand are used to compress sternum while the other hand is used to support the back of the body.

Method: Give chest compressions. Compress the lower half of the sternum but does not compress over the xiphoid.

- Depress the chest about one-third to one half anteroposterior diameter of chest.
- Push at the rate of 100 compressions per minute.
- Release completely to allow recoil of the chest by completely releasing the pressure minimum interruption.
- Two effective breaths should be given after 15 chest compressions by other person (rescuer).

Chest compressions for the child (1 year or above age)

- Place the heal of one hand over the lower half of the sternum lift your fingers to avoid pressing on the ribs.
- Further steps same as for infant.

Oxygen: Give oxygen supplementation so oxygen saturation remains SpO_2 <90% respiratory distress or <94% in without respiratory distress. If pulse oxymeter is not available, assess by clinical signs.

Circulation (Shock)

Assess circulation problem is as follows:

1. Warm hand—take the child's hand in your own, it feels warm, circulation is good.
2. Capillary refill time (CRT)—it is a simple test that assesses how blood returns to the skin after pressure is applied.

    Method: Apply pressure to the pink part of the thumb of hand or big toe of foot in a child and over the sternum or forehead in an infant for 3 seconds.

    Release the pressure capillary refill time (CRT) is the time form release of pressure to complete return of pink color.

    While checking is limbs lift the limb slightly above heart level. This helps in assessing arteriolar capillary refill and not venous stasis.

Normally, it is less than 3 seconds. If it is more than 3 seconds then it is prolonged.

Result: CRT is prolonged in shock because body tries to maintain blood flow to vital organ and returns the blood supply to less important part of body like the skin.

Cold room temperature may cause delayed capillary refill.

3. *Pulse*—weak or fast

    First the central pulse as at brachial artery, femoral artery or carotid artery.

    Pulse is fast if rate is >160/min in an infant and >140/min in children above 1 year.

Shock

Causes of shock are loss of fluid from circulation.

- Dehydration as in severe diarrhea
- Hemorrhage

Diagnosis—cold hand, CRT >3 seconds, fast and weak pulse

Fluids in children without severe acute malnutrition

Steps—rapid fluids

Give Ringer lactate or normal saline first bolus—20 ml/kg over 30–60 min.

Reassess child

For details *see* Flowchart 21.1.

Management

1. If child is bleeding apply pressure
2. Give oxygen
3. Establish IV assess

    Administer IV fluids—administration of fluid in shock is discussed under two heads.

1. Child without severe acute malnutrition.
2. Child with severe acute malnutrition (SAM).

Administration of fluid is child without SAM

Shock may be hypovolemic. Cardiogenic, distributive hypovolemic is leading cause in

Flowchart 21.1: Reassess child

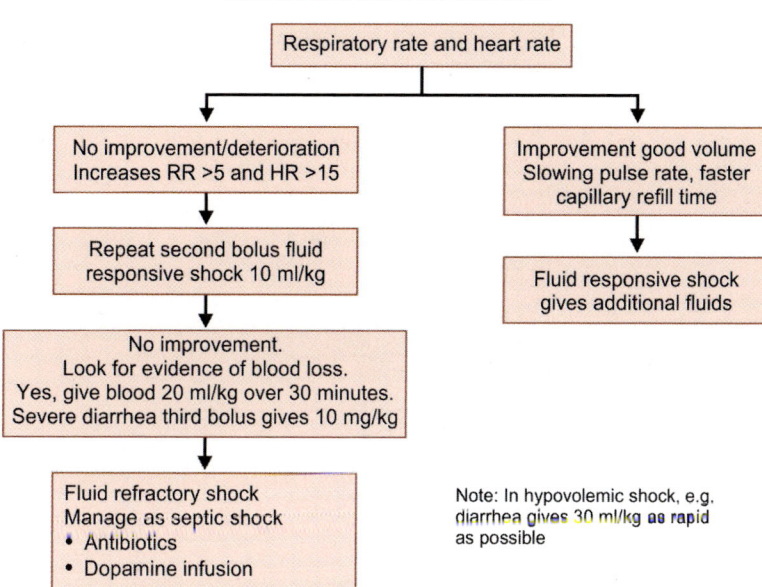

children which requires administration of intravenous fluids. Fluids are:

a. Isotonic crystalloid solutions, e.g. Ringer lactate or normal saline
b. Colloid solutions, e.g. hemocoel, 5% albumin, blood and fresh frozen plasma.

Fluid administration in SAM child

Child with severe malnutrition should not be treated by rapid IV infusion of fluid because in malnourished child heart becomes weak and may fail if it has to pump large volumes of fluid. Fluid accumulates in lungs resulting pulmonary edema which make breathing more difficult and child becomes worst. Oral fluid or fluid with nasogastric tube is choice of route for giving fluid if child is not conscious or not tolerate then only intravenous route is suggested.

Following ways are used for fluid administration (Flowchart 21.2).

Administration of IV fluid for shock in a child with severe acute malnutrition

Child is not in shock but shows sign of circulatory impairment such as in cold exposure child may have cold extremities and prolong capillary refill time. In pain pulse may be fast and weak so assess the child for other conditions also because in other conditions administration of fluid may be harmful, e.g. in SAM, high fever, pneumonia, etc.

Coma

The child who is unresponsive to voice (or being shaken) and to pain is considered unconscious.

Child who is not alert but responds to voice is lethargic.

Convulsions

Sudden loss of consciousness associated with uncontrolled jerky movements of limbs/or face.

Management of coma and convulsions

Child is placed in recovery position.
- Maintain airway
- Give oxygen
- Cheek and correct hypoglycemia
- Give IV calcium if infant <3 months
- If convulsions continue give anticonvulsants.

Flowchart 21.2

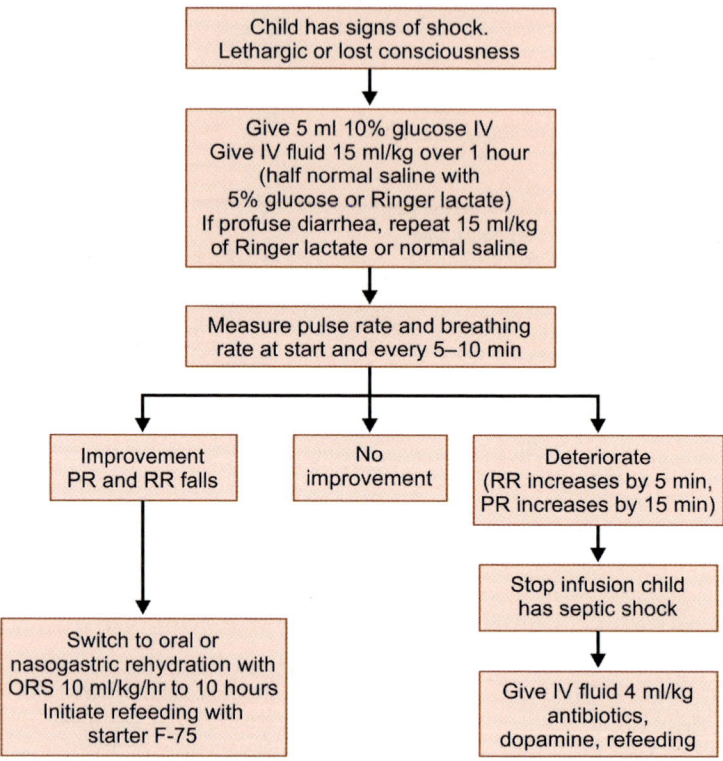

If neck trauma is suspected turn the child on the side to reduce risk of aspiration keep the neck slightly extended and stabilize by placing the cheek on one hand. Bend one leg to stabilize the body position.

Child is having convulsions, do not put anything in the child's mouth, in case child is vomiting turn him on side to avoid aspiration.

When convulsion has stopped and airway clear child can be placed in recovery position.

Insertion of an oropharyngeal (guedel) airway—oropharyngeal airway is used in an unconscious child to improve in airway opening. Guedel airways are available in 0 to 5 an appropriate sized airway goes from angle of mouth to the angle of jaw when laid on face with raised curved side up.

Procedure

a. Appropriate sized airway is selected.
b. Position the child to open the airway

c. Using a tongue depressor—depress the tongue and insert oropharyngeal airway.
   • In infant—convex side up
   • In children—concave side up, then rotate 180 and slide back over the tongue.
d. Recheck airway opening
e. Give oxygen.

Suction devices: Suctioning of secretions blood or vomitus is done best by large bore noncollapsible suction, joined with suction unit, appropriate sized suction catheters are used. Suction unit, it should have good suction power.

Diazepam: To control convulsions, diazepam is given intravenously directly slow at least in one minute, it can be given rectally also.

Dose: IV 0.25 ml/kg and rectally 0.1 ml/kg maximum 5 mg in children <5 year 10 mg in >5 year (diazepam solution 10 mg/2 ml) diazepam is administered per rectum by tuberculin syring with catheter hold the buttocks for a two minutes, flush the catheter with 2 ml of normal saline after administering diazepam.

If convulsions persist repeat the dose of diazepam 0.05 ml/kg–0.25 mg/kg IV infusion is running.

Do not give more than two doses of diazepam reassess breathing and airway because it may affect breathing.

Midazolam: It can be used in place of diazepam.

Dose: 0.15 mg–0.2 mg/kg IV, IM

0.3 mg/kg intranasal

Maximum 6 months to 5 years of age— 6 mg

- 6 years—10 mg

If seizures persist after second dose of diazepam.

IV valproate, phenobarbital or phenytoin can be used.

IV phenytoin 15–20 mg/kg, diluted in about 20 ml of saline not containing dextrose, or IV phenobarbitone 15–20 mg/kg in 20 ml dextrose

Slowly 1 mg/kg, or saline

Note: Valproate and phenytoin should not be given intramuscular while phenobarbitone can be given, if no IV assess.

Treatment of status epilepticus—*see* Chapter 11: Diseases of Central Nervous System.

High fever should be treated with cold sponging with room temperature water. Do not give oral medication till convulsions are controlled.

Dehydration treatment—as described in Chapter 8: Diseases of Gastrointestinal System.

Appendices

Appendix 1
Drug Dosage, Trade Names and Preparations

Drug and dose	Trade Names	Preparations
Acetaminophen (paracetamol) 25–50 mg/kg/day (O)	Pyregesic Crocin	Tab 500 mg Sy 125 mg/5 ml dr l0 mg/drop

Acetazolamide
  As diuretics 5 mg/kg/day (O, IM)
  Antiepileptic 8–30 mg/kg/day (O)
  also in cerebral edema, glaucoma
	Diamox	Tab 250 mg

Acetylsalicylic acid
  30–65 mg/kg/day (O) in divided doses
  65–130/mg/day (O) in rheumatic fever
	Disprin
	Micropyrin
		Tab 350 mg
		Tab 350 mg

Aminophylline
  3 mg/kg/dose (IV or IM)
  10 mg/kg/dose (O)
	Aminophylline	Tab l00 mg, 200 mg
		Inj 25 mg/ml

Adrenaline
  0.01 ml/kg/dose (SC)
  maximum 0.6 ml, repeat every 3–4 hr
	Adrenaline	1 mg/ml (1 in 1000
		aqueous solution)

ACTH 1.8 units/kg/day (SC, IM)		Inj 40 IU/vial, 60 IU/vial

Albendazole
  200 mg (up to 2 yr), 400 mg
  (after 2 yr) as a single dose
  In strongyloidosis, tapeworm given
  for 3 successive days
	Zentel
	
	Alba
		Tab 400 mg
		Sy 200 mg/5 ml

Albumin
  5% solution at the rate of 5–6 ml/minute
  25% solution given at the rate of 2 ml/minute
  10–15 ml given to premature 2–3 times in
    hypoalbuminemia
  50 ml (IV) in burn or edema
  100–150 ml on alternate day in nephrotic
    syndrome
	
	Albudac
		5% solution
		25% solution

Contd...

Drug and dose	Trade Names	Preparations

Amikacin
  15 mg/kg/day in 2 divided
    doses in neonate below 2 kg
  10 mg/kg/day in neonate above 2 kg
  30 mg/kg/day in neonate above 7 days
  15 mg/kg/day in 2–3 divided doses
    in older infant and children
	Amikacin
	Ivimicin
		Inj 100, 250, 500 mg/vial
		(2 ml)

Aluminum hydroxide 20–50 mg/kg/day in 4–5 divided doses	Aludrox	Tab 840 mg Gel 610 mg/10 ml
Aminosidine sulfate 10–20 mg/kg/day (IM) 2–3 divided doses	Gabromicina	Inj 500 mg/vial

Amodiaquine
  20 mg/kg/day (O) as single dose maintenance
  dose 8 mg/kg/day for 2 days
	Camoquin	Tab 200 mg

Amoxycillin 20–40 mg/kg/day	Wymox Moxidil	Cap 250, 500 mg Tab 125, 250 mg Sy 125/5 ml Inj 250, 500 mg/vial

Ampicillin
  50–400 mg/kg in 4 divided doses
  (higher limit is for septicemia, meningitis)
	Roscillin
	Campicillin
		Tab 125, 250 mg
		Cap 250 mg, 500 mg
		Inj 250, 500, 125 mg
		dr l00 mg per 1.2 ml
		Distab 125, 250 mg

Analgin (Novalgin) 100 mg/year/dose (O, IM)	Novalgin	Tab 500 mg Inj 500 mg/ml
Ascorbic acid 100–500 mg/day (O, IV)	Suckcee	Tab 50, 100, 500 mg dr l00 mg/20 drops
Astemizole 0.2 mg/kg as a single dose daily	Stemiz	Tab 10 mg Sy 5 mg/5 ml
Atropine sulfate 0.01 mg/kg/dose (SC) maximum 0.4 mg/dose	Atropine	Tab 0.3, 0.4, 0.6 mg Inj 0.6 mg/dose
BAL 2.5 mg/kg/dose IM	Dimercaprol	Inj 100 mg/2 ml
Bephenium hydroxynaphthoate 2.5 g for below 5 yr, 5 gm for above 5 yr	Alcopar	Granules 5 gm, providing 2. 5 gm base
Busulfan 0.06 mg/kg/day (O)	Myleran	Tab 0.5 mg, 2 mg

Calcium gluconate
  0.5 gm/kg/day (O) in divided doses,
  1–2 ml/kg/dose IV
	Calcium gluconate	Tab 0.5 gm
		Inj 137.5 mg/ml

Calcium chloride 0.3 gm/kg/day (O, IV)	Calcium chloride	Inj 100 mg/ml

Contd...

Drug and dose	Trade Names	Preparations
Captopril 0.1–0.4 mg/kg/day 1–4 times daily, maximum 2.0 mg	Acetein	Tab 25 mg
Carbamazepine 10–20 mg per kg/day (O)	Tegretol	Tab l00 mg, 200 mg, 400 mg Sy l00 mg/5 ml
Carbenicillin 50–400 mg/kg/day (IM, IV)	Carbelin	Inj 1 gm/vial
Cefadroxil 30 mg/kg/day in 2 divided dose	Cefadrox	Sy l25 mg/5 ml Tab and Cap 250, 500 mg
Cefalexin 25–100 mg/kg/day in 2–4 divided doses	Sporidex	Cap 250 mg, 500 mg Sy 125 mg/5 ml
Cephaloridine 15–30 mg/kg/day (IM, IV) in 2–3 divided doses—in serious gram-positive infection dose 40–60 mg/kg/day	Ceporan	Inj 1 gm, 0.5 gm per vial
Cefazolin 25–100 mg/kg/day (IM, IV) in 2–4 divided doses	Cefamejin Cefazin	Inj 250, 500 mg, 1000 mg, per vial
Cefotaxime 50–200 mg/kg/day (IM, IV) in 2 divided doses	Claforan	Inj 250 mg, 125 mg, 1 gm/vial
Ceftazidime Under 2 months 25–60 mg/kg/day (IM, IV) in 2 divided doses Above 2 months 30–100 mg/kg/day (IM, IV) in 2–3 divided doses	Fortum	Inj 250, 500, 1000 mg/vial
Ceftriaxone 20–80 mg/kg/day (IM, IV) in 1 or 2 doses	Monocef	Inj 250, 125, 1000 mg/vial
Cefuroxime 15–150 mg/kg/day (IM, IV) in 2–3 divided doses	Cefogen	Inj 250, 750 mg/vial
Cetzine Above 6 yr 10 mg daily Children (2–6 yr) 2.5 mg twice daily	Cetzine	Sy 5 mg/5 ml
Chloral hydrate 10–20 mg/kg/dose (O) hydrate 25 mg/kg/day as sedative, 50 mg/kg/day as hypnotic (max 2 gm/dose)	Chloral	Sy 200, 500 mg per 5 ml
Chlorambucil 0.1–0.2 mg/kg (O) as a single dose or in divided doses	Leukeran	Tab 2 mg, 5 mg
Chloramphenicol 50–100 mg/kg/day (O, IM, IV) in divided doses Neonates 25 mg/kg/day	Chloromycetin	Cap 250 mg, 500 mg Sy 125 mg/4 ml Inj 1 gm, 250 mg

Contd...

Drug and dose	Trade Names	Preparations
Chlordiazepoxide 0.5 mg/kg/day (O) is divided doses	Librium	Tab 10 mg

Chloroquine sulfate
  10–15 mg/kg/day (O)
  5 mg/kg/day (IM, IV)
	Nivaquin
	Lariago
		Tab 250 mg (150 mg base)
		500 mg
		Inj 40 mg/ml

Dosage by IV route
  See 'Malaria'
LM/SC route
  3.5 mg chloroquine base/kg every 6 hours
		Sy 100 mg/10 ml

Chlorpheniramine 0.35 mg/kg/day (O)	Corex	Sy 4 mg/5 ml as constituent)
Chlorothiazide 20 (7–40) mg/kg/day in 2 divided doses	Diuril	Inj 10, 100 mg/ml Tab 250, 500 mg

Chlorpromazine hydrochloride
  0.5–1 mg/kg/dose (O) IM
  2 mg/kg/day (O) in 4–6 divided doses
	Largectil	Tab 10 mg, 25 mg, 50 mg,
		100 mg, 200 mg
		Inj 25 mg/ml

Cemetidine 20–40 mg/kg/day in divided doses		Tab 200 mg

Ciprofloxacin
  10–30 mg/kg/day (O) in 2 divided doses
  5–10 mg/kg/day (IV) in 2 divided doses
	Cifran
	Ciprobid
		Cap 250, 500, 750 mg
		Inj 2 mg/ml infusion

Avoided in children as far as possible		

Clonazepam
  0.01–0.03 mg/kg/day increase
  0.3 mg/kg/day every 8 hours gradually
	Rivotril	Tab 05, 2 mg

Clonidine HCl 5–10 µg/kg/day	Catapres	Tab 100 mg
Cloxacillin 50–200 mg/kg/day (O, IV)	Klox	Cap 250, 500 mg Sy 125 mg/measure Inj 250, 500 mg/vial

Codeine
  1–1.5 mg/kg/day for cough
  3 mg/kg/day as sedative
		Sy 15, 30, 60 mg/ml

Colistin sulfate 5–8 mg/kg in divided doses (O)	Walamycin	Sy 12.5 mg/5 ml

Cortisone acetate
  2.5–10 mg/kg/day (O) in 3 divided doses
  Half of it as IM or IV
	Cortin	

Cotrimoxazole *See* trimethoprim with sulfamethoxazole		
Cromoglycate disodium 4–6 weeks	Cremolyn	Cap 20 mg

Contd...

Drug and dose	Trade Names	Preparations
Cyclophosphamide 2–3 mg/kg/day (O, IV) for resistant cases 4–8 mg/kg/day	Endoxan	Tab 50 mg Inj 100, 200, 500 mg 1 gm vial
Cycloserine 10 mg/kg/day in 2 divided doses	Cylorim	Cap 250 mg
Cyproheptadine HCl 0.25 mg/kg/day is 3–4 divided doses	Periactin	Tab 4 mg Sy 2 mg/5 ml
Daunorubicin 0.5–3 mg/kg as a single dose	Cerubidin	vial 20 mg
Desferrioxamine 8–32 mg/kg/dose (SC, IM, IV) max. 80 mg/kg/day (IV)	Deferal	Inj 500 mg/vial
Dextropropoxyphene 2–4 mg/kg/day in divided doses	Dexovan	Cap 70 mg
Diazepam 0.1–0.3 mg/kg/dose (IM, IV) or 1 mg/year of age (maximum 10 mg) 0.1–0.8 mg/kg/day (O) in 3–4 divided doses	Calmpose	Tab 2, 5 mg Sy 2 mg/5 ml Inj 5 mg/ml
Diazoxide 4–5 mg/kg/dose (IV)	Hyperstat	Inj 300 mg/20 ml
Diclofenac sodium 25–50 mg/day in 2 divided doses	Voveran	Tab 25, 50, 100 mg Inj 25 mg/ml
Diethylcarbamazine 10–12 mg/kg/day divided doses for ascariasis For filariasis—6 mg/kg/day (O) in 3 doses for 2–3 weeks	Hetrazan	Tab 50 mg, 100 mg Sy 50, 120 mg/5 ml
Digoxin 1–12 months age 0.08 mg/kg/24 hr after 1 year age 0.06 mg/kg/24 hr	Lanoxin	Tab 0.25 mg Inj 0.5 mg/2 ml Ped Sy 0.05 mg/ml
Diiodohydroxyquin 30 mg/kg/day in divided doses (O)	Didoquin	Tab 650 mg Sy 210 mg/5 ml
Diphenhydramine 4–6 mg/kg/day in divided doses	Benadryl	Sy 12.5 mg/5 ml Cap 25 mg, 50 mg
Dimethylpolysiloxane ¼–½ tab added to infant formula for burping	Dimol	Tab 40 mg
Diphenoxylate hydrochloride 0.3 mg/kg/day in divided doses (O, IM, IV)	Lomotil	Tab 2.5 mg
Doxycycline 5 mg/kg/day (O) in divided doses	Duracycline	Cap 100 mg
Diphenylhydantoin 3–8 mg/kg/day (O) as single or divided doses 10–15 mg/kg (IV, IM)	Epsolin	Tab 100 mg Inj 50 mg/ml

Contd...

Drug and dose	Trade Names	Preparations

Domperidone
  0.2–0.4 mg/kg
  3–4 times a day
	Domperon	Tab 10 mg
		dr 1 mg/ml

Dopamine HCl
  0.002–0.005 mg/kg/min
  Increased maximum up to 0.05 mg/kg/min
	Dopamine	Inj 200 mg/5 ml

Dexorubicin 1.2 to 2.4 mg/kg/dose (IV) every 3 weeks	Adriamycin	Inj 10 mg/vial
Doxycycline 5 mg/kg/day (O) in divided doses	Duracycline	Cap 100 mg
Ephedrine sulfate 3 mg/kg/day (O) in divided doses	Asmapax (As content)	Tab 25, 50 mg

Erythromycin
  30–50 mg/kg/day (O)
  15–20 mg/kg/day (IM, IV) in divided doses
	Althrocin	Tab 100, 125, 250, 500 mg
		Sy 125 mg, 250 mg/5 ml
		dr 100 mg/ml

Ethacrynic acid 25 mg (O) as a single dose	Edecrin	Tab 25, 50 mg Inj 50 mg
Ethambutol 15–25 mg/kg/day (O) as a single dose	Mycobutal	Cap 200, 400, 600, 800 mg
Ethionamide 10–20 mg/kg/day (O) in 2–3 divided doses	Ethomid	Tab 250 mg

Ethosuximide
  Below 6 years 250 mg/day (O)
  Above 6 years 500 mg/day (O)
  in divided doses
	Zarontin	Sy 250 mg/5 ml
		Cap 250 mg

Ethylestemol 0.06 mg (1 drop)/kg/day (O)	Orabolin	Tab 2 mg dr 1 mg per 15 drops

Ferrous sulfate
  6 mg/kg/day (O, IM, IV)
  1 mg/kg (O) prophylactic dose
	Fersolate
	Imferon (Inj)
		Tab 200 provide 40 mg of
		elemental
		Iron Inj 50 mg/ml

Frusemide
  1–3 mg/kg (O)
  0.5–1.5 mg/kg parenterally
	Lasix	Tab 40 mg
		Inj 10 mg/ml

Foli cacid
  5–20 mg/day (O)
  1 mg/day (IM) or 0.2 mg/kg/day
		Tab 5 mg, 10 mg

Furazolidone 5 mg/kg/day in divided doses	Furoxone	Tab 100 mg Sy 35.7 mg/5 ml

Gentamicin
  3–5 mg/kg/day (IM, IV) in divided doses
  (in newborn)
  7.5 mg/kg/day in divided doses—afterward
	Garamycin	Inj 40 mg/ml
		Pd Inj 10 mg/ml

Contd...

Drug and dose	Trade Names	Preparations
Globulin, Rh (D) immune. Human given to Rh negative mother 2 hours after delivery 350 µg optimal standard dose, 100 µg for abortion cases		Inj 100, 125, 350 mg
Griseofulvin 10–20 mg/kg/day (O) in 4 divided doses	Grisovin	Tab l25 mg
Guanethidine sulfate 0.2 mg/kg/day in 1–2 doses	Ismelin	Tab 10, 25 mg
Haloperidol 0.05 mg/kg/day	Serence	Tab 0.25, 1.5, 5, 10 mg dr 0.1 mg/drop Sy. 10 mg/5 ml Inj 5 mg/ml
Heparin 50 units/kg followed by 100 units per kg to be added to IV drip every 4 hourly		Inj 1.5, 7.5 thousands units/ml (1 mg is equivalent to 120 units)
Hydralazine 0.75 mg/kg/day in 4–6 divided doses	Aprosoline	Tab 10, 25, 100 mg Inj 20 mg/ml
Hydrochlorthiazide 2 mg/kg/day (O) in 2 divided doses	Esidrex	Tab 25, 50 mg
Ibuprofen 20 mg/kg/day in 3 divided doses	Brufen	Tab 200, 400, 600 mg Sy 100 mg/5 ml
Imipramine 1.5 mg/kg/day (O) in 2–4 divided doses	Dapsonil	Tab 25 mg
Indomethacin 3 mg/kg/day (O)	Indocap	Cap 25, 75 mg
Insulin 0.1 unit/kg/hour 0.5 unit/kg/day in 3 divided doses		40 IU, 80 IU/ml
Iron dextran		
Iron sorbitol 1.5 mg/kg/dose (IM)	Jectofer	Inj 50 mg/ml
Isoniazid 10–20 mg/kg/day (O) as a single dose or 2–3 divided doses	Isonex	Tab 50, 100, 300 mg Sy 50, 100 mg/TSF Inj 100 mg/ml
Isoproterenol 5–10 mg/dose (sublingual) 3–4 times daily		Tab 10, 15 mg

Iron dextran

$$\text{Dose } \frac{0.3 \times \text{weight in lbs} \times \text{Hb deficit \%}}{50} = \text{ml of injection imferon}$$

Add 20–30% for tissue iron store in above dose

Contd...

Drug and dose	Trade Names	Preparations
Kanamycin 10–15 mg/kg/day IM in 2 divided doses	Kancin	Inj 0.5, 1.0 gm, vial
L-asparaginase 50–200 units/kg/day by IV infusion	Leunase	Inj 10,000 units per vial
Levamisole 2.5–5 mg/kg in a single dose	Vermisol	Tab 50, 150 mg Sy 50 mg/5 ml
Lignocaine	Xylocaine	1%, 2% jelly, ointment, viscous
Lincomycin HCl 30–60 mg/kg/day (O) in 3 divided doses	Lincocin	Cap 500 mg Inj 300 mg/ml
Loperamide HCl 0.3 mg/kg/day; 0.1 mg/kg/dose	Lapamide	Tab 2 mg
Mannitol 7–10 ml/kg/day by drip		200 mg/ml (in 350, 500 ml bottles) providing 70 and 100 gm mannitol
Mebendazole 100 mg twice daily for 3 days	Wormin	Tab 100 mg Sy 100 mg/5 ml
Mepacrine 5 mg/kg/day (O) in 3 divided doses for 5–7 days for giardiasis 15 mg/kg (max 8 gm) as a single dose for tapeworms		Tab 100 mg
Mefenamic acid 20–25 mg/kg/day	Ineftal	Cap 250, 500 mg Tab 125 mg Sy 125 mg/5 ml
Melphalon 2–4 mg/day	Alkeran	Tab 2, 5 mg Inj 100 mg/vial
Mercaptopurine (6 MP purinethol) 2.5 mg/kg/day	Purinethol	Tab 50 mg
Metakelfin (see sulfamethopyrazine)		
Methandienone 0.04 mg/kg/day (O)	Dianabol	Tab 1, 5 mg dr 1 mg per 30 drops
Methenamine mandelate 50–100 mg/kg/day in 3 divided doses	Mandelamine	Tab 1 gm, 0.5 gm
Methicillin Newborn 100 mg/kg/day Children 100–400 mg/kg/day (IM, IV) in 6 divided doses	Staphicillin	Inj 900 mg/gm 1, 4, 6 gm vial

Contd...

Drug and dose	Trade Names	Preparations

Methotrexate
    0.12 mg/kg/dose (O),
    0.25–0.5 mg/kg/day (IT)
    3–5 mg/kg (IV) as a single dose every
    other week
	Methotrexate	Tab 2.5 mg
		Inj 5 mg/vial

Methyldopa
    10 mg/kg/day (O) 20–40 mg/kg/day IV
    for hypertensive crisis
	Alphadopa	Tab 250 mg

Metoclopramide HCl
    0.5 mg/kg/day in 3 divided doses
    up to 1 mg/kg/day
	Perinorm	Tab 10 mg
		Inj 5 mg/ml
		Sy 5 mg/5 ml

Metronidazole
    10–20 mg/kg/day (O) for 5–7 days
    in divided doses
	Flagyl	Tab 200, 400 mg
		Sy 100, 200 mg/5 ml
		IV 500 mg/100 ml

Minoxidil
    0.2 mg/kg/day as a single dose followed by
    stepwise increase to 0.25 to 1 mg/kg/day
	Loiten	Not avilable in India

Morphine 0.1–0.2 mg/kg/dose (SC)		Tab 60, 100 mg Inj 60 mg

Moxalactum
    Under 7 days 100 mg/kg/day in 2 divided doses
    Above 7 days 150 mg/kg/day in 3 divided
    doses
		Inj 250, 500/vial

Mustine HCl
    0.1–0.4 mg/kg/dose IV, for 3–4 days,
    maximum 8 mg
		Inj 10 mg/vial

Nalidixic acid 50 mg/kg/day (O) in 4 divided doses	Gramoneg	Tab 125, 500 mg Sy 300 mg/5 ml
Naproxen 10 mg/kg/day (O) in 2 divided doses	Artagen	Tab 250 mg
Neomycin 50–100 mg/kg day (O) in divided doses		Cap 350 mg

Niclosamide
    Dose under 2 years 500 mg/day
    2–6 year 1 gm/day
    6–12 years 1.5 gm/day
    Older children 2 gm/day
	Niclosan	Tab 500 mg

Nifedipine 0.2–0.7 mg/dose	Calcigard	Cap 5, 10, 20 mg

Nikethamide
    25 mg/kg/dose (IV, IM)
    Newborn 10 drops/dose
	Coramine	Tab 400 mg
		dr 25% soln
		Inj 250 mg/ml

Contd...

Drug and dose	Trade Names	Preparations
Netilmicin 6–9 mg/kg/day	Netromycin	Inj 25, 50, 100, 200, 300 mg/ml
Nitrazepam 0.12–0.2 mg/kg/day in a single or 2 divided doses	Nitrosun	Tab 5, 10 mg
Nitrofurantoin 6–10 mg/kg/day (O) in 3–4 divided doses	Furadantin	Tab 50,100 mg Sy 25, 50 mg/5 ml
Nitrogen mustard 0.4 mg/kg IV as a single or divided dose		Inj 10 mg
Nitroxazepine 25–50 mg at bed time	Sintarril	Tab 25, 75 mg
Nondrolone Infants 5 mg once a week or 10 mg once a fortnight Children 10–12.5 mg once every 10 days	Durabolin	Inj 10, 25 mg/ml
Norfloxacin 4–12 mg/kg/day (not recommended) in children	Norflox	Tab 200, 400, 800, 100 mg (DT)
Nystatin Newborn 4 lac units/kg/day (O) in divided doses Afterward 1–2 million units/day in divided doses	Mycostatin	Tab 5 lac units
Oflacin 4–16 mg/kg/day as a single or divided doses, (not recommended in children)	Tarvid	Tab 200 mg
Orciprenaline sulfate 0.02 mg/1 kg (IM) 3 mg/kg/dose (O) in 4 divided doses	Alupent	Tab 10, 20 mg Inj 1 ml have 0.5, 1.0 mg Sy 2 mg/ml
Oxacillin 50–100 mg/kg/day (O, IM, IV)		
Oxymetholone 0.1–0.8 mg/kg/day (O)		Tab 5 mg
Oxyphenonium bromide 2–6 yr 5–8 drops 1–3 times daily 6–12 yr 8–15 drops 1–3 times daily Older children 1–2 tab four times in a day	Artrenyl	Tab 5, 10 mg dr 10 mg/ml
Oxyphenylbutazone 5–10 mg/kg/day (O) in 4 divided doses		
Pancreatin 300–600 mg with each meal	Digeplex	Tab 0.15 gm
Paracetamol See acetaminophen		

Contd...

Drug and dose	Trade Names	Preparations

Paraldehyde
    0.1–0.2 ml/kg/dose or 1 ml/year/dose
    (O, IM, IV) 0.3 to 0.6 ml/kg/dose per rectal
		Inj 2, 5, 10 ml

Paromomycin 25–50 mg/kg/day in 3 divided doses	Humantin	Sy 125 mg/5 ml Cap 250 mg

Penicillin
    Oral 50 thousands units/kg/day in divided
    doses
	Crystapen	Tab 1, 2, 4, 8 lac units

Procaine penicillin
    Under 4 years 2 lac (IM) daily or twice a day;
    over 4 years 4 lac (IM) daily or twice a day
		vial 4 lac units

Crystalline penicillin
    50 thousands to 4 lac units/kg/day (IM, IV)
    in 4 divided doses
		vial 5, 10 lac units

Benzathine penicillin (Penidure LA 6, 12) 1 .2 mega units every 3 weeks		6, 12, 24 lac unit/vial
Pethidine 1–2 mg/kg/day (IM)		Tab 100 mg Inj 100 mg
Phananquone 5–10 mg/kg/day in divided doses	Entobex	Tab 50 mg
Pheniramine maleate 1–5 mg/kg/day (O, IM)	Avil	Tab 22.5, 45 mg Sy 15 mg/5 ml Inj 22.75 mg/ml

Phenobarbital
    3–5 mg/kg/dose (IM) for acute attack of
    convulsions
    3–5 mg/kg/day for maintenance
	Gardenal
	
	Luminal
		Tab 30, 60 mg
		
		Tab 15, 30 mg

Phenytoin sodium *See* diphenlhydantoin sodium	Dilantin	Cap 100 mg Sy 25 mg/ml

Piperazine citrate
    100–150 mg/kg/day as a single dose for
    ascariasis
    50–70 mg/kg/day (O) for 7 days for
    Enterobiasis
	Antepar	Tab 500 mg
		Sy 750 mg/5 ml

Potassium chloride
    1–3 mEq/day (IV) in hypokalemia
    2–5 mEq/day in kwashiorkor with diarrhea
	Potklor	Sy 1–3 g/15 ml
		Inj 0.15 g/ml

Prednisolone 2 mg/kg/day (O) in divided doses	Wysolone	Tab 5 mg
Primaquine *See* malaria		

Contd...

Drug and dose	Trade Names	Preparations
Primidone 40–50 rng/kg/day in divided doses	Mysoline	Tab 250 mg
Probenecid 25 mg/kg stat followed by 10 mg/kg 6–8 hourly	Procid, Benemid	
Prochlorperazine 0.5 mg/kg/day (O) in divided doses	Stemetil	Tab 5 mg, 25 mg Inj 12.5 mg/ml
Promethazine hydrochloride 0.5 mg/kg/dose (O, IM)	Phenargan	Tab 10, 25 mg Sy 5 mg/5 ml Inj 25 mg/2 ml
Propranolol HCl 0.15–0.25 mg/kg/dose (IV) for cyanotic spells 0.5–1 mg/kg/day (O) for arrhythmias	Ciplar, Inderal	Tab 10, 40, 80 mg Inj 1 mg/ml
Pseudoephedrine hydrochloride 3–5 mg/kg/day in 4 divided doses	Sudafed	Tab 30, 60 mg Sy 30 mg/5 ml
Pyrantel pyridokine 10 mg/kg (O) as a single dose	Expent	Tab 250 mg Sy 250 mg/5 ml
Pyritinol pyridoxine ½ Teaspoonful 1–3 times a day for infant ½–1 5 ml (or tab) 1–3 times a day for children	Encephabol	Tab 100, 200 mg Sy 100 mg/5 ml
Pyrvinium 5 mg/kg/day (O)	Vanpar	Sy 25 mg/5 ml
Quinine 25 mg/kg/day in 3 divided doses (O) 10 mg/kg/dose (IV) in slow infusion	Quininga	Tab 300 mg Inj 0.3 g/ml
Ranitidine 1–4 mg/kg/day (O, IM, IV) in 2–3 divided doses	Ranitidine Aciloc	Tab 150, 300 mg Inj 25 mg/ml
Reserpine 0.07 mg/kg/dose (IM)	Adelphane	Tab 0.1 mg
Rifampicin 10–20 mg/kg/day (O) as a single dose daily	R-Cin	Cap 150, 300 , 450 mg Sy 100 mg/teaspoonful
Salbutamol 0.2–0.4 mg/kg/day	Asthalin	Tab 2, 4 mg Sy 2 mg/5 ml
Sodium nitroprusside 0.5–8.0 µg/kg/min	Pruside	Inj 50 mg per 5 ml
Spironolactone 1.5–3 mg/kg/day (O) in 1–3 divided doses	Aldactone	Tab 25 mg
Streptomycin sulfate 20–50 mg/kg/day (IM) l–2 mg per kg/day (IT) 100 mg/kg/day (O)	Ambistryn S	Inj 1 gm, 0.75 g per vial

Contd...

Drug and dose	Trade Names	Preparations
Sucralfate 1 tab two times before food	Ulcerfae	Tab 1 gm

Sulfadiazine
    100–150 mg/kg/day (O) in divided doses
    100 mg/kg/day IV in divided doses
		Tab 500 mg
		Inj 250 mg/ml

Sulfamethopyrazine with pyrimethamine
    25 mg/kg (SMP) or 1 mg/kg
    (pyrimethamine) as a single dose
	Metakeltin	Tab SMP 500 mg
		         Pyr 25 mg

Sulfadoxine with pyrimethamine
    25 mg/kg (sulfadoxine) or
    1 mg/kg (pyrimethamine) as a single dose
	Melocide	Tab 500 mg sulfadoxine
		and 25 mg pyrimetha-
		mine

Sulfadimethoxine 25–50 mg/kg/day (O) as a single dose	Madribon	Tab 500 mg
Sulfaguanidine 150 mg/kg/day in divided doses		Tab 500 mg

Sulfisoxazole
    75–150 mg/kg/day (O) in divided doses
    50–100 mg/kg/day (IV) in divided doses
		Tab 500 mg
		Sy 500 mg/TSF

Terbutaline sulfate
    0.2 mg/kg/day (O), 0.005 mg/kg/dose
    (SC), intravenous in difficult cases
	Bricanyl	Tab 2.5, 5, 7.5 mg
		Sy 1.5 mg/TSF
		Inj (SC) 0.5 mg/ml

Tetrachloroethylene 0.1 ml/kg (O), max 3–4 ml		

Tetracyclines (oxytetracycline)
    25–50 mg/kg/day (O) in 4 divided doses
    15–25 mg/kg/day (IM) in 2 divided doses
    10–15 mg/kg/day (IV) in 2 divided doses
	Terramycin	Cap 250 mg
		Sy 100 mg/TSF
		dr 5 mg/drop

Tetracycline hydrochloride *See* oxytetracycline		
Chlorotetracycline *See* oxytetracycline		
Dimethylchlortetracycline 10 mg/kg/day (O) in 2–4 divided doses	Ledermycin	Cap 150 mg Sy 75 mg/5 ml dr 3–4 mg/drop

Rolitetracycline (reverin)
    15–20 mg/kg/day (IM, IV) as a single or
    two divided doses
		Inj 150, 350 mg
		275 mg vial

Doxycycline
    5 mg/kg/day (O) in divided doses on first day,
    then 2.5 mg/kg/day once daily
	Tetradox	Tab 100 mg
		Sy 25, 50 mg/5 ml

Tetramisole *See* levamisole		

Contd...

Drug and dose	Trade Names	Preparations
Theophylline 10–20 mg/kg/day (O) in 2–3 divided doses 5 mg/kg/dose (IM, IV, SC)	Deriphyllin	Tab 23 mg of theophylline and 77 mg of etophylline
Thiabendazole 50 mg/kg/day (O) in 2 divided doses	Mintezol	Tab 500 mg Sy 500 mg/5 ml
Thyroid 4 mg/day (O) as a single dose Infants 15 mg/day, Children 30 mg/day, increase gradually		Tab 15, 30 mg
Thyroxine 50–100 μg increase every 3–4 weeks by increments of 25–50 μg to about 200–300 μg	Eltroxin	Tab 100 μg, 75 μg, 50 μg
Tinidazole 50 mg/kg as a single dose for giardiasis 60 mg/kg/day on 3 days for amebiasis	Tiniba	Tab 150, 300 600, 1000 mg
Tobramycin Neonates under 7 days 4 mg/kg/day in 2 doses Neonates above 7 days 6 mg/kg/day in 3 doses	Tobacin	Inj 50 mg in 2 ml per vial 60 mg in 2 ml, 20 mg in 2 ml
Triflupromazine 0.05–0.2 mg/kg/day (O) 0.05 mg/kg/day (IM)	Siquil	Tab 10 mg Inj 10, 20 mg/ml
Trimeprazine tartrate 2.5–5 mg three or tour times daily as antipruritic 7.5–60 mg/day as sedative	Vallergan	Tab 10 mg Sy 7.5 mg/5 ml
Trimethadione Infant 300 mg 1–5 yr 600 mg 6–12 years 900 mg 12 years and above 1200 mg/day in 3–4 divided doses, or 40 mg/kg/day (O) in 3–4 divided doses		Tab 150, 300 mg
Trimethoprim with sulfamethoxazole (septran) 4–10 mg/kg/day (O, IV) in terms of trimethoprim		Tab l60 mg (TMP) Fed. Tab 20 mg (TMP) Sy 40 mg (TMP) Inj 80 mg (TMP)
Valethamate bromide 1–2 Tab twice or thrice daily	Epidosin	Tab 10 mg
Valproate Start with 15 mg/kg/day in 2–3 divided doses, increase gradually 5–10 mg daily up to max 30 mg/day	Valparin	Inj 8 mg/ml Tab 200 mg Sy 200 mg/5 ml
Vinblastine 0.1–0.2 mg/kg week IV	Velban	1 mg/ml

Contd...

Drug and dose	Trade Names	Preparations
Fluconazole 6–12 mg/kg as a loading	Cancap	Tab AF-150 mg Cap 150 mg Tab Dispursable 50 mg
Isosorbide dinitrate 0.1 mg/kg/day PO q 6–8 hr	Solosprin	Tab 150 mg
Ivermectin 200 μg/kg PO single dose contraindicated in less than 5 yr of age	Ivori	Tab 3 mg, 6 mg
Lactulose 10–15 ml q 12–24 hr	Laxan	607 mg/ml
Meconidazole 20–40 mg/kg/day PO q 8 hr		
Methyl prednisolone 0.5–1.7 mg/kg/day parenteral	Methyl-Prednicort	Vial 500 mg, 1000 mg Tab 4 mg, 16 mg
Nitizix 5–10 kg : 5 mg 10–20 kg : 10 mg <20 kg : 20 mg	Omeprazole	Ozo DS tab 20 mg. Cap 20 mg
Nitrazoxamide 1–4 yr 100 mg twice a day for 3 days 4–12 yr 200 mg twice a day for 3 days	Nitacure	FC tab 200 mg, 500 mg Sys 100 mg/5 ml Tab 500 mg
Piperacillin 1 month –12 yr 100–300 mg/kg daily in 3–4 divided IV route is preferred in dilution	Piperacil	Vial 2 gm, 4 gm
Ranitidine 10 mg/kg/day PO, IM, IV q 12 yr		Tab 150, 300 mg Inj 25 mg/ml
Tobramycin 6–7.5 mg/kg daily in 3–4 divided doses IV infusion	Tabacin	Vial 20, 60, 80 mg

Note: Consult and confirm drug dosage, preprations from literature supplied with drugs.

Abbreviation: O—oral; Inj—injection; Sy—syrup, Elixir, Liquid; Tab—Tablet; Cap—capsule;
IV—intravenous; IM—intramuscular; SC—subcutaneous; dr—drops

Appendix 2
Normal Values

Hematologic values during infancy and childhood

Age	Hb% (gm%)	Total WBC/cumm	Neutrophil (%)	Lymphocyte (%)	Eosinophil (%)	Monocyte (%)	Nucleated RBC (%)
Birth	16.8	18,000	61	31	2	6	7
2 weeks	16.5	12,000	40	48	3	9	0
3 months	12.0	12,000	.30	63	2	5	0
6 months	12.0	10,000	45	48	2	5	0
6–12 years	13.0	8,000	55	38	2	5	0
Adult: Male	14						
Female	16	7,500	55	35	3	7	0

Total RBC/cumm	4.5–5.0 million/cumm
Platelet count	1.5–4.0 lac/cumm
Bleeding time (BT)	2–5 minutes
Clotting time (CT)	2–8 minutes
Serum albumin	4.5 gm%/100 cc
Serum cholesterol	150–250 mg/100 cc
Serum alkaline phosphatase	20–140 U/L
Mean corpuscular volume (MCV)	78–98 cubic micron
Packed cell volume (PCV)	40–54%
Mean corpuscular hemoglobin concentration (MCHC)	32–38%
Blood urea	17–32 mg/100 ml

Cerebrospinal fluid	Normal value
Appearance	Clear, colorless
Pressure	60–150 mm of water
Protein	15–30 mg/100 ml
Glucose	50–70 mg/100 ml
Chloride	720–750 mg/100 ml
Cells	0–5 lymphocytes/cumm

Index

Drug and dose	Trade Names	Preparations
Vincristine 0.05–0.15 mg/kg/week	Cytocristin	Inj 1 mg/ml
Vitamin D *See* vitamin D		
Xylometazoline HCl Nasal drops 0.05% for pediatric use 1–2 drops to each nostrils once or twice daily		
Acyclovir 20 mg/kg up to 800 mg 4 times daily for 5 days IV 20 mg/kg every 8 hourly 7 days	Ocuvir	Tab 200, 400, 800 mg
Amphotericin 0.25 mg/kg/day	Myco	50 mg
Azithromycin 10 mg/kg/day PO once/day	Azithral	DT Tab 100 mg Tab 250, 500 mg Liqd 200 mg/5 ml
Betamethasone 0.06–0.25 mg/kg/day	Betnesol	FC tab 1 mg Q 6–12 hr Tab 0.5 mg DPS 0.5 mg Amp 4 mg/ml
Cefachlor 20–40 mg/kg 6–8 ml PO	Halocef	Cap 250, 500 mg
Cefepime 8–10 mg/kg IV		Vial 250 mg, 1 gm, 2 gm
Cefiprime 30–60 mg/kg 12 hr IM/IV	Cepime	1 gm/vial
Cefixime 8–10 mg/kg PO 12 hr	Taxim-o	Tab 50 mg, 100 mg sys 20 mg/5 ml Tab 100, 200 mg
Cefoperazone 40–80 mg/kg IV	Cefomycin	Vial 1 gm
Cefpodoxime 8–10 mg/kg Kid tab 50 mg 12 hr PO	Monocef-o	Tab 100, 200 mg Susp 50 mg/5 ml 100 mg/5 ml
Clarithromycin 15 mg/kg PO		Tab 250 mg
Dapsone 1–2 mg/kg/day PO	Dapsone	Tab 25, 50, 100 mg
Dexamethasone 0.01–0.25 mg/kg/dose (O) IV or IM 6 hr	Dexona	Tab 0.5 mg Inj 4 mg/ml
Femolidine 1–1.2 mg/kg/day PO 12 hr	Esotrax	Tab 20, 40 mg

Contd...